Crosslinguistic Encounters in Language Acquisition

COMMUNICATION DISORDERS ACROSS LANGUAGES

***Series Editors*:** Dr Nicole Müller, *University College Cork, Ireland* and Dr Martin Ball, *Bangor University, Wales*

The discipline of communication disorders has made great strides over the last 50 years and more. We now know much more about the nature and causes of breakdowns in speech and language, in both adults and children. We know more about how to classify these breakdowns, how to describe and analyze pathological speech and language and how to treat communication disorders. Unfortunately, a large proportion of this work is restricted to a small number of European languages; indeed, much of it is on and in English alone.

Research in communication disorders in languages other than English has seen a marked increase in recent years, as has the investigation of such disorders in speakers of more than one language, and in communities where bi- and multilingualism is the norm. This series serves to spotlight new and ongoing research in communication disorders across languages. We aim to do this by including studies of communication disorders (including assessment methods and guidelines for intervention) in particular multilingual communities, studies of the manifestations of specific types of disorder in a range of languages (particularly lesser researched languages), and studies of communication breakdown in bi- and multilingual speakers. Books in the series are used by practitioners, researchers and students, and they address a range of topics, including speech and language disorders in children, literacy, acquired speech and language disorders in adults, fluency and voice.

Full details of all the books in this series and of all our other publications can be found on http://www.multilingual-matters.com, or by writing to Multilingual Matters, St Nicholas House, 31–34 High Street, Bristol BS1 2AW, UK.

COMMUNICATION DISORDERS ACROSS LANGUAGES: 17

Crosslinguistic Encounters in Language Acquisition

Typical and Atypical Development

Edited by
Elena Babatsouli, David Ingram and Nicole Müller

MULTILINGUAL MATTERS
Bristol • Blue Ridge Summit

DOI https://doi.org/10.21832/BABATS9085
Library of Congress Cataloging in Publication Data
A catalog record for this book is available from the Library of Congress.
Names: Babatsouli, Elena, editor. | Ingram, David, 1944- editor. | Müller, Nicole, 1963- editor.
Title: Crosslinguistic Encounters in Language Acquisition: Typical and Atypical Development/Edited by Elena Babatsouli, David Ingram and Nicole Müller.
Description: Bristol; Blue Ridge Summit: Multilingual Matters, [2018] | Series: Communication Disorders Across Languages: 17 | Includes bibliographical references and index.
Identifiers: LCCN 2017035522| ISBN 9781783099085 (hbk : alk. paper) | ISBN 9781783099108 (epub) | ISBN 9781783099115 (Kindle)
Subjects: LCSH: Language acquisition. | Language and languages—Study and teaching. | Multilingualism.
Classification: LCC P118.3 .C76 2018 | DDC 401/.93—dc23 LC record available at https://lccn.loc.gov/2017035522

British Library Cataloguing in Publication Data
A catalogue entry for this book is available from the British Library.

ISBN-13: 978-1-78309-908-5 (hbk)

Multilingual Matters
UK: St Nicholas House, 31–34 High Street, Bristol BS1 2AW, UK.
USA: NBN, Blue Ridge Summit, PA, USA.

Website: www.multilingual-matters.com
Twitter: Multi_Ling_Mat
Facebook: https://www.facebook.com/multilingualmatters
Blog: www.channelviewpublications.wordpress.com

The policy of Multilingual Matters/Channel View Publications is to use papers that are natural, renewable and recyclable products, made from wood grown in sustainable forests. In the manufacturing process of our books, and to further support our policy, preference is given to printers that have FSC and PEFC Chain of Custody certification. The FSC and/or PEFC logos will appear on those books where full certification has been granted to the printer concerned.

Typeset by Nova Techset Private Limited, Bengaluru and Chennai, India.
Printed and bound in the UK by the CPI Books Group Ltd.
Printed and bound in the US by Edwards Brothers Malloy, Inc.

Contents

Part 3: Language Acquisition in the Presence of a Disorder

Acknowledgements

We are thankful to the authors for their contributions and to the chapter reviewers for their thorough and timely reviews. This volume would not have been possible without their willingness to share their work and knowledge, thus advancing research in typical and atypical language acquisition. We are appreciative to the Multilingual Matters reviewer for their thorough evaluation, comments and suggestions.

We also wish to express our gratitude to the book series editors, Nicole Müller and Martin J. Ball, who encouraged this project and hosted the volume in the Communication Disorders Across Languages series at Multilingual Matters.

Figures and Tables

Figures

Tables

Contributors

Georgia Andreou is a Professor in Neurolinguistics/Psycholinguistics and Director of the Laboratory of Bilingual Education at the Department of Special Education, University of Thessaly, Greece. She is the writer of one book, of six chapters in books and of more than 85 articles published in international journals and proceedings. Georgia has more than 800 citations and is a member of the editorial boards of 11 international journals and guest editor of the *International Journal of Disability, Development and Education*. Her research interests include, among others, bilingualism/multilingualism, language and communication impairment and cognitive development in developmental disorders.

Elena Babatsouli is the Director of the Institute of Monolingual and Bilingual Speech in Chania, Greece. She has a BA in English (University of London), an MA in languages and business (London South Bank University) and a PhD in linguistics (University of Crete). Her research interests are in typical and atypical speech acquisition by monolingual and bilingual children, as well as in second language acquisition. Elena chaired the organization of the *International Symposium of Monolingual and Bilingual Speech* 2015, and edited its *Proceedings*. She was guest editor at *Poznan Studies in Linguistics* and has co-edited the book *Phonology in Protolanguage and Interlanguage* in the series Studies in Phonetics and Phonology for Equinox Publishing.

Barbara May Bernhardt is a Full Professor in the School of Audiology and Speech Sciences at the University of British Columbia in Vancouver, Canada. She is also a speech-language pathologist. Her areas of specialization are language development, assessment and intervention with a focus on phonology and phonetics. Her major research area is the application of nonlinear phonology to phonological assessment and intervention, with a major recent cross-linguistic project (14 languages). Over the past decade Barbara has also focused on ultrasound in speech intervention, early prediction of language impairment and issues in service delivery to people of Aboriginal heritage in Canada.

Emily Danvers is a speech and language therapist, completing her community service year in 2016 at Umgeni Psychiatric Hospital in KwaZulu-Natal,

South Africa. She graduated from the University of Cape Town in 2015. Emily has a passion for working with communication difficulties relating to speech and articulation in children as well as helping improve communication through the use of assistive and alternative communication methods.

Aimée de Jager is a speech and language therapist at Zithulele Hospital in rural Eastern Cape, South Africa. She enjoys working in a culturally rich, rural setting. Aimee is currently working with teachers and partner NGOs to target phonological awareness and pre-literacy skills for monolingual isiXhosa, speakers in an illiterate community.

Barbara Dodd is retired, holding Honorary Professorships at the universities of Queensland, Melbourne, Curtin and Charles Sturt in Australia. She continues to collaborate on research projects and supervises postgraduate students. Barbara's recent research concerns the nature, assessment and treatment of articulation and phonological impairments in children. Current treatment case studies are evaluating a novel intervention approach for toddlers with phonological disorders, and analyses of cohort data are identifying types of speech impairments that fail to resolve by seven years.

Natania Esterhuizen graduated from the University of Cape Town in 2015, with an honours degree in speech-language pathology. In 2016 she is completing her community service year at Bill Pickard Hospital, a district hospital in the Northern Cape Province of South Africa.

Georgios Floros is Associate Professor of Translation Studies at the Department of English Studies, University of Cyprus, where he teaches translation theory and methodology. He received a PhD in translation theory from Saarland University, Germany, in 2001. His research interests include translation theory and translation ethics (especially culture in translation), secondary term formation, text linguistics and pragmatics, and interpreting theory and didactics. Georgios has written, co-authored and co-edited five books on translation theory, didactics and translation terminology, and has published a number of articles on translation, interpreting and text linguistics in international refereed journals.

Sue Franklin is Professor of Speech and Language Therapy at the University of Limerick, Ireland. She has many years of experience in working with people with aphasia and has more recently developed an interest in developmental speech and language disorders. Sue's research interests include the application of a cognitive neuropsychological approach to aphasia and SLT/teacher collaboration in post-primary language interventions. She is an executive member of the Cost Action 'Collaboration of Aphasia Triallists'.

Helen Grech is the Deputy Dean of the Faculty of Health Sciences and Head of the Department of Communication Therapy at the University of Malta. She is a registered audiologist and speech-language pathologist. Her research interests are related to speech acquisition and disorders in multilingual populations. Helen has been involved in a number of crosslinguistic research projects and COST Actions. She was awarded a Marie Curie Intra-European Research Fellowship by the European Commission, an Individual Mobility Grant, and received funding from the EU to coordinate a four-year FP6 project. She has also received several local research grants.

Kleanthes K. Grohmann is Professor of Biolinguistics in the Department of English Studies at the University of Cyprus and Director of the CAT Lab. He has published widely in the areas of syntactic theory, comparative syntax, language acquisition, impaired language and multilingualism. Among the books he has written and co-edited are *Understanding Minimalism* (with N. Hornstein and J. Nunes, 2005, CUP), *InterPhases* (2009, OUP), and *The Cambridge Handbook of Biolinguistics* (with Cedric Boeckx, 2013, CUP). Kleanthes is founding co-editor of the John Benjamins book series 'Language Faculty and Beyond', and editor of the open-access journal *Biolinguistics*.

David Ingram is Professor in the Department of Speech and Hearing Science at Arizona State University. He received his BS from Georgetown University and his PhD in linguistics from Stanford University. His research interests are in language acquisition in typically developing children and children with language disorders, with a crosslinguistic focus. The language areas of interest are phonological, morphological and syntactic acquisition. David is the author of *Phonological Disability in Children* (1976), *Procedures for the Phonological Analysis of Children's Language* (1981), and *First Language Acquisition* (1989). His most recent work has focused on whole word measures of phonological acquisition.

Maria Kambanaros is Associate Professor of Speech Pathology in the Department of Rehabilitation Sciences at the Cyprus University of Technology and Director of the Research Lab on Rehabilitation of Neurological Communication Disorders. She is an experienced speech pathologist focusing on multilingual populations, ranging from developmental language impairments and genetic syndromes to acquired language disorders and language breakdown. With more than 70 publications and over 100 conference presentations, her research is well received around the world. Maria is also the author of *Diagnostic Issues in Speech-language Therapy*, 2007 (in Greek), the standard textbook in the Greek language speech pathology curricula.

Jane Le Roux is a speech and language therapist and lecturer and clinical educator in the Division of Communication Sciences and Disorders at the University of Cape Town, South Africa. Her research focuses on language and literacy in the South African context.

Olebeng Mahura is a speech and language therapist and a lecturer in the Division of Communication Sciences and Disorders at the University of Cape

Town. Her research focuses on describing typical speech sound development in children acquiring Setswana, a Southern Bantu language. Olebeng is also interested in developing speech assessment tools which can be used by speech-language therapists working with children acquiring Setswana.

Nicole Müller is Professor and Head of Speech and Hearing Sciences at University College Cork, Ireland. She received an MA from Bonn University, Germany, and her doctorate from the University of Oxford. Her research interests are in clinical linguistics, bilingualism, and the consequences for communication of acquired neurological conditions such as dementia and aphasia. Among Nicole's current work is the analysis of bilingual encounters among nursing home residents. She is the co-editor of the journal *Clinical Linguistics and Phonetics*.

Chané Naidoo is a speech and language therapist at St Chads CHC, Ladysmith, South Africa. She studied at the University of Cape Town. Her particular interest is in paediatric dysphagia, as well as the importance of early intervention pertaining to neurological impairments in adults and children. Chané hopes to further her studies in her field of practice.

Mª Isabel Navarro-Ruiz is a part-time lecturer at the Department of Spanish, Modern and Classic Philologies of the University of the Balearic Islands. She obtained her PhD in Romanic philology from the University of Barcelona. She was trained as a speech and language therapist through the postgraduate course in language and audition at Santa Creu and Sant Pau Hospital in Barcelona She currently combines her academic career at the UIB with her professional career as a freelance language therapist. Her research interests include language pathology, specifically assessment and remediation of SLI, L1 acquisition and the development of metalinguistic skills.

Michelle Pascoe is a speech and language therapist and senior lecturer in the Division of Communication Sciences and Disorders at the University of Cape Town, South Africa. Her research focuses on typical and atypical speech, language and literacy acquisition. Michelle's particular interest is in speech development in the Bantu languages of Southern Africa, multilingualism, and ways to support clinicians when working with families from a range of language backgrounds.

Lucrecia Rallo Fabra is a tenure-track Associate Professor at the Department of Spanish, Modern and Classic Philologies of the University of the Balearic Islands. She holds a master's degree in rehabilitation of language and speech disorders from the Universitat Politècnica de Catalunya and a PhD in linguistics from the University of Barcelona. Her research interests include L1 and L2 learning, specifically perception and production of speech sounds. Lucrecia has published her research in different peer-reviewed international journals such as *Estudios de Fonética Experimental, Clinical Linguistics and Phonetics, Journal of Phonetics* and *Phonetica*.

Juliette Reynders graduated from the University of Cape Town in 2015, with her honours in speech-language pathology. In 2016 she is completing her community service year at Ngwelezane, a tertiary hospital in Kwa-Zulu Natal, South Africa. Juliette's special interests include childhood apraxia of speech and the assessment and management of dysphagia across all age groups.

Savannah Senior is a speech and language therapist who is currently practising in Bloemfontein, South Africa. Her research focuses on typical and atypical speech acquisition.

Froogh Shooshtaryzadeh received her MA degree from Ferdowsi University, Mashhad, Iran, and her PhD degree from Jawaharlal Nehru University, New Delhi, India. She joined the Farsi Teaching Centre at the International Imam Khomeini University, Gazvin, Iran, in 1995, where she taught Farsi to foreign students and English to Persian students. Froogh joined the English Language Department of that university in 2006, where she is currently an Assistant Professor of Linguistics. She has published articles and a chapter in a book on first and second language acquisition. Her research interests include bilingualism, multilingualism, language and communication impairment, and cognitive development in developmental disorders.

Anna Sosa is Associate Professor of Communication Sciences and Disorders at Northern Arizona University in Flagstaff, Arizona. She received a BA in Spanish and French linguistics from Pomona College, an MA in linguistics from the University of New Mexico, and a PhD in speech and hearing sciences from the University of Washington. Anna is Director of the NAU Child Speech and Language Lab and an ASHA-certified speech-language pathologist. Her research and clinical interests include pre-linguistic and early phonological development in infants, toddlers and pre-schoolers with typical and disordered speech and language development.

Dimitrios Sotiropoulos obtained a PhD at the University of California, San Diego and taught at Northwestern University before joining the Technical University of Crete where he is a Professor. His main area of research is acoustics from a multi-disciplinary perspective including speech. Dimitrios is well published in journals including the *Proceedings of the Royal Society of London*, the *Journal of the Acoustical Society of America* and the *Journal of Sound and Vibration*. His research also includes quantitative methods for evaluating phonetic and phonological errors in child typical and atypical speech development and in second language speech in adults.

Joseph Paul Stemberger is a Professor in the Department of Linguistics at the University of British Columbia, Canada. His research focuses on mental representations and the processing of phonological and morphological information during language production, addressing implications for both psychological models and linguistic theories. Much of his research focuses on the errors that occur in language production, both the infrequent non-systematic errors of adult (and child) production and the frequent systematic errors of child production. While Joseph began with research on English, current major projects address phonological development in Valley Zapotec and 14 other (especially European) languages.

Matina Tasioudi is a PhD candidate of the Department of Special Education, University of Thessaly, Greece. She graduated from the Department of Literature and Linguistics, Aristotle University of Thessaloniki, and holds an MA from the same department on 'Linguistic communication: teaching Greek as a second/foreign language'. Matina teaches Greek as a second/foreign language. She is the writer of 12 articles published in international journals and proceedings and has presented her studies at 15 national and international conferences. Her research interests are focused on language impairment in developmental disorders and L1/L2 acquisition.

Loukia Taxitari is a post-doctoral research associate at the Department of Rehabilitation Sciences, Cyprus University of Technology. She holds a DPhil in experimental psychology from the University of Oxford, where she conducted research in language development with infants. Her research interests focus on L1 acquisition in typical, and more recently also atypical, populations. Loukia is mainly interested in the acquisition of semantics and the formation of the lexicon at the early stages of word learning and the interaction with other cognitive, as well as linguistic abilities, such as categorization and grammatical development.

Eleni Theodorou received her PhD from the University of Cyprus with the thesis 'Diagnosing specific language impairment: the case of Cypriot Greek'. She holds a BSc in speech therapy from the Technological Institute of Patras and an MSc in language and communication impairment in children from the University of Sheffield, UK. Eleni has published papers investigating the language of typical and atypical Cypriot Greek children, the phonetics of Cypriot Greek and the use of augmentative and alternative communication systems in Cyprus. She is lecturer in speech pathology in the Department of Rehabilitation Sciences at the Cyprus University of Technology.

Amy van der Merwe is a speech and language therapist at Red Cross War Memorial Children's Hospital in Cape Town, South Africa. Amy studied at the University of Cape Town. Her professional interests include language, literacy and learning, paediatric dysphagia and neurology. She enjoys working with children and providing rehabilitation within a multidisciplinary team.

Marina Varnava is a PhD student at the University of Cyprus under the supervision of K.K. Grohmann. She has a BA in English language and literature from the University of Essex and an MA in applied linguistics from the University of Cyprus. Marina's current focus is on bilingualism.

Introduction

Elena Babatsouli, David Ingram and Nicole Müller

Developments in research have practical relevance for guiding early language intervention and thereby reducing the risk of poor language development in children with communication disorders. Given the variability involved in the acquisition of disparate languages in monolingual, bilingual and bi-dialectal settings, linguists deciphering the process of language acquisition are faced with the task of designing and coordinating studies where such acquisition can be legitimately compared. This has immediate repercussions for the work of clinical linguists and language pathologists, where a common challenge crosslinguistically is to validate the efficacy of assessment and screening tools that identify and differentiate *disordered* from *normal* linguistic behaviour in children. Owing to a lack of assessment materials in many languages, batteries standardized for use in one language (or dialect) are often utilized to assess another, and batteries designed for a monolingual population are utilized to assess language in bilingualism.

There are numerous books on child language acquisition, monolingual and bilingual, presenting clear and concise introductions to main concepts, issues and debates (e.g. Bhatia & Ritchie, 2012; Clark, 2009; Grosjean, 2010; Lust, 2006). Some recent titles address specific language impairment and communication disorders in children in general (e.g. Leonard, 2014) and in multilingual contexts (e.g. Armon-Lotem *et al.*, 2015; Patterson & Rodriguez, 2016). McLeod and Goldstein (2012) explored both multilingual and multicultural aspects of children with speech sound disorders. The focus in some of the existing books is on a specific major language, like Spanish (e.g. Grinstead, 2009) or on a specific language level, like phonology (e.g. Hua & Dodd, 2006) or morphology (e.g. Grohmann & Neokleous, 2014).

The present volume brings together a number of studies on typical and atypical language acquisition, purposefully turning diversity into a core theme. Diversity is underscored here in terms of linguistic typology, types of language acquisition, the language level examined, the language context, research methodologies and proposed assessment tools. This collection enhances and complements existing literature on recent developments in typical and atypical language acquisition with regard to typologically different languages that are relatively under-represented in the literature, such as Greek

(Andreou & Tasioudi; Kambanaros *et al.*; Taxitari *et al.* – Chapters 7, 8, 6); Icelandic, Mandarin, Granada Spanish, Slovene (Bernhardt & Stemberger – Chapter 4), Maltese (Grech *et al.* – Chapter 5), isiXhosa (Pascoe *et al.* – Chapter 1), Farsi (Shooshtaryzadeh – Chapter 10), different language levels, such as general language ability (e.g. Andreou & Tasioudi; Kambanaros *et* al.; Sosa – Chapters 7, 8, 2), phonology (e.g. Bernhardt & Stemberger; Grech *et al.*; Pascoe *et al.*; Shooshtaryzadeh – Chapters 4, 5, 1, 10), morphology (Andreou & Tasioudi; Navarro-Ruiz & Rallo Fabra; Taxitari *et al.* – Chapters 7, 9, 6), etc.; cases of SLI and communication disorder in under-researched languages (e.g. Andreou & Tasioudi; Kambanaros *et al.*; Navarro-Ruiz & Rallo Fabra – Chapters 7, 8, 9); bilingual and bi-dialectal combinations not much researched previously (e.g. Pascoe *et al.*; Taxitari *et al.* – Chapters 1, 6), and novel applications in methodology and assessment (e.g. Babatsouli *et al.*; Bernhardt & Stemberger; Grech *et al.*; Sosa – Chapters 3, 4, 5, 2).

While the chapters focus on different particular aspects of child language in development, authors explain why there is a particular focus on the aspects or structures in their analysis and how tasks were designed to elicit the target structures. In spite of the thematic disparity represented in the volume, nevertheless, the majority of studies here formulate guidelines for task design in typologically different languages. The volume unites language acquisition research in languages and contexts that are different with widespread implications and usefulness. This goal forms the general focus of the book.

On Typical Language Acquisition

This edited volume is concerned with language acquisition in childhood. The acquisition of language in childhood refers to how a single linguistic code is being acquired by a child, i.e. in monolingual acquisition, or how two (or more) linguistic codes are concurrently acquired by a child, as in bilingual (or multilingual) acquisition. We prefer the term *linguistic code* because it allows us to incorporate a distinction that is less frequently addressed in language acquisition research, one that distinguishes between languages and dialects.

There are several theoretical approaches that have been utilized to explain language acquisition in typically developing populations. Such approaches have overwhelmingly been influenced by a combination of *theory* and *evidence* from linguistics and psychology. This juxtaposition between abstract knowledge and evidence-based deductions has been the most fundamental point of contention in language acquisition, which is principally highlighted in the opposition of *nurture* and *nature*, or in more theoretically driven parlance, between *empiricism* and *nativism*. Overall, language is acquired via a blend of learning through experience, as this is tempered by human reaction to social interactions in the environment, and by genetically endowed competence (e.g. physical, cognitive) which is considered innate and thus is, to a certain extent, universally present. Examples of major works contributing to these lines of thought include Chomsky (1959), Piaget (1955), Skinner (1938) and Vygotsky (1962).

Developing a sound theoretical framework that can account for crosslinguistic and individual differences in language acquisition is the ongoing goal of theoretically driven language research. Such a theoretical framework needs to rely on actual evidence. Applied linguistics research, focusing on acquisition, is amassing crosslinguistic data-based evidence aiming to establish reliable sets of norms in language acquisition. Such norms include appropriate linguistic performance at a given point in the developmental path, as well as during the transition from one point to the next along this same developmental path longitudinally.

The delineation of norms across the world's languages will be deduced from a delineation of norms in individual languages crosslinguistically, because it is known that there are language-specific tendencies involved in acquisition (e.g. Ingram, 2012). Alongside these crosslinguistic norms, an account of what is normative in the acquisition of different dialects within a single language (e.g. Grohmann *et al.*, 2016) also lies within the general framework of what language acquisition involves. Lastly, linguists joining their efforts around the world still need to address the issue of individual differences in language acquisition; where individual children differ in their way of acquiring language may be equally telling for the ultimate theory of language acquisition, since individual differences fall well within the range of *normal*, even if they are not within the range of *normative*.

An optimal but not necessarily easy way to pull this together would be combining methodological resources, such as single-case and cross-sectional, naturalistic and task-elicited, age-specific and longitudinal for any group of participants in studies crosslinguistically. Such tactics would help discourage a one-sided focus in which we see the trunk, the leaves and the tree, but '… the "woods" […] remain always difficult to detect' (Kehoe, 2015: 163), or vice versa. As each methodological scheme has its drawbacks and advantages, an all-encompassing methodological stance would safeguard against specific research methodologies being considered less advantageous than others.

It may well be that fundamental steps towards getting closer to the ultimate goal of plotting thorough maps of language in development are to aim for '… detailed longitudinal records of many subjects (single subject designs multiply replicated)' (Bernhardt & Stemberger, 1998: 16), and to ensure that equivalent methodology is used across children and languages or dialects (e.g. Bernhardt & Stemberger, this volume: Chapter 4). Such an approach may yet be feasible. An indication favouring this approach is found in the methodological design of Navarro-Ruiz and Rallo Fabra (this volume: Chapter 9), where a cross-sectional design is combined with a longitudinal design to bypass the methodological limitation of testing a large group of children over nine years.

On Atypical Language Acquisition

The laborious ant race involved in collecting and documenting norms in human language acquisition serves to develop common yardsticks that sketch out *typical* language acquisition. It is primarily on these grounds that *atypical* phenomena are evaluated as such, that is, whether they meet the criteria of what is typical or not. Consequently, what does *atypical* mean in language acquisition?

The language faculty is not a separate independent entity but an integral part of human biology, and it is affected by a person's general wellbeing. As a result, it is no surprise that language has been referred to as an *organ*, much like the heart, or the lungs. Chomsky (1980) argues that the language acquisition device (LAD) is one of many interacting 'mental organs' which together with input data produce linguistic competence. Anderson and Lightfoot (2000) use the term 'language organ' which clearly expresses how alive and perishable language is, and that conscious effort is required to nurture it with proper use through life. It is therefore inevitable that the language faculty is affected by human pathology (e.g. Andreou & Tasioudi; Kambanaros *et al.*, this volume: Chapters 7, 8), and that linguists need to undertake the additional task of documenting how developmental language behaves under these atypical situations, where language impairment is a result of complications in genetics, anatomy, neurology, cognition, etc. In sum, language acquisition becomes a medical issue, as well.

Language disorder is determined by the same principal factors discussed earlier, that is, the interplay between abstract knowledge (which is partly innate and partly acquired) and more concrete factors (i.e. the speaker's physical condition or skill). 'There are no linguistic theories … of disordered language that do not start out as theories of normal language' (Müller & Ball, 2015: 29). The terms that are customarily used to differentiate children whose linguistic development conforms to the norm from those that do not are often seasoned by political correctness, or what is considered to be an acceptable standard across countries. For instance, *normal* versus *abnormal* may not be acceptable for some, though *typical* versus *atypical* may be. Pascoe (2015) briefly discusses issues of this terminology with regard to children's speech sound disorders.

When it comes to atypical patterns in the acquisition of the sound system of language (which combines phonology and phonetics), for example, Ingram *et al.* (2018) distinguish between phonological disorder (relating to abstract knowledge), articulatory disorder (involving physical condition and skill) and spectrum varieties that may involve both, at different degrees of influence. Alongside these, the age factor in language development is fundamental in distinguishing between acquisition that is completed on time or shows delay (also called protraction), and between performance that is either normal or shows evidence of a form of deviance. Overall, a combination of structural, articulatory, behavioural, biological and cognitive theories, among others, is used to make sense of children's speech sound disorders (Bowen, 2015: 26–50). Although the examples in the last two paragraphs have focused on phonology, the arguments are hardly specific to it; all main linguistic areas, like semantics (involving receptive and expressive vocabulary) or morphosyntax are concerned with the aspects just outlined.

Crosslinguistic Encounters of Typical and Atypical Language Acquisition

On practical grounds, developments in research on both typical and atypical language acquisition are hoped to have immediate repercussions on how to assess what is atypical, which in turn may guide speech-language intervention early on, and may help optimize language development in children with communication disorders or disorders affecting communication skills. By understanding and assessing how children with atypical language development communicate, we can tailor specific interventions. If this is successful, quality of life improves for them and for the people they associate with. In other words, the most meaningful payoff for all endeavours on both the typical and atypical fronts is a humanitarian one.

However, linking theoretical approaches to a comprehensive intervention approach that is common for those children showing the same type of speech-language disorder may not be sufficient. Knowing what individual variation entails in the acquisition of language is also crucial. It has been argued, at least with regard to speech sound disorders, that no single intervention approach should be used for all children, nor should intervention approaches necessarily be based on a single theoretical perspective (Ingram, 2015). Those working on theory (e.g. linguists) and those working on practice (e.g. therapists) need to collaborate closely (e.g. Duchan, 2001) to tailor theoretical knowledge and intervention practice to the specific needs of individual children with specific language problems.

Consequently, it may be necessary that more theoreticians adopt more hands-on approaches to simplify the theoretical implications of their research by making specific recommendations which are ready for practical use in the assessment and intervention of language pathology (e.g. Babatsouli, 2016; Babatsouli *et al.*, this volume). Then such material may need to be further modified for appropriate dissemination to practitioners. Many library books may never reach the practice room, especially when they are written in a language that is not the practitioner's native language.

Part 1: Typical Language Acquisition

The volume's first two chapters form the section on typical language acquisition. Although the majority of the studies in the volume combine a discussion on typical and atypical acquisition, these two studies differ in that they highlight the significance of the linguistic input in language development as part of social interaction. Specifically, the focus of one chapter is on infancy, making a clear differentiation between actual speech and infant speech volubility; the focus of the other is on bilingual acquisition of an English dialect and an under-represented language within a larger multilingual context.

Chapter 1: Speech Development in Three-year-old Children Acquiring isiXhosa and English in South Africa

Michelle Pascoe, Olebeng Mahura, Jane Le Roux, Emily Danvers, Aimée de Jager, Natania Esterhuizen, Chané Naidoo, Juliette Reynders, Savannah Senior and Amy van der Merwe

Chapter 1 focuses on an investigation of speech development in three-year-old bilingual children acquiring isiXhosa and South African English in a general multilingual or multi-dialectal context. Given that there are few studies documenting phonological development of isiXhosa-speaking children, the aim is to provide a yardstick of what is normative in these typically developing bilinguals to support the assessment of atypical speech assessment and intervention decisions of speech-language therapists in South Africa. Phonetic inventories and phonological processes are drawn up in this study, based on the speech data of 33 children published in previous studies. It is found that these children's development in English largely corresponds to known monolingual norms, while the development of both languages also exhibits specificity regarding some processes. Also, more variability is observed in both languages in younger children. The study emphasizes that future studies ought to take into consideration the dialectal influences present in the linguistic input of these bilingual children for a more accurate interpretation of bilingual phonological acquisition in these and similar contexts.

Chapter 2: The Impact of Parent Communication Patterns on Infant Volubility during Play with Books

Anna V. Sosa

This is the only study in this volume that investigates the relationship between the quality of social interaction and the quality of linguistic output in infancy. In particular, the study examines how parental communication patterns affect infant volubility in order to identify whether certain types of parental behaviour are likely to lead to increased speech volubility in infants aged between 0;10 and 1;4. The LENA Pro is used to analyze the linguistic behaviour of 27 parent-infant dyads during play sessions involving children's books. The results of the study show that parental verbal responsiveness was the only communicative behaviour that significantly correlated with increased infant volubility. The overall amount of adult input given did not correlate with infant volubility, as babies that regularly babbled more also did so during play sessions. These findings agree with previous ones in the literature, but it is argued here that parental contingent responsiveness could be employed as a strategy in atypical contexts to encourage more infant volubility which, in turn, supports better overall linguistic development, and could thus be used as an early intervention strategy to counteract language delay.

Part 2: Methods in Language Analysis and Assessment

The chapters in this section are grouped together because they propose novel tools and assessment practices with universal implications crosslinguistically, while also dealing with language-specific complications.

Chapter 3: On the Weight of Phones in Computing Phonological Word Proximity

Elena Babatsouli, David Ingram and Dimitrios Sotiropoulos

Within the tradition of measures that quantitatively evaluate speech performance in linguistic development, this study examines how computed phonological word proximity may be affected by the arbitrary relative weight between the phones in a word; this is investigated in the specific context of child speech productions of the same or different word samples. A mathematical expression for phonological word proximity is obtained in terms of PCC, the proportion of consonant phonemes, and the proportion of phonemes deleted. It is found that, although the difference between the weights of PCC, or the proportion of phones deleted, for different relative weights between the phones generally increases with the increasing proportion of phones, it remains effectively constant for a proportion of phones larger than 50%. The results have direct implications on assessing phonological word proximity in typical and atypical contexts. The study makes specific recommendations, directly employable in practice, on how to tailor assessment using the measure of phonological word proximity.

Chapter 4: Investigating Typical and Protracted Phonological Development across Languages

Barbara May Bernhardt and Joseph Paul Stemberger

Within the framework of universal and language-specific influences on phonological acquisition, Chapter 4 overviews methodological issues and some results emanating from an international study of crosslinguistic phonological development across 12 languages in the following families: Asian, Germanic, Romance, Semitic and South Slavic. The study combines investigations that aim to document differences in typical phonological development crosslinguistically, as well as to create resources for use in phonological assessment and intervention. The novel approach implemented here advances language acquisition research with the use of equivalent methodology across several well-studied and less investigated languages, highlighting the significance of the need to also account for dialectal variation. The methodological advances here enhance comparability across languages and emphasize the significance of this goal across different studies in the future.

Chapter 5: Bilingual Speech Assessment for Maltese Children

Helen Grech, Barbara Dodd and Sue Franklin

This chapter highlights a major pitfall in clinical assessment internationally whereby bilingual children are often evaluated and diagnosed with speech disorders using protocols standardized on monolingual, largely English-speaking populations. By reporting on the phonological development of 241 bilingual Maltese-English speaking children aged between 2;0 and 6;0, this study introduces a novel approach to an existing speech assessment tool for Maltese, i.e. the MESA: for all of the items investigated in the study, children respond in each language, thus reflecting the bilingual nature of the assessment in this population. The study expands previous methodological practices by including a subtest that assesses complex phonotactics such as those found in Maltese phonology. Results differentiate between articulatory ability and the effect of abstract phonological knowledge as this is evidenced in phonological processes. The methodology used and findings in this chapter provide clinicians with a better defined outlook on how to address divergence in typical development, speech protraction and speech deviation when assessing Maltese children.

Chapter 6: Early Language Development in a Bilectal Context: The Cypriot Adaptation of the MacArthur-Bates CDI

Loukia Taxitari, Maria Kambanaros, Georgios Floros and Kleanthes K. Grohmann

There are few studies crosslinguistically that aim to compare dialectal development in children. This chapter contributes in this direction by investigating lexical and morphological development in children who speak two dialects of Greek: Standard Modern Greek and Cypriot Greek. Additionally, the study introduces the MacArthur-Bates Communicative Development Inventory (CG-CDI) adapted for Cypriot Greek, and presents results from investigations based on toddlers aged 18–30 months old. Findings on a steady increase of vocabulary correspond to previous ones in the literature on lexical development, but also show that there is a noteworthy correlation between lexical and morphological development in Cypriot Greek. The adapted tool for Cypriot Greek is significant for language assessment of typically developing children in Cyprus which also gives insights into early bilectal (bi-dilectal) development, with implications on the development of the Greek language in general.

Part 3: Language Acquisition in the Presence of a Disorder

This section summarizes contributions in language acquisition in the presence of disorder: obstructive sleep apnoea syndrome (OSAS) in Standard Modern Greek; self-repair mechanisms in specific language impairment (SLI) in Spanish; 22q11.2 deletion syndrome in Cypriot Greek; and local assimilation patterns in the typical and atypical phonology of two groups of Persian children acquiring Farsi.

Chapter 7: Obstructive Sleep Apnoea Syndrome: Does It Really Affect Language Acquisition during Early Childhood?

Georgia Andreou and Matina Tasioudi

The chapter investigates how obstructive sleep apnoea syndrome (OSAS) affects linguistic development in early childhood, since little is known about whether language is fundamentally affected by OSAS. The particular emphasis is on which linguistic domains are affected and to what degree. The focus is on Standard Modern Greek, where there are no previous studies reporting on the performance of different language levels in children with OSAS. The study involved a total of 50 aged-matched children (mean age: 5;6): 25

children with OSAS, and a control group of typically developing children. The standardized psychometric language test L-a-T-o I, developed for Greek, was used to evaluate general language ability, phonology, morphosyntax and semantics. Children with OSAS are found to show significant difficulties with all tasks, but mostly with phonology and morphosyntax. The performance of the OSAS group on general language ability was lower than in the TD group, though not so in their non-verbal ability. The results of this study extend findings in other languages by focusing on which language areas are the most problematic in children with OSAS and suggest that medical treatment should be combined with early language intervention in order to avoid the risk of poor language development during childhood and adolescence, i.e. the critical ages of brain growth and development.

Chapter 8: Language Impairment in 22q11.2 Deletion Syndrome: A Case Study from Cyprus

Maria Kambanaros, Loukia Taxitari, Eleni Theodorou, Marina Varnava and Kleanthes K. Grohmann

Chapter 8 contributes to research that assesses how cognitive abilities affect linguistic ones. It does so with a case study on the Cypriot Greek linguistic profile of a six-year-old male child with 22q11.2 deletion syndrome, an autosomal dominant genetic disorder. The child's data are compared with those of pre-school children with SLI and a control group. Language testing involved comprehension of complex structures, clitic production and a narrative retell task. The study concludes that the language impairment attested in the child with 22q11.2 deletion syndrome differs qualitatively from the patterns of both his peers with SLI and the control group. His impairment was evident on the receptive and expressive measures of complex language, which did not hold for the age-matched group with SLI. While similar in terms of below-TLD performance, his inferior language abilities in comprehending complex language are different from the patterns in SLI. With regard to clinical implications, the study provides a first gauge for differentiating language disability in SLI and 22q11.2DS in Cypriot Greek, but also with direct implications for other languages.

Chapter 9: The Emergence and Development of Self-repair: A Longitudinal Case Study of Specific Language Impairment from 3;0 to 6;10 Years

Mª Isabel Navarro-Ruiz and Lucrecia Rallo Fabra

This study utilizes a longitudinal design to examine self-repair development in Spanish, comparing a child with SLI with a control group of 40 typically developing children (aged between 1;10 and 10 years). The results of the study show that self-repairs in the control group follow a U-shaped pattern of reorganization, but do not emerge simultaneously at all linguistic levels. The phonological level is the one that is mostly affected beginning around age 1;10, while pragmatic self-repairs are the most common type. The child with SLI shows fewer self-repairs, which appear at a later age (4;3) and are morphological and syntactical, rather than phonological. The authors argue that the linguistic levels that show many errors but few self-repairs correspond to the more affected language levels with less metalinguistic information. They suggest that linguistic competence is influenced by metalinguistic functions. The study fills in a gap in the literature on language disorders in Spanish: the data provide information on which language levels are more affected during self-repairs in specific language impairment. In practical terms, the results provide a perspective on designing customized plans for specific language impairment, utilizing metalinguistic intervention approaches. Lastly, it is shown that social integration has positive effects on the general wellbeing of the child with SLI, including language skills.

Chapter 10: Local Assimilation in Children Acquiring Farsi: A Case Study of Typical versus Atypical Phonological Development

Froogh Shooshtaryzadeh

This chapter, on the development of typical and atypical Farsi, compares local assimilation patterns in the speech of two groups of Persian children, and further compares their speech patterns with published literature. In particular, the developing speech of five children with functional phonological disorder (PD) is compared to that of 10 typically developing (TD) peers. The data, which were elicited using a picture-naming task of 132 items, show qualitatively different assimilation patterns between adjacent segments in the two groups. The results of the study are viewed from the theoretical perspective of optimality theory (e.g. Prince & Smolensky, 1993) with reference to phonetic approaches, where relevant. The investigation shows significant differences in the local assimilation patterns of the Farsi-speaking children and known patterns in other languages, as well as differences between the acquisition patterns of the TD children and those of the PD group. While results in the TD group are straightforward, the children with PD show more complex assimilation patterns. Findings of this study have implications for clinical assessment and intervention, and add to the cross-linguistic knowledge base on phonological development.

Concluding Remarks

The present book documents recent developments in typical and atypical language acquisition. While the focus in the related literature so far has mostly been on major languages, like English, much less is known about language acquisition and the language skills of children in development across different languages, in different bilingual combinations, and in gradient varieties such as dialects of the same language. Also, little is known about how typically developing populations crosslinguistically, and in the aforementioned contexts, compare with atypical populations. A number of linguistic levels, e.g. lexical, phonological, morphological and metalinguistic, are represented here, contrasting and comparing typical with atypical, and often focusing on which linguistic levels are mostly affected by a given disorder. Overall, this book with its divergent chapters asks questions and seeks to formulate answers on how the evidenced diversity may inform language and communication development in the presence or absence of disorder.

The book addresses these issues by presenting studies in typologically different languages, some of which are not widely studied, like Farsi, Greek, isiXhosa, Maltese, and some of which are in combinations with a major language in a bilingual or bi-dialectal context, e.g. English-Maltese, isiXhosa-South African English, Modern Greek-Cypriot Greek. The volume enhances the literature by addressing disorder in language acquisition also from the perspective of human pathology, i.e. what to expect in linguistic development in the presence of under-studied syndromes, such as obstructive sleep apnoea syndrome (OSAS) and 22q11.2 deletion syndrome. Direct comparisons are made not only with the typical populations but also with patterns common in SLI. Lastly, this collection of studies advances methodological and assessment issues in language development research, discussing the effectiveness of current methodologies. Furthermore, it proposes and applies new assessment tools and batteries, some of which target equivalence of assessment across different languages and across different dialects of the same language, while others are more language specific.

As a flashback to the earlier discussion on methodology, comparisons of single-case and cross-sectional developmental language data are utilized in the book, exploiting both approaches, sometimes separately and sometimes combining them. This edition highlights a need for language research to draw a clear picture of patterns in typical language acquisition, not only by zooming in on the petiole (the part of the leaf that connects the blade to the stem) or by roughly making out the shape of the woods, but combining simultaneous efforts on both fronts. To bring up Leopold's (1954) metaphor: 'children's language learning' may be better depicted 'with the detail of a slow-motion picture and the speed of a fast-motion picture' (Leopold, 1954: 14). Working in this direction will also contribute towards delineating norms and individual differences in atypical child language, which will in turn better facilitate customized evaluation and intervention for children exhibiting a specific communication difficulty or combinations of them. Daunting as this may seem, ants are known to collect and save for the winter.

Overall, this edition advances further the increasing awareness for the need of a lot more sharing and collaboration on many levels, the kind of sharing that will save time and duplication of efforts on the research methodologies used, on the specifics of existing methodological and intervention adaptations crosslinguistically, which may prove useful in similar contexts, on data sharing and, last but not least, on narrowing the gap between academia, clinicians, the children and their families. All of this brings us back to where we started. Where do typical and atypical language development meet crosslinguistically? They meet where the child is, and that is where the future lies.

References

Anderson, S.R. and Lightfoot, D. (2000) The human language faculty as an organ. *Annual Review of Physiology* 62, 697–722.

Armon-Lotem, S., de Jong, J. and Meir, N. (2015) *Assessing Multilingual Children: Disentangling Bilingualism from Language Impairment*. Bristol: Multilingual Matters.

Babatsouli, E. (2016) Added syllable complexity in a child's developmental speech and clinical implications. *Clinical Linguistics and Phonetics* 30 (8), 628–648.

Bernhardt, B. and Stemberger, J. (1998) *Handbook of Phonological Development from the Perspective of Constraint-based Nonlinear Phonology*. San Diego, CA: Academic Press.

Bhatia, T.K. and Ritchie, W.C. (eds) (2012) *The Handbook of Bilingualism and Multilingualism* (2nd edn). Malden, MA: Wiley-Blackwell.

Bowen, C. (2015) *Children's Speech Sound Disorders* (2nd edn). Oxford: John Wiley.

Chomsky, N. (1959) A review of B.F. Skinner's verbal behavior. *Language* 35 (1), 26–58.

Chomsky, N. (1980) *Rules and Representations*. Cambridge, MA: MIT Press.

Clark, E.V. (2009) *First Language Acquisition* (2nd edn). Cambridge: Cambridge University Press.

Duchan, J.F. (2001) *A History of Speech-Language Pathology in America*. See http://www.acsu.buffalo.edu/~duchan/history.html

Grinstead, J. (2009) *Hispanic Child Languages: Typical and Impaired Development*. Amsterdam/Philadelphia, PA: John Benjamins.

Grohmann, K.K. and Neokleous, T. (2014) *Developments in the Acquisition of Clitics*. Newcastle-upon-Tyne: Cambridge Scholars.

Grohmann, K.K., Kambanaros, M., Leivada, E. and Rowe, C. (2016) A developmental approach to diglossia: Bilectalism on a gradient scale of linguality [In E. Babatsouli and D. Ingram (guest eds) Special issue on 'Monolingual and Bilingual Speech across Languages']. *Poznan Studies in Contemporary Linguistics* 52 (4), 629–662.

Grosjean, F. (2010) *Bilingual: Life and Reality*. Cambridge, MA: Harvard University Press.

Hua, Z. and Dodd, B. (2006) *Phonological Development and Disorders in Children: A Multilingual Perspective*. Bristol: Multilingual Matters.

Ingram, D. (2012) Prologue: Cross-linguistic and multilingual aspects of speech sound disorders in children. In S. McLeod and B. Goldstein (eds) *Multilingual Aspects of Speech Sound Disorders in Children* (pp. 3–12). Bristol: Multilingual Matters.

Ingram, D. (2015) The role of theory in SSD. In C. Bowen (ed.) *Children's Speech Sound Disorders* (2nd edn) (pp. 42–45). Oxford: John Wiley.

Ingram, D., Williams, L. and Scherer, N.J. (2018, January) Are speech sound disorders phonological or articulatory? A spectrum approach. In E. Babatsouli and D. Ingram (eds) *Phonology in Protolanguage and Interlanguage* (pp. 27–48). Sheffield: Equinox.

Kehoe, M. (2015) Cross-linguistic interaction: A retrospective and prospective view. In E. Babatsouli and D. Ingram (eds) *Proceedings of the International Symposium on Monolingual and Bilingual Speech 2015* (pp. 141–167). See http://ismbs.eu/publications

Leonard, L.B. (2014) *Children with Specific Language Impairment*. Language Speech and Communication. Cambridge, MA: MIT Press.

Leopold, W.F. (1954) Patterning in children's language learning. *Language Learning* 5, 1–14.

Lust, B. (2006) *Child Language: Acquisition and Growth*. Cambridge: Cambridge University Press.

McLeod, S. and Goldstein, B.A. (2012) *Multilingual Aspects of Speech Sound Disorders in Children*. Bristol: Multilingual Matters.

Müller, N. and Ball, M. (2015) Clinical linguistics (and phonetics). In C. Bowen (ed.) *Children's Speech Sound Disorders* (2nd edn) (pp. 28–31). Oxford: John Wiley.

Pascoe, M. (2015) Going between intervention for children's speech sound difficulties from an international perspective. In C. Bowen (ed.) *Children's Speech Sound Disorders* (2nd edn) (pp. 12–14). Oxford: John Wiley.

Patterson, J.L. and Rodriguez, B.L. (2016) *Multilingual Perspectives on Child Language Disorders*. Bristol: Multilingual Matters.

Piaget, J. (1955) *The Language and Thought of a Child* (trans. M. Gabain). Cleveland, OH: Meridian Books.

Prince, A. and Smolensky, P. (1993) *Optimality Theory: Constraint Interaction in Generative Grammar*. Oxford: Blackwell.

Skinner, B.F. (1938) *The Behavior of Organisms: An Experimental Analysis*. Cambridge, MA: B.F. Skinner Foundation.

Vygotsky, L.S (1962) *Thought and Language*. Cambridge, MA: MIT Press.

Part 1

Typical Language Acquisition

1 Speech Development in Three-year-old Children Acquiring isiXhosa and English in South Africa

Michelle Pascoe, Olebeng Mahura, Jane Le Roux, Emily Danvers, Aimée de Jager, Natania Esterhuizen, Chané Naidoo, Juliette Reynders, Savannah Senior and Amy van der Merwe

Introduction

This chapter focuses on bilingual children simultaneously acquiring English and isiXhosa in Cape Town, South Africa. We aim to describe the typical speech acquisition of three-year-old children acquiring both these languages. The chapter starts by providing background regarding the language and demographics of South Africa, together with a rationale for why it is important, but challenging, to identify children with speech sound disorders in this context. This is followed by a description of the two languages. We then move into a review of the literature on monolingual acquisition of isiXhosa and South African English before considering our data from bilingual children.

South Africa is characterized by a culturally and linguistically diverse population. Our progressive constitution recognizes 11 official languages and advocates equal status for them all. These 11 languages include nine indigenous Bantu languages: isiZulu, isiXhosa, Sepedi, Setswana, Sesotho, Xitsonga, Siswati, Tshivenda and isiNdebele, together with the West Germanic languages of English and Afrikaans. Of course there are many more languages and dialects spoken beyond the officially recognized ones, especially by people who have immigrated to South Africa from neighbouring countries. Multilingualism is common in South Africa, with the exact combinations of languages and dialects spoken varying from region to region. In the Western Cape, the main languages spoken are Afrikaans (spoken by 49.7% of the population), isiXhosa (spoken by 24.7%) and English (spoken by 20.3%) (Statistics South Africa, 2011).

The rich linguistic diversity of Southern Africa offers many exciting research opportunities, yet the study of speech acquisition in this context remains relatively unresearched. Some of the Bantu languages, such as Sesotho, isiXhosa and isiZulu, now have small datasets and several papers documenting typical speech acquisition. Much of this work has focused on monolingual children, and where bi- or multilingual children have been investigated, the children's language exposure and abilities across all their languages have not been well documented. This focus on monolingual children is understandable since researchers wish to investigate these under-researched languages in their purest forms, uninfluenced by other languages. There are rural parts of the country where it is common to find children acquiring one language with little exposure to other languages. However, in cities in South Africa, monolingualism is less common and children will typically be exposed to multiple languages (Posel & Zeller, 2016). There are relatively few studies that have focused on the typical acquisition of multiple phonologies at the same time. According to Gxilishe (2004) and Tuomi *et al.* (2001), the interplay between the languages is often ignored.

Around the world, children with speech sound difficulties (SSDs) comprise a large proportion of speech-language therapists' caseloads. SSDs may affect more children than any other developmental communication disorder and, if left untreated, can result in long-term academic and psychosocial difficulties (Broomfield & Dodd, 2004; Fox & Dodd, 2001). The World Health Organization's (2007) *International Classification of Functioning, Disability and Health* considers activity and participation to be profoundly affected by speech impairments. Although the prevalence of speech difficulties in South Africa has not yet been documented, in the United States it is estimated to be 7.5% of children between the ages of three and 11 years (Ruscello, 2008) and UK figures suggest that at least 48,000 children are referred for speech difficulties each year (Broomfield & Dodd, 2004).

For speech and language therapists working in South Africa, the lack of knowledge about typical speech development presents a challenge. Clinicians need to identify children with SSDs and assist them and their families. Being able to identify and manage such children requires a baseline of normative data, collected from the same population as that of the child. There are few speech assessments relevant for use with local indigenous languages (van der Merwe & Le Roux, 2014; van Dulm & Southwood, 2015). Many of the English assessments currently used by speech and language therapists in South Africa have been normed on different populations, e.g. monolingual

British children, which could possibly result in therapists *pathologizing* children who are in fact typical (Holm *et al.*, 1999). We are beginning to build knowledge about typical monolingual acquisition of isiXhosa and South African English, but knowledge about the nature of typical bilingual acquisition is limited. As a prelude to a description of current knowledge about phonological development in South Africa, the following sections provide a description of the phonology of isiXhosa and South African English, in turn.

isiXhosa

isiXhosa is a Southern Bantu language belonging to the Nguni group of languages (Mesthrie *et al.*, 2004). The isiXhosa phonological system is made up of 46 phonemes; five vowels (/a, i, u, e, ɛ/), 38 consonants, and three basic clicks (/|, ||, !/). The three basic clicks have 12 allophones, which occur when the clicks combine with guttural, nasal and palatal sounds. Consonantal features which are characteristic of the isiXhosa sound system include ejective plosives (/p'/), bilabial implosive (/ɓ/), velar and lateral fricatives (/x, ɬ/) and voiced affricate (/ʤ/) (Mowrer & Burger, 1991). Light /l/ is used. Consonant clusters are rarely found in isiXhosa and only occur in the form of borrowed words, e.g. ***ibr**ushi* 'brush'; ***igr**eyivi* 'gravy' (Demuth, 2003; Mohammed, 2001). isiXhosa is a tonal language, i.e. the meaning of a word can be altered by using contrastive tone, and consists of open syllables (syllables ending in vowels) (Mosaka, 2000). Lexical stress is not a feature of the isiXhosa sound system. The penultimate syllable of a word is, however, often lengthened (Mosaka, 2000).

isiXhosa is characterized by a number of dialects described in detail by Gxilishe (1996). These include the Thembu, Gcaleka, Bomvana, Mpondomise, Mpondo, Hlubi, Xesibe, Ntlangwini, Cele and Bhaca dialects. Each dialect is linked to a specific geographical region of the country. Although mutually intelligible, the differences between the dialects can be marked and there is a need to undertake further research into dialectal differences and to consider the dialect being spoken when working with children acquiring isiXhosa.

South African English

As with other varieties of English, dialectal variation is common in South African English (Mesthrie *et al.*, 2004). As a result of South Africa's past, marked by racial segregation after the institution of Apartheid in 1948, distinct varieties of South African English have developed (de Klerk, 1999; Lass, 2004). The two main varieties of South African English commonly spoken in the Western Cape are termed *Black South African English* (BSAE) and *White South African English* (WSAE). BSAE refers to the dialect of English spoken by first language speakers of Bantu languages such as isiXhosa, in addition to being a regional dialect of some first language English speakers (de Klerk, 1999; de Klerk & Gough, 2004; van Rooy, 2000). Defining features of BSAE include reduced contrasts between tense and lax vowels due to neutralization, the use of fewer central vowels and lengthened duration of diphthongs. Consonant features include the realization of the dental fricatives /θ, ð/ as plosives /t, d/; and palatal fricatives /ʃ, ʒ/ realized as alveolars /s, z/ (de Klerk & Gough, 2004; Van Rooy, 2000). Devoicing processes, particularly word final and velar plosive devoicing, are frequently reported as defining characteristics of BSAE (Lass, 2004; Van Rooy, 2000).

WSAE is the dialect of English spoken by first language English speakers in South Africa (Bowerman, 2008). According to this model, the dialect of those with high socio-economic status (SES) (known as the conservative variety, Dialect 1) most closely resembles British Received Pronunciation (Bowerman, 2008; Lass, 2004). Dialect 2, most commonly associated with the middle class in terms of SES, shares many features with Received Pronunciation. A third variety (Dialect 3) is often associated with the lower SES groups and many Afrikaans speakers.

One of the defining features of WSAE is the pronunciation of vowels. South African English is characterized by the *kit/bit* split: in South African English the /ɪ/ in *kit* is closer and more frontal than in other varieties, where it is more centralized (Lass, 2004). In no other variety of English do the words *kit* (produced [kɪt]) and *bit* (produced [bət]) not rhyme (Lass, 2004). Defining consonant features include distinct contrasts between voiced and voiceless consonants, with consistently unaspirated voiceless variants (e.g. /t/ in *tune* realized as [tj]) in all three categories. In most varieties of South African English, light and dark /l/ are used as allophones. The influence of Afrikaans is particularly evident in Dialect 3. For example, where Dialects 1 and 2 produce [ɹ] (as in *rat*), speakers of Dialect 3 use an alveolar trill [r] (Bowerman, 2008; Lass, 2004). The tendency for /θ/ to be produced as /f/ in the final word position is a further distinctive feature of Dialect 3 (Bowerman, 2008; Lass, 2004). In light of the variations within South African English, and the features that define it as a variety distinct from other varieties of English, including those in which the majority of standardized tests are normed, it is essential that assessment and therapy materials are adapted for the South African context.

isiXhosa speech acquisition in monolingual children

Although information on speech sound development in isiXhosa is limited, a number of studies have investigated the acquisition of isiXhosa segmental phonology in monolingual children. Children acquiring isiXhosa appear to develop most phonemes early (Gxilishe, 2004; Mowrer & Burger, 1991; Pascoe & Smouse, 2012; Tuomi *et al.*, 2001). The small group of published studies that have focused on monolingual children's acquisition of isiXhosa are summarized in Table 1.1.

Most of the studies presented in Table 1.1 used small samples that cannot be generalized to the population (Gxilishe, 2004; Pascoe *et al.*, 2016;

Table 1.1 Speech acquisition studies focusing on monolingual children acquiring isiXhosa

Author(s)	*Participants*	*Areas investigated*	*Main findings*
Mowrer and Burger (1991)	70 children aged 2;6–6;0 years	Consonants	2;6–3;0 years: Fricatives /x, ɣ, ɦ, f, v, z/ and dental /ǀ/ and palatal /!/ clicks are acquired.[a] 3;0: Most consonants have been acquired. 3;0–3;6: /s/ is acquired. 3;6–4;0: /ʃ/ and lateral click /ǁ/ acquired. 4;0–5;0: Trilled /r/. 5;0–5;6: /ʧ'/ 6;0 and beyond: /cʰ, ɟ/.
Tuomi *et al.* (2001)	10 children aged 1;0–3;0 years	Consonants and vowels	1;6 years: Five isiXhosa vowels are acquired.[b] 1;6–2;0: Sibilants /s, z/ are acquired. 2;7–3;0: Clicks are frequently produced correctly. 3;6–3;11: All basic clicks /ǀ, ǁ, !/ are acquired.
Gxilishe (2004)	10 children aged 1;0–3;0 years	Acquisition of clicks	1;0–1;6 years: All basic clicks emerge, although correct production only occurred at 70% accuracy. The dental click /ǀ/ is acquired[c] first, followed by the palatal /!/ and lateral /ǁ/ clicks.
Pascoe *et al.* (2016)	Two children aged 2;5 and 2;8 years	Comparison of naming, repetition and auditory processing	Both children were approximating adult levels of accuracy in their speech output, but were constrained by limited vocabulary.

Source: Based on Pascoe and Smouse (2012).
Notes: [a]When 80% of children accurately produced the sound in word-medial position on one occasion.
[b]When 75% of the children in a given age range produced the phoneme correctly at a criterion frequency of 66.6%.
[c]Produced accurately four times.

Tuomi *et al.*, 2001). These studies specified monolingual exposure to isiXhosa as inclusion criteria for their participants so that the influences of other languages did not confound results. Mowrer and Burger (1991) studied a relatively large sample of children, with the phonology of 70 monolingual isiXhosa children contrasted with that of a smaller group of monolingual English-speaking children for the phonemes shared across languages. Together, these studies highlight the early acquisition of vowels, a trend similar to that reported for children acquiring English (Dodd *et al.*, 2003). Affricates and complex clicks appear to only develop after nasals, liquids, glides and plosives. The basic clicks, even though produced accurately at a low frequency rate, seem to emerge between 1;0 and 1;6 years (Tuomi *et al.*, 2001). These clicks follow a specific order of acquisition: the dental click occurs first, often followed by the palatal, with the lateral being the last of the basic clicks to be acquired (Gxilishe, 2004; Mowrer & Burger, 1991; Tuomi *et al.*, 2001).

Maphalala *et al.* (2014) carried out an investigation of 24 isiXhosa-speaking children aged three to six years. The children were typically developing and exposed to isiXhosa (as a first language) and English through their family, community and day care environment. Maphalala *et al.* (2014) describe the way in which many children in this study did not name pictures as expected for isiXhosa. For example, a picture expected to elicit the response *uyatyhala* 's/he is pushing' was named as *uyapusha* (*uya*: isiXhosa, s/he is; *push(a)*: English verb *pushing*/ verb*a* indicates present stem in isiXhosa) by many of the participants. Maphalala *et al.* (2014) found that aspirated plosives and affricates were still developing in the five-year-old children in their sample, i.e. these consonants may be some of the last acquired in isiXhosa. Five- and six-syllable words appeared to continue to develop beyond six years. The paper by Maphalala *et al.* (2014) is one of few isiXhosa acquisition studies to have included bilingual children, and in this chapter we draw on some of the data from that project.

South African English in monolingual children

In contrast to adult South African English, children's acquisition of South African English has been minimally studied. Sociolinguistic literature documents dialectal features of this variety of English and the way in which it is influenced by other local languages such as Afrikaans and isiXhosa (Mesthrie *et al.*, 2004; van Rooy, 2008) (see discussion above about BSAE and WSAE). This knowledge can inform research with a developmental focus, as knowing about acceptable adult targets allows for better understanding of what is typical for children. Knowledge of adult production of South African English suggests that the following might be observed in children acquiring SAE:

- Alveolar trill /r/ and post-vocalic /r/.
- Word final devoicing (e.g. *dok* for *dog*).
- Reduced contrasts between long and short vowels (*seat*/*sit*); fewer central vowels and avoidance of schwa. Schwa may be produced as /a/ in open syllables; and some diphthongs are reduced to monophthongs.

- Vowel raising (English L1 speakers), e.g. *yis* for *yes*; *Efrica* for *Africa*.
- A *kit/bit* split, i.e. the words *kit* [kɪt] and *bit* [bət] do not rhyme. [ɪ] is used when it occurs before or after velars, after /h/, before /ʃ/, and word initially. [ə] is used elsewhere.
- Production of *bath* with a low and fully back /ɑː/.

The Current Study

Given the lack of knowledge about children's mono- and multilingual speech development in South Africa, and the need for assessments to identify children with speech difficulties, the present study focused on building knowledge about speech acquisition in isiXhosa and South African English.

The challenge of carrying out reliable, valid, culturally relevant assessment is a worldwide issue beyond South Africa and, in general, studies of bilingual speech acquisition are limited. The International Expert Panel on Multilingual Children's Speech has drafted a position paper setting aspirational standards for ways in which professionals working with multilingual children might best serve them. These include to:

> … generate and share knowledge, resources, and evidence to facilitate the understanding of cultural and linguistic diversity that will support multilingual children's speech acquisition … acknowledge and respect [children's] existing competencies, cultural heritage, and histories … assessment and intervention should be based on the best available evidence. (International Expert Panel on Multilingual Children's Speech, 2012: 2)

This chapter aims to respond to this call through focusing on the specific needs of South Africa. As clinicians we must identify children with SSDs as early as possible, offer evidence-based treatment and prevent negative sequelae linked to speech difficulties. Here we focus on bilingual preschool children (ages 3;0–3;11) acquiring isiXhosa and South African English in Cape Town. Knowledge of the typical acquisition of these two languages in bilingual children is urgently required from a clinical perspective. These data can also contribute to debates about bilingual phonological acquisition. Interaction between two phonological systems may result in positive or negative transfer. Positive transfer indicates that a bilingual child will show phonological skills commensurate with or beyond those of his/her monolingual peers (Goldstein & Bunta, 2011). For example, Grech and Dodd (2008) found that children who spoke both Maltese and English had a higher percentage consonants correct score than their monolingual peers, and Fabiano-Smith and Goldstein (2010) found that children acquiring both English and Spanish had age-appropriate consonant accuracy in both languages when compared with monolingual norms. This often occurs when there are common characteristics between two languages; the frequent use of these structures can allow the child's knowledge in one language to aid acquisition in the other (Kehoe, 2015). In contrast to this, negative transfer may occur where phonological acquisition in bilingual children appears slower than that of monolingual peers. For example, Gildersleeve-Neumann *et al.* (2008) found children acquiring both English and Spanish presented with more errors in their English speech than their monolingual peers, while Goldstein and Washington (2001) found Spanish-English bilingual children had less accurate production of fricatives, flap and trill phonemes in Spanish. Given the limited research undertaken with bilingual children acquiring isiXhosa and English, it is difficult to make predictions about the relationship between the two phonological systems. The languages are quite distinct in terms of phonology, so it may be that there is little opportunity for positive transfer to occur. What seems clear from the literature is that the nature of phonological development differs in bilingual children as opposed to children who are only acquiring one language.

Method

Aims and objectives

The study aimed to describe the development of speech in bilingual three-year-old children simultaneously acquiring South African English and isiXhosa. More specifically, the objectives were to describe the children's consonant and vowel inventories, and phonological processes for each language, with a view to supporting speech and language therapists in their clinical decision making about what is typical for bilingual children.

Participants

We describe two datasets with a total of 33 bilingual English-isiXhosa children.

Dataset 1 consisted of speech productions from 25 bilingual English-isiXhosa speaking children (10 males, 15 females; mean age 3;6) whose English phonology was documented by Pascoe *et al.* (2015). These children were studied as part of a larger project documenting the typical development of South African English in monolingual, bilingual (English-Afrikaans; English-isiXhosa) and trilingual (English, Afrikaans and isiXhosa) speakers. For the purpose of this chapter we focus on the subset of bilingual English-isiXhosa children. Although these children were bilingual, only their English was assessed. Most of the children came from families where isiXhosa was the main language spoken at home, but children had been exposed to English from the time they attended day care from just a few months old.

Dataset 2 consisted of recordings of eight bilingual English-isiXhosa speakers (five males; three females; mean age 3;7) whose isiXhosa was described by Maphalala *et al.* (2014). These children were studied as part of a larger project documenting typical isiXhosa speech development in children aged three to six years. For the purpose of this chapter we focus only on the small subset of children aged three years who were reported as being bilingual. Although these children were bilingual, only their isiXhosa was assessed. Like the children in the first group, most of these children came from families where isiXhosa was the main language spoken at home, but children had been exposed to English from the time they attended day care from just a few months of age.

All participants were aged between 3;0 and 3;11 years and were acquiring South African English and isiXhosa in Cape Town. They were judged to be developing typically by their teachers and parents. Unfortunately each of the datasets focused on just one language. Although it would have been ideal to assess each bilingual child's English and isiXhosa, given the original purpose of these projects, this was not the case. However, as the children were bilingual, in this chapter we try to build a composite understanding of typical speech development in the two languages based on the data available. Children were recruited from a range of different areas in Cape Town representing a variety of socio-economic backgrounds. Children were excluded from the study where languages other than English or isiXhosa were spoken, since these other languages may have impacted the results. Children were also excluded if information about their language background could not be obtained. Table 1.2 provides an overview of the participants.

isiXhosa assessment

Masincokoleni ('Let's chat together') (Maphalala *et al.*, 2014) is an assessment designed to evaluate the speech of isiXhosa-speaking children between the ages of three and six years. It was developed as part of a study aimed at

Table 1.2 Total number of participants by age and gender ($n = 33$)

	Younger group 3;0–3;5	*Older group 3;6–3;11*	*Total (n)*
Male			15
Dataset 1	4	6	10
Dataset 2	3	2	5
Female			18
Dataset 1	5	10	15
Dataset 2	1	2	3
Total (*n*)	13	20	33

describing phonological development in children acquiring isiXhosa as a first language in Cape Town. It consists of a picture book and a recording sheet. The picture book consists of 46 coloured illustrations, two of which are practice items. The pictures used to elicit words are culturally relevant and the vocabulary used is selected for pre-school children. *Masincokoleni* is designed to elicit 53 words used to assess all 54 isiXhosa consonants, as well as the five vowels. The types of words used include nouns and verbs. To elicit nouns, children were asked *Yintoni le?* 'What is this?'; to elicit verbs they were asked *wenza ntoni?* 'what is s/he doing?' for the singular, and *benza ntoni?* 'what are they doing?' for the plural. *Masincokoleni* allows for word repetition in cases where the child does not know a word (Maphalala *et al.*, 2014).

Unlike assessments of English phonology which typically focus on consonants in word-initial, -medial and -final position, the phonotactic characteristics of isiXhosa necessitated a slightly different approach. isiXhosa nouns always begin and end with a vowel (e.g. ***i**langa* 'sun'); thus assessments do not test for target consonants in the word-initial or -final positions. The target consonants were assessed in the penultimate syllable, which is often lengthened in isiXhosa (e.g. /ibʰa**n**ana/ 'banana'); and the final syllables of disyllabic words (e.g. /i**t**i/ 'tea'). Consonant phonemes were also targeted at the initial position of a lexical root (e.g. /pʰ/ in /uja**pʰ**ɛka/ 's/he is cooking'). The click /ŋk|/ was elicited in an earlier syllable (e.g. /uja**ŋk|**ɛŋk|ɛʃɛla/ 's/he is watering'), as it does not occur in the other positions described (Maphalala *et al.*, 2014). Target phonemes were only elicited once in these positions, but do occur in other contexts (e.g. /bʰ/ occurs in /**ibʰ**ɔla/ 'ball' and in /i**bʰ** anana/ 'banana'). Each phoneme appeared at least twice. Consonants clusters were not assessed since there are none noted in isiXhosa, except in some borrowed words.

The five vowels found in the isiXhosa phonetic inventory were also assessed in different contexts (e.g. /isiʧʰ**a**ɓa/ 'crown', /ibʰ**ɔ**la/ 'ball') (Maphalala *et al.*, 2014). The length of words used to target phoneme production in *Masincokoleni* ranges between two and six syllables (e.g. /i-ti/ 'tea'; /u-ja-ŋk|ɛ-ŋk|ɛ-ʃɛ-la/ 's/he is watering'). The vowels were assessed word medially, e.g. *ibh**o**la* 'ball' and word finally, e.g. *inj**a*** 'dog'.

Masincokoleni is in the early stages of validation and psychometric evaluation (for further information about the development and validation of this assessment, please refer to Maphalala *et al.*, 2014). Several measures have been taken to ensure that the assessment is suitable for use with pre-school children, and that results obtained from the assessment are reliable. Some of these include making use of an expert panel (which included speech and language therapists, linguists and pre-school educators) to check the meaning and relevance (age and cultural) of the words selected (Maphalala *et al.*, 2014). The assessment was developed to address clinical need and continues to undergo refinement. It has been designed to be user friendly for clinicians who do not have isiXhosa as a first language (as is frequently the case in Cape Town). A brief explanation of isiXhosa phonology is included to enable clinicians to familiarize themselves with the structure of the isiXhosa sound system before administering the assessment. Information on how the test should be administered and descriptions of complex phonemes are provided (e.g. 'the occurrence of /n/ next to a basic click means that the click becomes nasalised'). In addition to what the clinician is required to say, this assessment consists of extra cues which can be given to a child if s/he does not produce the target word. For instance, for the word /ip'ap'a/ 'porridge', the clinician can ask the child *yintoni u-ku-tya kwa-se-ku-se-ni?* 'what do you eat in the morning?', if s/he has difficulty identifying the picture.

South African English assessment

The *Diagnostic Evaluation of Articulation and Phonology* (*DEAP*; Dodd *et al.*, 2002) is an English speech assessment for children aged 3;0–6;11 years. It was standardized in 2001/2002 using a sample of 144 monolingual Australian children and 584 monolingual British children. Eighty-three bilingual Punjabi/Mirpuri/Urdu-English speaking children aged 3;9–6;11 were also involved in the standardization project.

The *DEAP* facilitates classification of children into the categories of Dodd's (2005) differential diagnostic framework. As speech difficulties are heterogeneous in nature, a theoretical framework is useful for understanding and classifying them. Children acquiring a range of different languages can be described using this framework, which appears to hold true for both mono- and multilingual groups (Holm *et al.*, 1999). A comparison of English, Cantonese, Putonghua, Spanish and German children showed similar results for all these languages (Waring & Knight, 2013). The distribution of diagnostic categories is fairly constant across languages, estimated at approximately 50% of children with phonological delay: 25% in the consistent atypical disorder category; and the remaining children split equally between articulation (12.5%) and inconsistent phonological disorder (12.5%) (Broomfield & Dodd, 2004).

Since there are no locally developed assessments specifically designed to evaluate the acquisition of South African English, the *DEAP* was used in this study. The articulation (30 single words) and phonology (50 single words) subtests were administered. The articulation subtest has each English consonant assessed in word-initial and -final positions. The phonology subtest probes for phonological processes in a child's speech, and makes comparisons between single word and connected speech production. For further information about the *DEAP*, please refer to Dodd (2005) and Dodd *et al.* (2002).

Comparison of the two assessments used

Masincokoleni and the *DEAP* are similar assessments in many ways: they both require children to name pictures, and have been created to allow each vowel and consonant of the languages to be produced in specific contexts, on multiple occasions. The tests are different in many ways too. The *DEAP* contains separate subtests to evaluate articulation and phonology, whereas *Masincokoleni* aims to assess both these areas in one test. *Masincokoleni* was designed specifically for use with South African children. It is an unpublished test in the early stages of development with a very small set of normative data associated with it. The *DEAP* was not designed for children in South Africa, although we did adapt scoring in keeping with recommendations in the test manual, and it has been standardized for other populations using a large sample of children. It is important to be mindful of the differences between these assessments because they may affect the results obtained.

Procedure

Children were individually assessed in quiet rooms at schools. Both English and isiXhosa speech tests required children to name pictures and produce short strings of connected speech. For all picture-naming tasks, a hierarchy of cues was used when children could not give a relevant response. Semantic cues in either English or isiXhosa, depending on which test was being used (e.g. *You use it to tell the time*) were provided first, followed by forced choice within category (e.g. *Is it a watch or a phone?*), then imitation cues. Short breaks were taken to ensure concentration levels were maintained. One or two speech and language therapy students engaged with each participant, and real-time transcription took place, along with audio-recordings, which were used for later re-transcription. The recordings were taken using an Olympus VN-721 audio-electronic device (Dataset A) and a Sony mini-disc digital audio-recorder (MZ-R38) (Dataset B) with an external microphone (ECM-MS907) placed about 30 cm from the child's mouth. First language English speakers undertook the English assessment; a fluent isiXhosa speaker undertook the isiXhosa assessment. A short questionnaire was given to parents to obtain information about each child's language abilities and exposure to the different languages, as well as general developmental information (see Maphalala *et al.*, 2014; Pascoe *et al.*, 2015, for further details of procedures).

Data analysis

Live transcriptions were cross-checked with recordings, and 20% of the data was transcribed again by an independent speech and language therapist familiar with the respective languages. Inter-rater reliability was found to be 93%. The discrepancies between the two transcribers were discussed and resolved by a process of consensus. In most cases the difficulties related to vowel transcription. Results from each child's individual assessment were analysed quantitatively and qualitatively, in accordance with the *DEAP* manual (Dodd *et al.*, 2002) for English and the guidelines for *Masincokoleni* (Maphalala *et al.*, 2014) for isiXhosa. Accuracy judgements were based on perception.

Quantitative analysis used the indices of percentage consonants correct (PCC) and percentage vowels correct (PVC) to capture the degree of accuracy that children exhibit in their production of speech segments in words (Shriberg *et al.*, 1997). For these indices we counted the multiple components of any consonant clusters as individual units. We included consonants in all word positions for both languages, i.e. not just those that were targeted in particular contexts. Unstressed vowels of isiXhosa were not considered and slight deviations in place and voicing were considered acceptable.

The descriptive analysis was in the form of phonetic inventory analysis and descriptions of phonological processes. A 90% criterion was used to determine whether a phoneme had been acquired by the participants in each group, i.e. where 90% of the children in a group/age-band used the phoneme on at least one occasion that phoneme was considered to have met the criterion for being in the phonetic inventory. These criteria for independent analysis were based on guidelines from Hua (2002) and Hua and Dodd (2006). For the relational analysis, Dodd *et al.* (2003) suggested criteria for a phonological process when a process occurs five or more times in an individual's speech sample obtained using the *DEAP* (or more than twice in the case of weak syllable deletion). These guidelines were also used in our analysis. We compared results for the indices (PCC, PVC), consonant and vowel inventories, and phonological process repertoires across languages, and made comparisons for each language with published literature regarding monolingual speech production in the two languages.

We expected to find features of typical South African English in the English productions of the children in our sample based on what is known about the speech production of adult models. Bearing in mind these common adult productions, we modified *DEAP* scoring so that children would not be considered atypical if they showed these features. Dodd *et al.* (2003) have cautioned that dialectal variation should be considered when interpreting the results of a speech sample.

Results and Discussion

Consonant inventories

Table 1.3 shows the mean PCC score for each language. The PCC for isiXhosa is higher than for English, suggesting that three-year-old bilingual children have higher levels of accuracy in isiXhosa. The isiXhosa data cannot

Table 1.3 Mean percentage of consonants correct (PCC) by language for three-year-old bilingual children

PCC (English) (*n* = 25)	*PCC (isiXhosa)* (*n* = 8)
83.5 (*SD* 5.4)	94.125 (*SD* 6.19)

be compared to data obtained from other studies since there is none available. However, authors such as Gxilishe (2004) and Tuomi *et al.* (2001) suggest that the consonants of isiXhosa are acquired relatively early in comparison to English. The English data are comparable to those found in other studies of monolingual English children (e.g. Dodd *et al.*, 2003).

For English, the younger group of children (aged 3;0–3;5) had acquired all the phonemes of the language with the exception of five consonants: /θ, ð, ʒ, r, ʤ/. These phonemes did not meet the 90% criterion level. The older group (3;6–3;11) had acquired /ʤ/, but the other four consonants /θ, ð, ʒ, r/ were still being developed. In comparison to monolingual data for English three-year-olds this shows relatively advanced acquisition, although given the difference between the assessments, datasets and generally small sample size this is a speculative suggestion. Pascoe *et al.* (2015) investigated monolingual three-year-olds acquiring South African English in Cape Town. They found that the monolingual English children in the study had a slightly larger set of outstanding consonants than their bilingual counterparts. The monolingual English children were still acquiring the set of consonants already detailed above, but in addition they had yet to acquire /ʃ/ and did not achieve the criterion level for /ʤ/ by the age of 4;0. Published norms of monolingual children's phonological inventories also suggest that the bilingual children in our study may be slightly ahead of expected norms in their English. For example, Dodd *et al.* (2003) note that /ʤ/ and /ʒ/ are acquired at 4;0 and /θ, ð, r/ only after this point.

isiXhosa has a larger consonantal inventory than English and includes some 38 consonants and a further three basic clicks with 12 allophones. Ejectives and aspirated plosives are other consonants occurring in isiXhosa that do not occur in English, but there are also many consonants common to both languages. When considering the isiXhosa of the three-year-old bilingual children, we found that although they had acquired a substantial proportion of the inventory (e.g. many plosives, fricatives, all nasals, the implosive, most laterals and glides) they were yet to acquire several consonants. There was a difference between the younger (3;0–3;5) and older (3;6–3;11) three-year-olds participating in the study, suggesting rapid development at this age. For example, the older group showed acquisition of four affricates /ts', dz, $tʃ^h$, dʒ/ of the total eight used in isiXhosa. The younger group had not acquired any of these. Affricates have been noted in several studies focusing on Bantu language acquisition to be a late-acquired sound category (Maphalala *et al.*, 2014; Mowrer & Burger, 1991; Pascoe *et al.*, 2016). The older three-year-old children added two aspirated consonants to their inventory (with three plosives still to be acquired), and completed fricative acquisition by acquiring /s, z, x, ɣ/. Four clicks were added by the older three-year-old group so that only one click remained to be acquired after four years of age. Table 1.4 summarizes the consonant acquisition for English and isiXhosa in three-year-old bilingual children.

Table 1.4 English and isiXhosa consonant acquisition by three-year-old children in our sample

	English		*isiXhosa*	
	Acquired	*Still to acquire*	*Acquired*	*Still to acquire*
Plosives	p, b, t, d, k, g		p′, pʱ*, b, t′, d, k′, kʱ*, g, c′	tʰ, cʰ, ɟ
Nasals	m, n, ŋ		m, n, ŋ, ɲ	
Implosive			ɓ	
Fricatives	f, v, s, z, ʃ, h	θ, ð, ʒ	f, v, s*, z*, ʃ, x*, ɣ*, ɦ	
Affricates	tʃ, dʒ*		ts′*, dz*, tʃʱ*, dʒ*	tɬ, tʃ′, kx′, tsʰ
Trill		r		r
Approximant		ɹ		ɹ
Lateral	l		l, ɮ, ɬ*	
Glides	w, j		w, j	
Clicks			ǀ, ǀʰ, ŋkl, ǀg˚, !, ŋ!, ŋ!ʱ, !g˚, ǁʰ, ǁg˚ ŋǀ*, ŋǀʱ*, ǁ*, ŋǁ*, ŋǁʱ*	!ʰ

Notes: *Only the older children in the study (3;6–3;11) had acquired these consonants.

Table 1.4 shows the larger consonant inventory of isiXhosa in relation to English. Although three-year-old children have more consonants to acquire beyond age three for isiXhosa, the proportions of what has been acquired and what is still to be acquired are roughly comparable across the languages. There are consistencies between the two languages, as would be expected, e.g. nasals, glides and lateral /l/ were acquired by age three for both languages. The fricatives that were yet to be acquired in English are ones that are not found in isiXhosa. The affricates and plosives that were yet to be acquired in isiXhosa are consonants specific to that language. Mowrer and Burger (1991) found similar results in their study of monolingual children, although they noted that /s/ is acquired in the period 3;0–3;6 and /ʃ/ in the period that follows (3;6–3;11). For our study this appeared to be reversed, with /ʃ/ acquired in the earlier period and /s/ emerging in the 3;6–3;11 period.

The trill [r] and approximant [ɹ] were still to develop in both languages. As noted previously, the trill is a dialectal variant used in South African English by some participants for /ɹ/. Normative data associated with the *DEAP* derives from British and Australian children, and Dodd *et al.* (2003) have cautioned that dialectal variation should be considered when interpreting the results of a speech sample. We consulted literature regarding adult production of varieties of South African English to assist with interpretation (e.g. Bowerman, 2008; de Klerk & Gough, 2004; Lass, 2004; Mesthrie *et al.*, 2004; van Rooy, 2008). The different productions of /r/ were expected, given what is known about adult productions, and we thus modified the *DEAP* scoring so that children would not be considered atypical if they showed these features. Mowrer and Burger (1991) noted in their study of monolingual isiXhosa speakers that the trill /r/ is acquired after the age of four.

Although the study did not focus specifically on consonant clusters in English, individual participant analysis showed that clusters were emerging for many children, especially where they had acquired both elements of the cluster (e.g. swing; glove; queen), could produce some elements of a three-element cluster (e.g. [kweə] for *square*) and were using processes such as gliding within a cluster (e.g. [fwɔg] *frog*).

Looking more closely at the consonant inventory data, we found that the English data from the bilingual children are slightly more advanced compared to equivalent data from monolingual children reported in a related study (Pascoe *et al.*, 2015) and more generally in the literature on monolingual consonant acquisition in English. English may be *bootstrapped* by isiXhosa so that positive transfer occurs from isiXhosa to English phonological development in bilingual speakers. There are about 12 consonants that bilingual isiXhosa-English three-year-olds must still acquire beyond this age: one that is common to both languages (/r/); and three fricatives in English and eight consonants for isiXhosa including a click, affricates and some plosives. Again, as noted above, the proportion of acquired consonants looks fairly equivalent between languages in spite of the difference in inventory sizes.

Vowel inventories

Table 1.5 shows the mean PVC scores for each language. As in the case of consonants, the PVC scores for isiXhosa were higher than for English. isiXhosa has a simple five-vowel system, and other studies (e.g. Tuomi *et al.*, 2001) have suggested that vowels are acquired before the age of two. The results for English fit broadly with monolingual data for three-year-olds reported in the literature. For example, James *et al.* (2001) reported figures of between 88% and 94% for the Australian children in their study, but British (e.g. Dodd *et al.*, 2003) and some American data (e.g. Pollock & Berni, 2003) give higher estimates.

Table 1.5 Mean percentage vowels correct (PVC) by language for three-year-old bilingual children

PVC (English) *(n = 25)*	*PVC (isiXhosa)* *(n = 8)*
89.3 (*SD* 7.1)	98.37 (*SD* 1.32)

For isiXhosa, the children in the sample were able to produce all five vowels with a high level of accuracy which exceeded the 90% criterion for acquisition. The vowel system of South African English, with its larger set of vowels and diphthongs, appears to be reinterpreted by isiXhosa speakers as a five-vowel system. The children showed reduced contrasts between long and short vowels, used fewer central vowels and avoided use of schwa. Given that these are expected features of the dialect, it was important to modify the scoring criteria of the *DEAP* and not consider vowel differences as pathological.

South African English has some specific features associated with it, which have been documented in the literature focusing on adult productions. Some of these features were noted by the bilingual children in our study and included: (1) vowel raising; (2) the *kit/bit* split where these words are produced so that they do not rhyme. There are several different dialects of South African English spoken in Cape Town and thus these features and the extent to which they were noted in the children's speech depended on the models of English to which they are exposed, location and SES. Table 1.6 provides a

Table 1.6 English and isiXhosa vowel acquisition by three-year-old children in our sample

Types		*English*	*isiXhosa*	*Comments*
Front	High	i, iː, ɪ	i	Long short distinction between /i/ and /iː/ may be lost, e.g. *sit* and *seat* may both be produced as *sit*.
	Mid	e	e	Vowel raising may occur when *yes* for example is produced more like *yis*.
	Low	æ		Vowel raising may occur when *tan* for example is produced more like *ten*.
Mid	Mid	ə		Schwa (and other central vowels) may be avoided.
	Low	ɜ	a	
Back	High	u, ʊ	u	
	Mid	ɔ, ɔː, ʌ	o	Long short distinction between /ɔ/ and /ɔː/ may be lost, e.g. *cot* and *court* may both be produced as *cot*.
	Low	ɑ, ɒ		
Diphthongs		aɪ, aʊ, ɔɪ, ɪə, ɔə, ʊə, eə, əʊ, eɪ, oʊ		

summary of vowel acquisition for English and isiXhosa three-year-olds which indicates expected variations that may occur as part of typical acquisition in our context.

Note that the dialect and transfer issues concerning vowels are not straightforward since there is considerable variety in the different South African English dialects to which children are exposed. Where children have adult BSAE models from whom they learn English they are likely to speak like the adults in their environment. We suggest that speech and language therapists should not consider dialect features as problematic and that their scoring protocols should reflect this. Where bilingual children are learning English from speakers who speak a different (non-BSAE) variety of South African English they may well not exhibit the features noted. Thus what appears to be a phenomenon of transfer inherent in the relationship between the two languages may not actually be so. It may simply reflect the language models to which children are exposed. Awareness of dialectal vowel variations is essential to prevent over-diagnosis.

Phonological processes

Phonological processes are descriptions of general patterns of difference between child and adult targets. In this study we considered a process to be present when it appeared five or more times in the speech sample, or more than twice for weak syllable deletion (Dodd *et al.*, 2003). Common and uncommon processes were identified using the *DEAP* guidelines and guidelines from *Masincokoleni*. Table 1.7 summarizes the main processes occurring in both languages. Processes noted in more than 10% of children are shown (following Goldstein & Iglesias, 1996; So & Dodd, 1995). Devoicing was observed in 16% of the children speaking English in this study, e.g. children were noted to say *pik* for *pig* and *frok* for *frog*. This devoicing was not noted as a developmental phonological process in Table 1.7 because adults often devoice final consonants in South African English.

Gliding and stopping were the most widely occurring phonological processes when considering both languages. Both of these processes appeared frequently in both of the languages, although there was more gliding in isiXhosa and more stopping in English. The main process in English was cluster reduction, seen in more than half of the children. isiXhosa has no clusters in it, apart from borrowed/loan words from English and Afrikaans. Some weak syllable deletion, backing and final consonant deletion were also noted in the English sample, although to a much smaller extent than the other processes. Final consonant deletion is not expected in isiXhosa because this language typically has open syllables. Although backing has been noted as an atypical or unusual process sometimes indicative of disordered speech (Dodd *et al.*, 2003), for children who also speak isiXhosa, backing might be considered to be a common developmental process. Pascoe *et al.* (2015) contend that since isiXhosa has a

Table 1.7 Developmental phonological processes in English and isiXhosa

	English and isiXhosa (n = 33)	*English (n = 25)*	*isiXhosa (n = 8)*	*Examples*
	*Percentage of children from each group using each process**			
Gliding	33.3	28	50	English: [fwɒg] for *frog*; isiXhosa: [ujakx'azu**j**a] for/ ujakx'azu**l**a/ 'to tear'.
Stopping	42.4	48	25	English: [dɪs] for *this;* isiXhosa: [i**t**ele] for / isele/ 'frog'.
Deaspiration	15.2	0	62.5	isiXhosa: [uja**k**aɓa] for /ujaykʰaɓa/ 'kicking'.
Cluster reduction	39.4	52	0	English: [tɔ:bwi] for 'strawberry'.
Deaffrication	12.1	0	50	isiXhosa: [inɬɔkɔ] for /in**tɬ**oko/ 'head'.
Depalatalization	9.1	0	37.5	isiXhosa: [i**dz**asi] for / i**ɟ**asi/ 'coat'.
Dentalization	9.1	0	37.5	isiXhosa: [ama**ð**iɲɔ] for /ama**z**iɲɔ/ 'teeth'.
Denasalization	6.1	0	25	isiXhosa: [iɮeɓe] for / i**nɮ**eɓe/ 'ear'.
Weak syllable deletion	12.1	16	0	English: [mɑtoʊ] for *tomato*.
Backing	12.1	16	0	English: [kubwʌʃ] for *toothbrush*.
Final consonant deletion	9.1	12	0	English: [laɪ] for *knife*.

Notes: *Processes were considered to be used by a child when they were used more than five times in the assessment (or twice for weak syllable deletion) based on Dodd *et al.* (2003).

Devoicing of word-final consonants (e.g. *dock* for *dog*) was not considered as a developmental process given that this is a common dialectal feature observed in adult speakers.

high frequency of velar phonemes (Niesler *et al.*, 2005) these children may favour a posterior place of articulation, making backing more prevalent.

For isiXhosa, deaspiration was the most widely used process, being shown by more than 60% of the three-year-olds. Aspirated plosives were noted to be challenging when considering consonant acquisition, so it is not surprising to see that this process is prevalent. Research suggests that aspirated plosives in isiXhosa have voice onset time (VOT) values which are relatively long when compared to other languages, and that closure duration tends to be shorter in aspirated plosives than for other categories (Jessen, 2002).

There are few studies that have investigated the phonological processes of young children acquiring isiXhosa. Normative data from studies of monolingual children acquiring English suggest that our data for the bilingual children fit broadly with what is known about monolingual English acquisition (Cohen & Anderson, 2011). Grunwell (1987) suggests that stopping, fronting and gliding are the main processes evident at this age. Dodd *et al.* (2003) note that gliding, deaffrication, cluster reduction, weak syllable deletion and stopping (up to 3;6) are processes to be expected. We noted processes common to both languages (e.g. gliding, stopping), and processes specific to each language related to the particular structure of the language, e.g. no final consonant deletion was noted for isiXhosa which does not typically use final consonants; no cluster reduction was observed in isiXhosa which does not contain clusters.

Similar to other languages, young bilingual isiXhosa-English speaking children presented with more phonological processes than older children. The younger group of children (3;0–3;5) consistently showed a wider range of phonological processes in both languages than the older group (3;6–3;11). The younger children showed seven different processes for isiXhosa, and six different processes for English, in contrast with four processes used by the older children in both languages. In the larger study by Maphalala *et al.* (2014) with its multiple age bands, four- and five-year-old children presented with even fewer processes (see Maphalala *et al.*, 2014).

Limitations and future work

This chapter drew retrospectively on two datasets collected as part of other projects, which resulted in several limitations. In future it would be important to collect data that describe both languages within the same bilingual children. Using a well-designed prospective study would allow for more rigorous comparisons to be made between the two languages without exposure to confounding variables. More detailed information could also be obtained about the children's two languages and the amount of exposure and opportunity to use each one. For example, the acquisition of tone might be considered in isiXhosa. The two datasets described here made a small sample, and since the two groups were not of equal numbers comparisons were difficult to make (25 English versus eight isiXhosa samples). Both South African English and isiXhosa comprise many different dialects. The children studied in this project were most likely exposed to many different dialectal influences, which were not systematically detailed. There is a great need to consider these influences and resulting variations in future projects.

Despite these limitations, this chapter was able to offer some tentative suggestions which might contribute towards building a *clinical blueprint* of how typically developing bilingual children acquiring isiXhosa and English might present. Although this blueprint will need to be developed and tested further, Tables 1.3–1.7 presented here may be useful for speech and language therapists working with children who speak these languages and want to make decisions about their next steps. The type of process followed to construct these tables could be undertaken for a range of different language combinations, in keeping with the call of the International Expert Panel on Multilingual Children's Speech and authors such as de Lamo White and Jin (2011).

Building knowledge about the typical development of bilingual children acquiring isiXhosa and English is an important first step. This project focused on three-year-olds, but clearly there is further work to be done with children of different ages so that a developmental trajectory can be mapped out. A diagnostic framework such as Barbara Dodd's (2005) has been shown to apply to a range of languages and language combinations. Future work will consider isiXhosa in light of the framework and aim to detail the nature and prevalence of speech disorders in this language, for both mono- and bilingual children. *Masincokoleni* could be refined further in line with this or other frameworks such as constraint-based nonlinear phonology.

Conclusion

Research has shown that bilingual children are able to differentiate between their phonological systems from a young age (Genesee *et al.*, 1995). These systems interact with each other, creating a pathway for the bilingual child which can differ in some ways from that of a monolingual child. Findings from this analysis illustrate this interaction. In this chapter we showed how the consonant and vowel inventories of the two languages were similar and different and how they possibly influenced one another. We emphasized the need to consider local adult models when making clinical judgements about what should be considered common or uncommon for children in a given context. For isiXhosa this work is preliminary and it remains for further studies to determine the nature of common and uncommon phonological processes, and the ages by which the processes are typically suppressed. This study was driven by clinical need to provide normative data about children's speech development. It represents only a small fragment of the language complexity in South Africa and will be strengthened by work that investigates a larger sample of children across a range of age groups using a prospective design. Children with speech difficulties in South Africa – and the clinicians who work with them – urgently need to benefit from this knowledge.

References

Bowerman, S. (2008) White South African English: Morphology and syntax. In R. Mesthrie (ed.) *Varieties of English* (pp. 472–487). Berlin and New York: Mouton de Gruyter.

Broomfield, J. and Dodd, B. (2004) Children with speech and language disability: Caseload characteristics. *International Journal of Language & Communication Disorders* 39 (3), 303–324.

Cohen, W. and Anderson, C. (2011) Identification of phonological processes in preschool children's single word productions. *International Journal of Language & Communication Disorders* 46 (4), 481–488.

de Klerk, V. (1999) Black South African English: Where to from here? *World Englishes* 18, 311–324.

de Klerk, V. and Gough, D. (2004) Black South African English. In R. Mesthrie (ed.) *Language in South Africa* (pp. 356–380). Cambridge: Cambridge University Press.

de Lamo White, C. and Jin, L. (2011) Evaluation of speech and language assessment approaches with bilingual children. *International Journal of Language & Communication Disorders* 46 (6), 613–627.

Demuth, K. (2003) The acquisition of Bantu languages. In D. Nurse and G. Philippson (eds) *The Bantu Languages* (pp. 209–222). Richmond: Curzon Press.

Dodd, B. (2005) *Differential Diagnosis and Treatment of Children with Speech Disorder* (2nd edn). London: Whurr Publishers.

Dodd, B., Hua, Z., Crosbie, S., Holm, A. and Ozanne, A. (2002) *Diagnostic Evaluation of Articulation and Phonology*. London: Psychological Corporation.

Dodd, B., Holm, A., Hua, Z. and Crosbie, S. (2003) Phonological development: A normative study of British English-speaking children. *Clinical Linguistics & Phonetics* 17 (8), 617–643.

Fabiano-Smith, L. and Goldstein, B. (2010) Phonological acquisition in bilingual Spanish-English speaking children. *Journal of Speech, Language, and Hearing Research* 68, 160–178; doi:10.1044/1092-4388(2009/07-0064.

Fox, A.V. and Dodd, B. (2001) Phonologically disordered German-speaking children. *American Journal of Speech Language Pathology* 10 (3), 291–307.

Genesee, F., Nicoladis, E. and Paradis, J. (1995) Language differentiation in early bilingual development. *Journal of Child Language* 22, 611–631.

Gildersleeve-Neumann, C., Kester, E.S., Davis, B.L. and Peña, E.D. (2008) English speech sound development in preschool-aged children from bilingual English-Spanish environments. *Language, Speech and Hearing Services in Schools* 39, 314–328; doi:10.1044/0161-1461(2008/030).

Goldstein, B. and Bunta, F. (2011) Positive and negative transfer in the phonological systems of bilingual speakers. *International Journal of Bilingualism* 16, 388–401; doi:10.1177/1367006911425817.

Goldstein, B.A. and Iglesias, A. (1996) Phonological patterns in normally developing Spanish-speaking 3- and 4-year-olds of Puerto Rican descent. *Language, Speech and Hearing Services in Schools* 27 (1), 82–90.

Goldstein, B. and Washington, P.S. (2001) An initial investigation of phonological patterns in typically developing 4-year-old Spanish-English bilingual children. *Language, Speech and Hearing Services in Schools* 32, 153–164.

Grech, H. and Dodd, B. (2008) Phonological acquisition in Malta: A bilingual language learning context. *International Journal of Bilingualism* 12 (3), 155–171.

Grunwell, P. (1987) *Clinical Phonology* (2nd edn). London: Croom Helm.

Gxilishe, D.S. (1996) The dilemma of dialect in the classroom: A case for Xhosa. *Per Linguam* 12 (1), 1–14.

Gxilishe, S. (2004) The acquisition of clicks by isiXhosa-speaking children. *Per Linguam* 20 (2), 1–12.

Holm, A., Dodd, B., Stow, C. and Pert, S. (1999) Identification and differential diagnosis of phonological disorder in bilingual children. *Language Testing* 16 (3), 271–292.

Hua, Z. (2002) *Phonological Development in Specific Contexts: Studies of Chinese Speaking Children*. Trowbridge: Cromwell Press.

Hua, Z. and Dodd, B. (2006) A multilingual perspective on phonological development and disorders. In Z. Hua and B. Dodd (eds) *Phonological Development and Disorders in Children: A Multilingual Perspective* (pp. 3–14). Clevedon: Multilingual Matters.

International Expert Panel on Multilingual Children's Speech (2012) Multilingual children with speech disorders. Position paper, Charles Sturt University, Bathurst, NSW. See http://www.csu.edu.au/research/multilingual-speech/position-paper.

James, D.G., Van Doorn, J. and McLeod, S. (2001) *Vowel Production in Mono-, Di- and Polysyllabic Words in Children Aged 3;0 to 7;11 years*. Melbourne, Vic: Speech Pathology Australia.

Jessen, M. (2002) An acoustic study of contrasting plosives and click accompaniments in Xhosa. *Phonetica* 59, 150–179.

Kehoe, M. (2015) Cross-linguistic interaction: A retrospective and prospective view. In E. Babatsouli and D. Ingram (eds) *Proceedings of the International Symposium on Monolingual and Bilingual Speech 2015* (pp. 141–167). Chania, Greece: Institute of Monolingual and Bilingual Speech.

Lass, R. (2004) South African English. In R. Mesthrie (ed.) *Language in South Africa* (pp. 104–126). Cambridge: Cambridge University Press.

Maphalala, Z., Pascoe, M. and Smouse, M.R. (2014) Phonological development of first language isiXhosa-speaking children aged 3;0–6;0 years: A descriptive cross-sectional study. *Clinical Linguistics & Phonetics* 28, 174–194.

Mesthrie, R., Schneider, E., Burridge, K., Kortmann, B. and Upton, C. (2004) *A Handbook of Varieties of English*. Berlin: Mouton de Gruyter.

Mohammed, M.A. (2001) *Modern Swahili Grammar*. Nairobi: East African Educational Publishers.

Mosaka, N.M. (2000) Stress assignment in syllabic structures in Xhosa and Tswana. *South African Journal of African Languages* 20, 177–185.

Mowrer, D.E. and Burger, S. (1991) A comparative analysis of phonological acquisition of consonants in the speech of 21/2–6-year-old Xhosa- and English-speaking children. *Clinical Linguistics & Phonetics* 5 (2), 139–164.

Niesler, T., Louw, P. and Roux, J.C. (2005) Phonetic analysis of Afrikaans, English, Xhosa and Zulu using South African speech databases. *Southern African Linguistics and Applied Language Studies* 23, 459–474.

Pascoe, M. and Smouse, M. (2012) Masithethe: Speech and language development and difficulties in isiXhosa. *South African Medical Journal* 102, 469–471.

Pascoe, M., Le Roux, J., Mahura, O. *et al.* (2015) Three-year-old children acquiring South African English in Cape Town. In E. Babatsouli and D. Ingram (eds) *Proceedings of the International Symposium on Monolingual and Bilingual Speech 2015* (pp. 277–287). Chania, Greece: Institute of Monolingual and Bilingual Speech.

Pascoe, M., Rossouw, K., Fish, L., Jansen, C., Manley, N., Powell, M. and Rosen, L. (2016) Speech processing and production in two-year-old children acquiring isiXhosa: A tale of two children. *South African Journal of Communication Disorders* 63, 1–15; doi:10.4102/sajcd.v63i2.134.

Pollock, K.E. and Berni, M.C. (2003) Incidence of non-rhotic vowel errors in children: Data from the Memphis Vowel Project. *Clinical Linguistics & Phonetics* 17, 393–401.

Posel, D. and Zeller, J. (2016) Language shift or increased bilingualism in South Africa: Evidence from census data. *Journal of Multilingual and Multicultural Development* 37, 1–14.

Ruscello, D.M. (2008) *Treating Articulation and Phonology Disorder in Children*. St. Louis, MO: Elsevier Health Sciences.

Shriberg, L.D., Austin, D., Lewis, B.A., McSweeny, J.L. and Wilson, D.L. (1997) The percentage of consonants correct (PCC) metric extensions and reliability data. *Journal of Speech, Language, and Hearing Research* 40, 708–722.

So, L.K. and Dodd, B.J. (1995) The acquisition of phonology by Cantonese-speaking children. *Journal of Child Language* 22, 473–495.

Statistics South Africa (2011) *Pretoria* (pp. 23–25). See http://www.statssa.gov.za/Census2011/Products/Census_2011_Census_in_brief.pdf.

Tuomi, S., Gxilishe, S. and Matomela, L. (2001) The acquisition of isiXhosa phonemes. *Per Linguam* 17, 14–23.

van der Merwe, A. and Le Roux, M. (2014) Idiosyncratic sound systems of the South African Bantu languages: Research and clinical implications for speech-language pathologists and audiologists. *South African Journal of Communication Disorders* 61 (1), 1–8.

van Dulm, O. and Southwood, F. (2015) Child language assessment and intervention in multilingual and multicultural South Africa: Findings of a national survey. *Stellenbosch Papers in Linguistics* 42, 55–76.

van Rooy, B. (2000) The consonants of BSAE: Current knowledge and future prospects. *South African Journal of Linguistics* 18, 35–54.

van Rooy, B. (2008) Black South African English: Phonology. In R. Mesthrie (ed.) *A Handbook of Varieties of English* (pp. 177–187). Berlin: Mouton de Gruyter.

Waring, R. and Knight, R. (2013) How should children with speech sound disorders be classified? A review and critical evaluation of current classification systems. *International Journal of Language & Communication Disorders* 48, 25–40.

World Health Organization (2007) *Classification of Functioning, Disability and Health. Version for Children and Youth*. Geneva: World Health Organization.

2 The Impact of Parent Communication Patterns on Infant Volubility during Play with Books

Anna V. Sosa

Introduction

In his seminal paper in the field of child phonology, Jakobson (1941/1968) referred to the prelinguistic period of vocal development (babble) as, 'the purposeless egocentric soliloquy of the child' and as 'biologically oriented "tongue delirium"' (Jakobson, 1968: 24). Both expressions reflect a general opinion, which may have been widely held at the time, that babble is unrelated to language and that the study of language development should begin at the point when children begin producing true words. Over the past several decades, however, researchers in the area of language development in general and child phonology in particular have investigated the phonetic similarities between babble and early words and have identified important relationships between prelinguistic vocalization and later language ability.

Continuity between Babble and Speech

One of the major findings in this area is the observation of continuity between prelinguistic vocalization and the later period of meaningful speech. A number of studies have shown that the phonetic characteristics of early words are similar to the phonetic characteristics of babble: simple syllable shapes with stops, nasals and glides dominate in both babble and early speech (Stoel-Gammon, 1998b). This continuity between babble and early words has also been observed at the level of the individual child in that specific sound pattern preferences in babble have been found to carry over into meaningful speech, forming the building blocks for an individual child's early lexicon (Vihman, 1993). For example, one child studied by Ferguson and Farwell (1975) showed a marked preference for acquiring words with sibilant consonants, while another child described by Stoel-Gammon and Cooper (1984) had a disproportionate number of words with velar stops in his early expressive vocabulary. These observations suggest that the prelinguistic and early linguistic stages of vocal development are not discrete, separable stages, but are rather part of a continuous developmental trajectory in which speech production ability acquired during babbling is used by the child as he begins to produce true words that approximate the adult target.

Predictive Value of Babble

If prelinguistic vocalizations are the precursors or building blocks of meaningful speech, then it follows that children who are better babblers may have an advantage as they begin to acquire their first true words and may become advanced talkers when compared to infants who babble less or have a more restricted use of different sounds and syllable shapes during the prelinguistic period. This hypothesis is supported by numerous studies that have found an association between babble 'ability' and later speech and language skills, with 'better' babblers, as determined by a variety of different measures, becoming 'better' talkers.

One notable prelinguistic milestone that has been linked repeatedly to later language development is the age-of-onset of canonical babble. Canonical babble is defined as any vocalization that consists of a well-formed syllable with at least one full vowel and at least one consonant-like element, the two of which are linked by a rapid formant transition (Oller *et al.*, 1999). These canonical syllables sound very speech-like and the appearance of these syllables marks an important milestone in a child's trajectory towards meaningful use of language. Parents easily identify the onset of use of canonical babble and these vocalizations are often interpreted by parents as attempts at real words (e.g. [dada] produced by an 11-month-old is interpreted as an attempt to say *daddy*). In typical development, canonical babble emerges often by six months of age and lack of canonical babble by 10 months is considered delayed onset (Oller *et al.*, 1999). A number of studies have found that age-of-onset of canonical babble is closely associated with later language development and that delayed onset may be an important early indicator of later speech and language disorder. An early study (Stoel-Gammon, 1989) found that atypical babbling, including late onset of canonical babble, was associated with delayed acquisition of meaningful speech in two late-talking toddlers. Later, results of a large-scale screening project of high-risk infants found that those with delayed onset of canonical babble (i.e. no canonical babble by 10–12 months) showed significant delays in expressive vocabulary development at 18, 24 and 30 months compared to those infants who had reached the canonical babble stage by 10–12 months (Oller *et al.*, 1999). Oller and colleagues conclude that late onset of canonical babble is an indicator of future communication deficits and should be included in screening batteries to assist with early identification and intervention.

In addition to age-of-onset of canonical babble, other quantitative and qualitative measures of babble ability have been linked to later language development. Measures of babble complexity, including proportional use of consonantal versus vowel babble, consonant inventory, and use of a variety of different syllable shapes have all been linked to future language outcome. For example, in one study that investigated predictors of language growth in a group of 37 two-year-olds with severe expressive language delay, the proportion of consonantal babble to vowel babble at approximately 28 months was the strongest predictor of expressive language outcome five months later (Whitehurst *et al.*, 1991). Similarly, several studies have found that toddlers with expressive language delay vocalize less and demonstrate reduced phonetic inventories, including limited use of a variety of different syllable shapes, compared to typically developing peers (Pharr *et al.*, 2000; Rescorla & Ratner, 1996). More recently, the same patterns have been observed in Italian-learning late talkers and pre-term infants. Fasolo *et al.* (2008) found that a child's Mean Babbling Level (Stoel-Gammon, 1989) at 18–20 months, a measure that quantifies syllabic and consonantal complexity of prelinguistic vocalizations, predicted expressive vocabulary size at 24 months in a group of children with slow expressive language development. In a study of Italian-learning infants born prematurely, consonant inventory and use of canonical babble at 12 months predicted vocabulary size at 18 months (d'Odorico *et al.*, 2011).

The same predictive relationship between prelinguistic vocalization and general language outcome has been observed in other populations of children at risk for communication impairment. These include studies of children with global developmental delay (McCathren *et al.*, 1999), children with cochlear implants (Walker & Bass-Ringdahl, 2008) and children with cleft palate (Chapman *et al.*, 2003; Scherer *et al.*, 2008). McCathren *et al.* (1999) found that overall volubility as well as rate of vocalizations with consonants were related to later expressive vocabulary size in 58 toddlers with mild to moderate developmental delay of mixed aetiology. Interestingly, neither degree of developmental delay nor overall cognitive level were associated with later expressive vocabulary, suggesting that quantity and quality of prelinguistic vocalization are more predictive of later language outcome than general cognitive developmental level in this population. In a study of 19 children with prelingual deafness who use cochlear implants (Walker & Bass-Ringdahl, 2008), researchers found that Mean Babbling Level six and nine months post implantation was predictive of general speech and language outcome at four years of age. Similar patterns have been observed in children with cleft palate. Chapman *et al.* (2003) found significant correlations between prelinguistic vocalization ability immediately post surgical palate repair (13 months) and later vocabulary development, while Scherer *et al.* (2008) observed a relationship between overall volubility at six months and vocabulary size at 30 months.

In spite of earlier held beliefs that babble and language were unrelated, there is now overwhelming evidence demonstrating that the prelinguistic and linguistic stages of communication development are intricately connected. It has been demonstrated repeatedly that various measures of prelinguistic vocalization ability including onset of canonical babble, overall volubility and complexity of babbled utterances are highly predictive of later language outcome in a variety of populations. This relationship has been observed in children with typical development, children with delayed expressive communication, children born prematurely, children with global developmental delay, children who use cochlear implants and children with cleft palate. The findings are extremely robust and clearly demonstrate that observation and evaluation of prelinguistic vocalization patterns, particularly in populations at risk for communication disorders, should play an important role in any clinical screening and evaluation programme.

Why are Babble and Language So Closely Connected?

Several reasons for the observed relationship between babble and later speech and language development have been discussed. Stoel-Gammon (1998a, 2011) describes words as having two components, sound and meaning. That is, in order to produce a word, a child must be able to produce a relatively stable phonetic form that approximates an adult target word and use it consistently with an intended meaning. The physical aspect of producing the word is described by Stoel-Gammon as having a skill component, similar to other types of motor behaviour (Bybee, 2003), and that with more practice comes greater control and precision of the movement. These practised motor routines become automatic and thereby easier for the child to produce, making them readily available phonetic forms to which meaning can be attached to produce a word. Thus, babies who babble more and produce a wider variety of phonetic forms during the prelinguistic stage will have an advantage in word learning because they have a larger repertoire of practised syllables that can be used meaningfully (Vihman, 1992) once they have developed the cognitive-linguistic ability to connect meaning to sound.

When they vocalize, babies receive both kinaesthetic and auditory input. That is, they can both feel and hear their own vocal productions. Production of sounds and syllables in babble facilitates mapping of specific movement patterns to the resulting acoustic output, allowing infants to refine their movement patterns in order to produce an intended output. This feedback process has been highlighted by a number of researchers (Fry, 1966; Stoel-Gammon, 2011) and is often referred to as the auditory-articulatory feedback loop. With this auditory-articulatory feedback, infants can then begin to recognize similarities between their own productions and words in the ambient language, which facilitates development of stored lexical and phonological representations that are needed to produce words (Stoel-Gammon, 1998a). Thus, babies who babble more and use a wider variety of sounds and syllable shapes get more auditory and articulatory feedback experience, allowing them to learn new words at an accelerated pace compared to babies who babble less frequently.

In addition to the auditory and articulatory feedback they receive from their own productions, babies also receive social feedback from caregivers in response to their vocalizations. When a baby produces a vocalization in the presence of a caregiver, they may receive some type of verbal or behavioural feedback that then influences subsequent infant vocalizations. This mutual influence of infant vocalization on parent behaviour and parent behaviour on infant vocalization has been referred to as the social feedback loop for speech development (Warlaumont *et al.*, 2014). There is substantial evidence showing that parental responsiveness to infant vocalizations facilitates language development. For example, the number of conversational turns a child participates in and the responsiveness of caregivers is highly predictive of current and later language ability as well as the attainment of major language milestones (Tamis-LeMonda *et al.*, 2001; Zimmerman *et al.*, 2009). Tamis-LeMonda *et al.* (2001) found that a higher rate of maternal responsiveness at nine and 13 months was predictive of earlier attainment of five major language milestones: use of imitations, spontaneous use of first words, attainment of first 50 words, use of combinatorial speech and use of language to talk about past events. Zimmerman *et al.* (2009) found that the number of conversational turns a child engaged in (i.e. back and forth verbal interactions between infant and parent) was predictive of later measures of language development. Because parent responses and conversational turns can only occur in the presence of an infant's vocalization and because the number of responses or conversational turns a baby experiences positively influences later language development, it follows that babies who babble more would be expected to show advanced language development simply due to the fact that the more a baby babbles, the more opportunities there are for parent responses.

Beyond just the number of opportunities for parent responses due to overall volubility, there is also evidence to suggest that babies who use more complex babble receive more and different responsive feedback from caregivers. This reflects the point in the proposed social feedback loop where the nature of a child's vocalization influences the type of response they receive. If an infant produces a vocalization that contains speech or speech-like properties, they are more likely to receive a positive contingent response from an adult than if their utterance is not speech-like (Warlaumont *et al.*, 2014). Further, the type of response they are likely to receive is contingent on the phonetic properties of their utterance (Gros-Louis *et al.*, 2006). Gros-Louis *et al.* (2006) found that mothers responded differently to different types of infant vocalizations. Specifically, mothers responded to canonical babble with more imitations/expansions and language-oriented responses than they did to vocalizations that contained only vowel sounds. These findings suggest that the use of more advanced vocalizations on the part of an infant influences a parent's response in ways that are known to promote language development. Taken together, the findings from these studies indicate that babies who babble more and use more complex phonetic forms would be likely to experience a higher quantity and better quality of parental responsiveness compared to babies who are less vocal or who use simpler phonetic forms when they babble.

The most immediate observable effects of the impact of prelinguistic vocalization on language ability are likely to be in the early stages of language development (i.e. age of use of first words or early vocabulary growth). Not surprisingly, this has been the focus of the majority of the studies described here. However, it is reasonable to suspect, and there is some empirical evidence to support the hypothesis, that delays in expressive vocabulary growth associated with late and limited babbling may set off 'a cascade' (Oller *et al.*, 1999) of negative consequences impacting future development of morphology, syntax, and even literacy. To provide just one example, there is substantial evidence showing that grammatical development is significantly mediated by lexical development; that is, attainment of morphological and syntactic milestones is largely dependent on the size of a child's expressive vocabulary (Bates *et al.*, 1995; Marchman & Bates, 1994). Thus, children with slower expressive vocabulary growth in the second year of life subsequent to delayed babble in the first year of life may also exhibit delays in morphological and syntactic development in the third and fourth years of life. This possibility further emphasizes the importance of evaluating and monitoring the use of prelinguistic vocalizations in children at risk for communication disorder.

Child-internal and External Factors that Influence Babble

Given the empirical evidence as well as the theoretical rationale for the association between prelinguistic vocalization and later language development, it follows that interventions focusing on increasing and expanding babble repertoire may be relevant for young children who are exhibiting or who are at risk for language delay. For example, if a child with a history of pre-term birth has not begun to produce canonical babble by 10 months, an intervention programme focusing on the development and use of canonical syllables may be warranted. In order to implement this type of intervention, however, an understanding of the factors that influence infant vocal production is necessary. To date, researchers have looked at child-internal factors as well as environmental and interactional factors, external to the child, that influence prelinguistic vocalization.

Several child-internal factors are known to affect the quantity and quality of babble. These include language delay (Rescorla & Ratner, 1996), global developmental delay (Thiemann-Bourque *et al.*, 2014), autism spectrum disorder (ASD) (Patten *et al.*, 2014; Paul *et al.*, 2011; Warlaumont *et al.*, 2014), cleft palate (Scherer *et al.*, 2008), childhood apraxia of speech (CAS) (Overby & Caspari, 2015) and hearing status (Oller & Eilers, 1988). In some populations, for example infants with Down syndrome, differences in quantity and quality of babble appear to be quite minimal (Abbeduto *et al.*, 2007). In others the differences are more pronounced. For example, the finding of reduced volubility and reduced complexity of prelinguistic vocalization in infants at high risk for or diagnosed with ASD is quite robust. Warlaumont *et al.* (2014) report reduced volubility, fewer speech-like vocalizations and reduced parent–infant vocal interaction in children with ASD than in a control group. Similarly, Patten *et al.* (2014), using retrospective video analysis, report delayed onset of canonical babble, reduced volubility and limited use of canonical syllables relative to other types of vocalizations. Finally, Paul *et al.* (2011) found that infant siblings of children with ASD used fewer speech-like vocalizations, had smaller consonant inventories and used fewer different syllable types than a control group. These findings demonstrate that in these populations of children known to be at high risk for communication disorder, indicators of future delay are present in the prelinguistic stage, well before delays in the development of expressive vocabulary, morphology or syntax are identifiable. This represents important clinical information for healthcare professionals involved in the screening and evaluation of infants, particularly for disorders that are not identifiable on the basis of recognizable physical differences (e.g. ASD and CAS).

In addition to child-internal factors, a variety of child-external factors have been investigated in an attempt to identify environmental or interactional variables that may influence prelinguistic vocal development. One environmental factor that has been found to impact babble is socio-economic status (SES). While children living in low SES households typically develop canonical babble within the expected timeframe (i.e. by 10 months), infants living in extreme poverty may demonstrate reduced overall volubility compared to infants living in higher SES households (Oller *et al.*, 1995). An explanation for this observation may be found in the social feedback loop proposed by Warlaumont *et al.* (2014). As mentioned previously, adult contingent responsiveness has been found to influence subsequent infant vocalizations (Franklin *et al.*, 2014; Goldstein & Schwade, 2008; Goldstein *et al.*, 2003;

Warlaumont *et al.*, 2014). In an experimental study in which parents' response contingency to infant vocalizations was manipulated, Goldstein *et al.* (2003) found that positive contingent responses by parents served to increase the frequency and complexity of infant vocalizations. At the same time, there is evidence showing that children living in low SES households hear less child-directed speech overall than their higher SES peers (Hart & Risley, 1995, 2003; Rowe, 2008; Vanormelingen & Gillis, 2016) and that they may experience fewer verbal responses that are contingent on their own vocalizations (Vanormelingen & Gillis, 2016). In a recent study of the influence of SES on child-directed speech in Dutch-speaking families, Vanormelingen and Gillis (2016) found that mothers from low SES backgrounds produced fewer utterances and responded significantly less frequently to their children's utterances than mothers from mid- to high SES backgrounds. The social feedback loop predicts that both reduced volubility and reduced responsiveness would result in decreased infant volubility, as reported in Oller *et al.* (1995).

In addition to general contingent responsiveness, another parental verbal behaviour that has been linked to increased infant volubility is parent imitation of a child's preceding utterance. In a review of 22 studies looking at the effect of various types of adult responsiveness on infant vocalizations, Dunst *et al.* (2010) conclude that imitation of an infant's vocalization is the most effective reinforcement for increasing infant volubility. The authors caution, however, that the studies reviewed were experimental studies and that the effectiveness of imitation as a reinforcer may fade if it is used for an extended period of time in a natural setting without varying the response type. Nonetheless, in an intervention setting, encouraging use of both general responsiveness as well as imitation of a child's utterance may represent an important starting point.

Other contextual and interactional factors that have been found to influence prelinguistic vocalization include the presence of a television that is on and the type of activity the child is engaged in. Several studies have found that television/video viewing, whether viewed directly by the infant or just present in the background during an interaction, negatively impacts the quantity and quality of adult language produced and has a negative influence on parent–child social interaction (Courage *et al.*, 2010; Masur *et al.*, 2016; Pempek *et al.*, 2011; Tanimura *et al.*, 2007). Most of these studies did not directly analyze the impact of television viewing on infant vocal behaviour, but one study did find that audible television exposure was associated with reduced child vocalization rates (Christakis *et al.*, 2009). In studies looking at the effect of activity type on parent–infant communication, results show that the activity they are engaged in does impact the quantity of adult language produced and the number of conversational interactions. In particular, play with books or 'storytime' is consistently associated with significantly more adult words produced than other types of activities (Gilkerson *et al.*, 2015; Soderstrom & Wittebolle, 2013; Sosa, 2016), but it is not necessarily associated with infant volubility per se. One exception is the finding by Sosa (2016) that infants vocalized significantly more during book reading than during play with electronic toys. Thus, the type of activity parents and infants are engaged in appears to have a large effect on parental verbal behaviour but a smaller effect on infant vocal behaviour itself.

During natural interactions, parents use a variety of interactional and communicative behaviours to engage their infants. These behaviours include sound effects, songs, questions, directives, etc. While the studies reviewed have shown that verbal responsiveness and imitation do serve to promote infant vocalization in experimental settings, little is known about the impact of these and other parental communicative behaviours during naturally occurring parent–infant play. If behaviours that encourage infant vocalization can be identified, these behaviours may be used in interventions provided by parents and clinicians to increase infant volubility in children who are at risk for or who are already exhibiting signs of communication delay.

The Current Study

The purpose of this investigation was to explore the relationship between parent communicative behaviours and infant volubility during short parent–infant play sessions with age-appropriate books. The goal was to identify naturally occurring parent behaviours that are associated with increased vocalizations by the child. It was hypothesized that parents who talk more, maintain their child's interest through use of animated and engaging expressions, and who are consistently responsive to their child's vocalizations would have children who are themselves more vocal during interactions. While many studies have identified relationships between parent–infant communication and later language development (Gilkerson & Richards, 2009; Hart & Risley, 1995, 2003; Tamis-LeMonda *et al.*, 2001) and between infant vocalization and later language development (see previous discussion), few have investigated the relationship between naturally occurring parent communicative behaviours and concurrent infant volubility. The results of this study will add to that knowledge base and may offer detailed information regarding recommendations for intervention strategies that may promote rate of prelinguistic vocalizations.

Method

Participants

The data analyzed for the current study are taken from a larger project investigating the effect of the type of toy used during play on the quantity and quality of parent–infant communication (Sosa, 2016). Data for the current study are from 27 parent–infant dyads recruited through the posting of flyers in areas frequented by families with young children. The infant participants were between 10 and 16 months (Mean = 12.98) at the time of the study; 12 were male and 15 were female. The parents who participated in the study along with their children included 25 biological mothers and two biological fathers. American English was reported as the primary language used in the home. All parents had at least a high school degree and 23 parents had completed four or more years of post-secondary education. Racial/ethnic information was gathered at the time of enrolment. Of the 27 participating families, 25 self-reported as non-Hispanic white, one was Hispanic, and one was Native American.

Data collection

As part of the larger study, parent–infant dyads participated in three days of data collection taking place in their homes. Over the course of these three days, parents engaged in six 15-minute play sessions with their babies using three different toy sets, which were provided by the researchers. The toy sets included traditional toys (blocks, puzzles and shape-sorters), electronic toys (baby laptop, electronic baby cell phone and talking farm) and books (five stiff board books with animal, colour and shape themes), all designed and marketed for children in this age range. Parents engaged in two 15-minute play sessions with each toy set. Data for the current investigation are taken from the first 15-minute play session with books only. The decision to use the play session with books for the current investigation was based on the results of the larger study which found that parents talked the most and were most responsive to their infants during book play than during play with other toys. Furthermore, infants vocalized significantly more during play with books than during play with electronic toys. Based on these findings, it was felt that both parents and infants were highly engaged and interactive during book reading and that the impact of parental behaviour on infant vocalization might be more easily identified during these interactions. The set of books consisted of five books: two books had a farm animal theme; two books had a shapes theme; and one book had a colour theme. Parents were free to choose when during the day to play with the toys and were not directed to minimize natural distractions of the home environment. Therefore, there were sometimes other children, pets or other adults present during the play session.

Play sessions were recorded using the LENA Pro (Language Environment Analysis [LENA Foundation, Boulder, CO]) System. The system includes a small digital recording device called a digital language processor, which is placed in a pocket in a vest worn by the child. The processor records up to 16 hours of recorded sound and is worn continuously by the child for at least 10 hours. The accompanying LENA software conducts automatic analyses of the recordings and generates estimates of the amount of speech produced by adults in the child's environment, the number of child vocalizations, the number of adult–child conversational turns, and the amount of exposure to electronic noise (e.g. television). The software generates percentile scores relative to the normative sample for number of adult words and number of child vocalizations produced, as well as Automatic Vocalization Assessment (AVA) scores which reflect general expressive communication ability based on analysis of the child's vocalizations (Gilkerson & Richards, 2009). Parents were instructed to turn on the recording device when the baby woke up in the morning and keep it running until the baby went to bed in the evening, resulting in recordings that were between 10 and 14 hours long. Because the recordings were done by the parents using the LENA Pro system, researchers were not present in the home during the play sessions. This was done in order to increase the naturalness of the parent–infant interaction and thereby increase the ecological validity of the study findings.

Parents also completed the *Lena Developmental Snapshot* before the first day of recording. This measure is a parent questionnaire which is completed together with the researcher and asks questions about expressive and receptive communication development. Based on parent responses, a standard score is generated, providing a quick estimate of overall communication development.

Data coding

Using information provided by parents in daily logs regarding start and stop times of individual play sessions, the audio-recordings of the 15-minute book play sessions were extracted from the longer recordings for coding and analysis. All parent utterances from the play sessions were orthographically transcribed by graduate student research assistants. These parent utterances were coded to generate seven different measures of parent communicative behaviour. These parental behaviours were included because most have been identified as factors that may influence language development. The category of engaging and excited expressions (EXC) was included as an attempt to quantify the overall animation and engagement of the parent. It was thought that these types of interesting and animated expressions may serve to maintain the infant's interest in the interaction and thereby promote vocalizations. The most frequent behaviours in this category were animal sounds (e.g. *moo*), gasping (i.e. short audible inhale by the parent interpreted as an attempt to gain the child's attention before speaking), and *baby-words*, which were primarily diminutive forms (e.g. *piggy*). The measures are given, along with definitions and examples, in Table 2.1.

Infant volubility (VOL) was determined by calculating the number of infant vocalizations produced per minute during the play session. Only speech-like utterances were counted in determining infant volubility. Speech-like utterances were defined as vocalizations that met the minimum

Table 2.1 Description of measures of parent communicative behaviours that were analyzed

Measure of parent behaviour	*Definition*	*Example*
Adult words per minute (AW)	All words produced by the parent during the play session	'You're such a big girl.' (AW = 5)
Questions per minute (QUEST)	Questions produced by the parent during the play session	'Who says quack?' 'Does this look like your little chick?'
Directives per minute (DIR)	Utterances produced by parents that were interpreted as an attempt to direct or redirect the child's attention or behaviour	'Come here.' 'Can you make the sound of the snake.'
Rejections/ negations per minute (REJ)	Utterances produced by parent that included a rejection of the child's utterance or behaviour	'That one's not the dog ...' 'No, nope, you cannot take my glasses.'
Engaging/excited expressions per minute (EXC)	Parent productions of animal sounds, sound effects, gasps, claps, singing, baby games, interjections, nursery words or baby's name	'Quack quack' 'Oops' 'Bang'
Verbal responsiveness (RESP)	Parent verbal response to child vocalization produced within 5 seconds of child utterance (calculated as a proportion by dividing the total number of parent responses per minute by the total number of child vocalizations per minute)	Child: (babbled utterance) Parent: 'Oh yeah'
Imitation of child vocalizations per minute (IMIT)	Utterances produced immediately following a child vocalization that includes an imitation of the child's babbled or linguistic utterance. (Utterances that included an imitation of the child's vocalization and also expanded on it were also counted as imitations; see example.)	Child: (vocalization that approximates 'bye bye') Parent: 'oh bye bye books'

requirements of a Level I babble based on Stoel-Gammon's Mean Babbling Level classification system (Stoel-Gammon, 1989). According to Stoel-Gammon's criteria, a Level I babble consists of a voiced vowel, a syllabic consonant, or a CV syllable in which the consonant is a glottal stop, a glide or [h]. Cries, grunts and vegetative noises were not coded as infant vocalizations.

This is consistent with Oller's definition of 'protophones', which he describes as specific precursors to speech that are unique to humans (Oller *et al.*, 1999). Additional analysis was conducted using some of the measures derived from the LENA automatic analyses. The measures used included the adult word count (AWC) and the child vocalization (CV) percentile scores generated from all three days of recording. These measures reflect quantity of adult language heard by the child and overall volubility of the child (with percentile scores generated from normative data).

Results

As part of the larger study, reliability coding was conducted by a second research assistant for 15 of the participants. Reliability coding was conducted for number of adult words produced (AWC), child vocalizations (CV), and parental verbal responses (RESP). For all measures analyzed, reliability was high: Pearson-product moment correlations between coder 1 and coder 2 for these measures averaged $r = 0.981$ (range = 0.925–0.999). Reliability for the other measures was not performed.

The study children's mean standard scores, range, and standard deviation for the *Developmental Snapshot* and the *Automatic Vocalization Assessment* (AVA) are presented in Table 2.2. The mean standard score for these measures, based on normative data, is 100 while the standard deviation is 15. The AVA measure reflects overall level of expressive communication derived from acoustic analysis of infant vocalizations and the *Developmental Snapshot* score reflects both expressive and receptive communicative development based on parent report. Group means for both measures were within one standard deviation of the mean, suggesting that, as a group, the children were demonstrating typical communication development. On an individual level, all children had scores within one standard deviation of the mean on the *Developmental Snapshot* and only one child scored more than one standard deviation below the mean on the AVA (standard score of 83).

Mean, range and standard deviation for each coded parent communicative behaviour as well as for number of child vocalizations produced during the 15-mintue play session are presented in Table 2.3. All values, with the exception of verbal responsiveness rate and imitation rate, are presented in

Table 2.2 Mean, range and standard deviation Automatic Vocalization Assessment (AVA) standard score and Developmental Snapshot (DS) standard score

Measure	*Mean*	*Range*	*Standard deviation*
DS standard score	100.75	86–123	12.66
AVA standard score	97.54	83–114	8.64

Table 2.3 Mean, range and standard deviation for parent communicative behaviours and infant volubility

Behaviour	*Mean*	*Range*	*Standard deviation*
AW	66.28	33.84–108.13	20.55
QUEST	4.88	2.52–9.59	1.87
DIR	2.24	0.31–6.07	1.29
REJ	0.73	0.00–1.38	0.43
EXC	8.18	2.93–16.6	3.45
RESP	0.53	0.15–1.00	0.19
IMIT	0.05	0.00–0.18	0.05
VOL	4.1	0.27–9.63	2.43

Notes: AW = words produced by parent during play session per minute; QUEST = questions per minute; DIR = directives per minute; REJ = rejections per minute; EXC = engaging/excited expressions per minute; RESP = rate of parent responses to infant vocalizations; IMIT = rate of parent imitation of infant vocalization; VOL = infant vocalizations per minute.

occurrences per minute. Parent verbal responsiveness and parent imitation are directly related to the frequency of child vocalizations; that is, there is only an opportunity for a response or an imitation immediately after a child vocalization. In order to account for this, responsiveness and imitations are not reported in terms of absolute frequency of occurrence, but rather as the rate with which a parent responded verbally or imitated a child vocalization (e.g. a responsiveness rate of 0.5 indicates that the parent responded verbally to the child's vocalizations 50% of the time). Inspection of the range and standard deviation shows that there was considerable variability between participants in terms of frequency of the parent communicative behaviours as well as infant volubility. For instance, the number of adult words produced per minute ranged from only 33 all the way to a high of 108 words per minute. Similarly, one infant produced only 0.27 vocalizations per minute (which would be approximately only four vocalizations during the entire play session), while another infant produced almost 10 vocalizations per minute (approximately 150 vocalizations in the same time period). Imitations were noticeably infrequent, with an average imitation rate of 0.05 (this corresponds to parents imitating an average of only 5% of their child's utterances).

In order to investigate the concurrent relationship between parent communicative behaviours and infant volubility during play with books, a series of correlational analyses were conducted. The correlations between seven parent communicative behaviours and infant volubility (i.e. child vocalizations per minute) are presented in Table 2.4. As evident in the table, there were no significant correlations between parent communicative behaviours and infant volubility.

Table 2.4 Correlations between parent communicative behaviours and infant volubility

	AW	*QUEST*	*DIR*	*REJ*	*EXC*	*RESP*	*IMIT*
VOL	−0.08	0.03	0.13	−0.08	−0.27	0.12	0.23

Since none of the measures of parent communicative behaviour was correlated with concurrent infant volubility during the play sessions, the question arose as to whether infant volubility may be more closely related to a child's overall language environment, rather than to specific communicative behaviours present during a brief interaction. To explore this question, the automatic LENA measures generated from the three days of recording were analyzed to determine the relationship between general language environment and overall infant volubility during the three days, as well as infant volubility and adult words per minute during the play sessions. The measures of general language environment that were used in the analysis include AWC and CV and are expressed as percentile scores. The correlation matrix showing the relationship between these measures is presented in Table 2.5.

As can be seen in Table 2.5, the general language environment of the child in terms of the number of adult words heard over the course of three days is not associated with either overall infant volubility or the number of vocalizations produced during the play sessions. There are, however, two significant relationships. Infant volubility during the play sessions is significantly correlated (at the $p < 0.01$ level) with the child's general volubility as measured by the child vocalization percentile. Similarly, the number of adult words produced by the parent during the play sessions is significantly correlated (also at the $p < 0.01$ level) with overall adult words produced as measured by the adult word percentile. These results seem to indicate that generally vocal babies are also quite vocal during book sharing and generally talkative parents are also quite talkative during book sharing.

In spite of a general pattern of considerable variability in the number of child vocalizations produced ($M = 4.1$, $SD = 2.43$, range = 0.27–9.63), three children stood out as outliers in terms of their volubility during the play

Table 2.5 Correlations between adult and infant volubility during the play sessions (AW and VOL) and over the three days of recording (AWC and CV)

	CV	*AW*	*AWC*
VOL	0.54**	−0.08	0.11
CV		0.02	0.27
AW			0.54**

Notes: **Correlation is significant at the 0.01 level. VOL = infant volubility during the play sessions; CV = overall infant volubility over three days of recording; AW = adult words per minute during the play sessions; AWC = overall adult word percentile over three days of recording.

Table 2.6 Correlations between parent communicative behaviours and infant volubility with outliers removed

	AW	*QUEST*	*DIR*	*REJ*	*EXC*	*RESP*	*IMIT*
VOL	0.25	0.29	0.19	−0.11	−0.34	0.47*	0.09

Notes: *Correlation is significant at the 0.05 level.

session. Three infants had a vocalization rate of less than one vocalization per minute (i.e. almost two standard deviations below the mean) and one infant vocalized almost 10 times per minute (i.e. more than two standard deviations above the mean). Since these extreme values may have strongly influenced the results of the preliminary analysis, it was decided to run the correlational analyses again with these four outliers removed. The results of this analysis are presented in Table 2.6. With the outliers removed there was one significant relationship: rate of parent verbal responsiveness was positively associated with infant volubility. A scatter plot showing the relationship between rate of parent verbal responsiveness and infant volubility for the 23 parent–infant dyads is given in Figure 2.1.

Discussion

The purpose of the current study was to determine which, if any, parent communicative behaviours during a parent–infant play session were

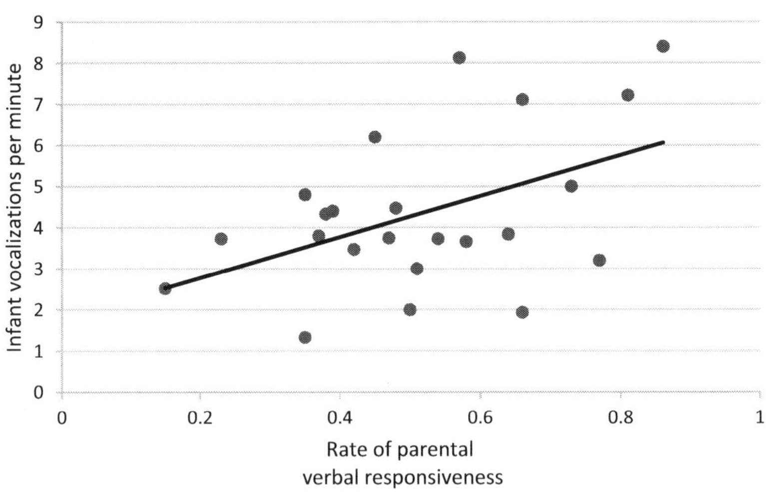

Figure 2.1 Scatter plot showing the relationship between verbal responsiveness and infant volubility (four outliers removed)

associated with infant volubility during the same session. Correlational analysis showed that the only parent behaviour that was significantly associated with infant volubility was verbal responsiveness. Children of parents with higher rates of verbal responsiveness vocalized more during the play session. There was no consistent relationship between quantity of language produced by the parent or any of the measures of communication style (e.g. use of questions, directives, engaging/excited expressions, etc.). Surprisingly, there was also no consistent relationship between overall amount of adult language heard by the child (as measured over three full days of recording) and infant volubility, either during the play session or over the three days of recording. There were, however, positive correlations between infant volubility during the play sessions and overall infant volubility as well as between adult words produced during the play sessions and overall counts of adult words produced. In other words, overall 'talkative' babies babbled more during the play sessions and overall taciturn babies babbled less, regardless of their parent's communicative behaviours, with the exception of verbal responsiveness. Similarly, overall talkative parents (i.e. those who produced more words heard by their child over three days of recording) were those who produced the most words during the play sessions.

The lack of a concurrent relationship between the number of words produced by parents and infant volubility is consistent with the results of Franklin *et al.* (2014), who also found no relationship between parent and infant volubility during play sessions in a laboratory. Similarly, data from the LENA Natural Language Study which analyzed child vocalizations and the language environment of over 300 children (Gilkerson & Richards, 2009) show that at early ages, infants of talkative parents and infants of taciturn parents have similar rates of vocalizations. The effect of parent talk on child vocalization rates was not evident until the children were older. Thus, while increased parent talk has consistently been associated with better language outcome for young children, this is the third study that has found that increased parent talk is not necessarily associated with concurrent infant volubility. It seems that the relationship between overall quantity of language input heard by infants and language development only emerges over an extended period of time, not at a single measurement point.

The results of the current study are also consistent with previous work showing that contingent responsiveness by the parent (both verbal and nonverbal) shapes infant vocalization (Dunst *et al.*, 2010; Goldstein & Schwade, 2008). A number of recent studies have concluded that in addition to just the quantity of language input, the quality of the communicative interaction (e.g. parental responsivity) is an important factor in language development (Zimmerman *et al.*, 2009). And, unlike just the quantity of adult words produced, parent responsiveness does seem to impact infant volubility during a single interaction, as well as over time. Taken together, these results emphasize that parental contingent responsiveness is a strategy that should be encouraged in order to increase infant volubility and to support overall language development. Imitation of the child's vocalization by the parent is another parental behaviour that has been found to increase and shape babble during parent–infant interactions (Dunst *et al.*, 2010). Parent imitation of a preceding infant vocalization was very infrequent in the data analyzed here. In fact, the parent who imitated the most, imitated their child's utterances only 18% of the time (approximately 0.87 times per minute) and eight of the parents did not imitate at all. While it is possible that the parents imitated their children's utterances more during other activities and interactions, the limited number of imitations observed here suggests that this is likely to be a relatively infrequent behaviour. Thus, imitation as a strategy to increase infant volubility may need to be directly taught to and practised by parents of children who are at risk for language delay.

A final, and important, consideration is that infant vocalization may shape parental communicative behaviour as much as parent behaviour shapes infant vocalization. Consistent with predictions based on the social feedback loop, parents' interaction and communication style may change based on how much – or little – their child vocalizes. The direction of the change in parent communication, however, may vary depending on the parent and the specific behaviours of the child. For example, a parent of a child who naturally babbles very little may also reduce the amount of input they provide because they are not 'pulled in' to communicative interactions by their child. On the other hand, a parent who observes that their child is not vocalizing very much may increase their overall language input as well as their use of engaging and excited expressions in an attempt to encourage more babbling. This bidirectional influence may explain why the hypothesized relationship between most of the parent communicative behaviours studied and infant volubility was not observed. Evidence for this possibility is found in the observation that the mother who produced the greatest number of words during the play session had an infant who produced only 0.29 vocalizations per minute, the second lowest of all the infants. Similarly, the mother of the infant who babbled the most during the play session produced very few words per minute, the third lowest of all the parents.

While the results of the current study are in many ways consistent with previous work, it is important to consider limitations that may have impacted results. An important limitation of the present work is the relatively small sample size; caution should be used in generalizing results based on just 27 parent–infant dyads. Furthermore, data are based on a volunteer sample of relatively highly educated and ethnically homogenous participants and results based on a more diverse sample might have been different. Additionally, the activity of playing with books is known to influence the communicative interaction (Gilkerson *et al.*, 2015) and different results might be found if interaction during different activities is analyzed. Future work should explore this possibility. Another limitation of the current analysis is that the complexity of the infants' vocalizations was not considered. It is possible that while the parent behaviours may have had little impact on the total number of vocalizations produced, certain parent behaviours (e.g. imitation) may have a larger effect on the complexity of those vocalizations. Finally, any clinical implications of the current findings rest on the assumption that increasing infant volubility during the prelinguistic stage of development will have a direct, positive influence on language development and growth. To this author's knowledge, empirical evidence for this assumption is not available and remains to be explored in future work.

Conclusion

The results of the current study contribute to the evidence showing that parental contingent responsiveness plays an important role in language development, influencing both concurrent infant volubility as well as later language growth. The other parental communicative behaviours investigated did not have an obvious impact on infant volubility. The results suggest that, in working with families of children who are at risk for or who are already exhibiting communication delay, emphasis should be placed on increasing parental responsivity rather than on increasing the overall quantity of parent talk. Additionally, a previously identified strategy for encouraging babble, imitation of child vocalizations, was used infrequently by the parents during the play sessions analyzed. An important implication of this finding is that imitation is a strategy that may need to be explicitly taught to and practised by parents in order to become established as a consistent part of their communicative repertoire.

References

Abbeduto, L., Warren, S.F. and Conners, F.A. (2007) Language development in Down syndrome: From the prelinguistic period to the acquisition of literacy. *Mental Retardation and Developmental Disabilities Research Reviews* 13 (3), 247–261.

Bates, E., Dale, P.S. and Thal, D. (1995) Individual differences and their implications for theories of language development. In P. Fletcher and B. MacWhinney (eds) *The Handbook of Child Language* (pp. 96–151). Oxford: Blackwell.

Bybee, J. (2003) *Phonology and Language Use*. Cambridge: Cambridge University Press.

Chapman, K.L., Hardin-Jones, M. and Halter, K.A. (2003) The relationship between early speech and later speech and language performance for children with cleft lip and palate. *Clinical Linguistics & Phonetics* 17 (3), 173–197.

Christakis, D.A., Gilkerson, J., Richards, J.A. *et al.* (2009) Audible television and decreased adult words, infant vocalizations, and conversational turns: A population-based study. *Archives of Pediatrics & Adolescent Medicine* 163 (6), 554–558.

Courage, M.L., Murphy, A.N., Goulding, S. and Setliff, A.E. (2010) When the television is on: The impact of infant-directed video on 6- and 18-month-olds' attention during toy play and on parent–infant interaction. *Infant Behavior and Development* 33 (2), 176–188; doi:10.1016/j.infbeh.2009.12.012.

d'Odorico, L., Majorano, M., Fasolo, M., Salerni, N. and Suttora, C. (2011) Characteristics of phonological development as a risk factor for language development in Italian-speaking pre-term children: A longitudinal study. *Clinical Linguistics & Phonetics* 25 (1), 53–65.

Dunst, C.J., Gorman, E. and Hamby, D.W. (2010) Effects of adult verbal and vocal contingent responsiveness on increases in infant vocalizations. *Center for Early Literacy Learning* 3 (1), 1–11.

Fasolo, M., Majorano, M. and D'Odorico, L. (2008) Babbling and first words in children with slow expressive development. *Clinical Linguistics & Phonetics* 22 (2), 83–94.

Ferguson, C.A. and Farwell, C.B. (1975) Words and sounds in early language acquisition. *Language* 51, 419–439.

Franklin, B., Warlaumont, A.S., Messinger, D. *et al.* (2014) Effects of parental interaction on infant vocalization rate, variability and vocal type. *Language Learning and Development* 10 (3), 279–296.

Fry, D.B. (1966) The development of the phonological system in the normal and deaf child. In F. Smith and G. Miller (eds) *The Genesis of Language* (pp. 187–206). Cambridge, MA: MIT Press.

Gilkerson, J. and Richards, J. (2009) The power of talk: Impact of adult talk, conversational turns, and TV during the critical 0–4 years of child development. LENA Foundation Technical Report ITR-01-2, Boulder, CO.

Gilkerson, J., Richards, J.A. and Topping, K.J. (2015) The impact of book reading in the early years on parent–child language interaction. *Journal of Early Childhood Literacy*; doi:10.1177/1468798415608907.

Goldstein, M.H. and Schwade, J.A. (2008) Social feedback to infants' babbling facilitates rapid phonological learning. *Psychological Science* 19 (5), 515–523; doi:10.1111/j.1467-9280.2008.02117.x.

Goldstein, M.H., King, A.P. and West, M.J. (2003) Social interaction shapes babbling: Testing parallels between birdsong and speech. *Proceedings of the National Academy of Sciences of the USA* 100 (13), 8030–8035; doi:10.1073/pnas.1332441100.

Gros-Louis, J., West, M.J., Goldstein, M.H. and King, A.P. (2006) Mothers provide differential feedback to infants' prelinguistic sounds. *International Journal of Behavioral Development* 30 (6), 509–516.

Hart, B. and Risley, T.R. (1995) *Meaningful Differences in the Everyday Experience of Young American Children.* Baltimore, MD: Paul H. Brookes.

Hart, B. and Risley, T. (2003) The early catastrophe. *American Educator* 27 (4), 6–9.

Jakobson, R. (1968) *Child Language, Phonological Universals and Aphasia* (trans. A. Keiler). The Hague: Mouton. (Original work published 1941 as *Kindersprache, aphasie und allgemeine Lautgesetze.*)

Marchman, V.A. and Bates, E. (1994) Continuity in lexical and morphological development: A test of the critical mass hypothesis. *Journal of Child Language* 21 (2), 339–366.

Masur, E.F., Flynn, V. and Olson, J. (2016) Infants' background television exposure during play: Negative relations to the quantity and quality of mothers' speech and infants' vocabulary acquisition. *First Language* 36 (2), 109–123.

McCathren, R.B., Yoder, P.J. and Warren, S.F. (1999) The relationship between prelinguistic vocalization and later expressive vocabulary in young children with developmental delay. *Journal of Speech, Language, and Hearing Research* 42 (4), 915–924.

Oller, D.K. and Eilers, R.E. (1988) The role of audition in infant babbling. *Child Development* 59, 441–449.

Oller, D.K., Eilers, R.E., Basinger, D., Steffens, M.L. and Urbano, R. (1995) Extreme poverty and the development of precursors to the speech capacity. *First Language* 15 (44), 167–187.

Oller, D.K., Eilers, R.E., Neal, A.R. and Schwartz, H.K. (1999) Precursors to speech in infancy: The prediction of speech and language disorders. *Journal of Communication Disorders* 32 (4), 223–245.

Overby, M. and Caspari, S.S. (2015) Volubility, consonant, and syllable characteristics in infants and toddlers later diagnosed with childhood apraxia of speech: A pilot study. *Journal of Communication Disorders* 55, 44–62.

Patten, E., Belardi, K., Baranek, G.T., Watson, L.R., Labban, J.D. and Oller, D.K. (2014) Vocal patterns in infants with autism spectrum disorder: Canonical babbling status and vocalization frequency. *Journal of Autism and Developmental Disorders* 44 (10), 2413–2428.

Paul, R., Fuerst, Y., Ramsay, G., Chawarska, K. and Klin, A. (2011) Out of the mouths of babes: Vocal production in infant siblings of children with ASD. *Journal of Child Psychology and Psychiatry* 52 (5), 588–598.

Pempek, T.A., Demers, L.B., Hanson, K.G., Kirkorian, H.L. and Anderson, D.R. (2011) The impact of infant-directed videos on parent–child interaction. *Journal of Applied Developmental Psychology* 32 (1), 10–19.

Pharr, A.B., Ratner, N.B. and Rescorla, L. (2000) Syllable structure development of toddlers with expressive specific language impairment. *Applied Psycholinguistics* 21 (4), 429–449.

Rescorla, L. and Ratner, N.B. (1996) Phonetic profiles of toddlers with specific expressive language impairment (SLI-E). *Journal of Speech, Language, and Hearing Research* 39 (1), 153–165.

Rowe, M.L. (2008) Child-directed speech: Relation to socioeconomic status, knowledge of child development and child vocabulary skill. *Journal of Child Language* 35 (1), 185–205.

Scherer, N.J., Williams, A.L. and Proctor-Williams, K. (2008) Early and later vocalization skills in children with and without cleft palate. *International Journal of Pediatric Otorhinolaryngology* 72 (6), 827–840.

Soderstrom, M. and Wittebolle, K. (2013) When do caregivers talk? The influences of activity and time of day on caregiver speech and child vocalizations in two childcare environments. *PloS One* 8 (11), e80646.

Sosa, A.V. (2016) Association of the type of toy used during play with the quantity and quality of parent–infant communication. *JAMA Pediatrics* 170 (2), 132–137.

Stoel-Gammon, C. (1989) Prespeech and early speech development of two late talkers. *First Language* 9 (6), 207–223.

Stoel-Gammon, C. (1998a) Sounds and words in early language acquisition: The relationship between lexical and phonological development. *Exploring the Speech-Language Connection* 8, 25–52.

Stoel-Gammon, C. (1998b) The role of babbling and phonology in early linguistic development. In A.M. Wetherby, S.F. Warren and J. Reichle (eds) *Communication and Language Intervention. 7: Transitions in Prelinguistic Communication* (pp. 87–110). Baltimore, MD: Paul H. Brookes.

Stoel-Gammon, C. (2011) Relationships between lexical and phonological development in young children. *Journal of Child Language* 38 (1), 1–34.

Stoel-Gammon, C. and Cooper, J.A. (1984) Patterns of early lexical and phonological development. *Journal of Child Language* 11 (2), 247–271.

Tamis-LeMonda, C.S., Bornstein, M.H. and Baumwell, L. (2001) Maternal responsiveness and children's achievement of language milestones. *Child Development* 72 (3), 748–767.

Tanimura, M., Okuma, K. and Kyoshima, K. (2007) Television viewing, reduced parental utterance, and delayed speech development in infants and young children. *Archives of Pediatrics & Adolescent Medicine* 161 (6), 618–619.

Thiemann-Bourque, K.S., Warren, S.F., Brady, N., Gilkerson, J. and Richards, J.A. (2014) Vocal interaction between children with Down syndrome and their parents. *American Journal of Speech-Language Pathology* 23 (3), 474–485.

Vanormelingen, L. and Gillis, S. (2016) The influence of socio-economic status on mothers' volubility and responsiveness in a monolingual Dutch-speaking sample. *First Language* 36 (2), 140–156.

Vihman, M.M. (1992) Early syllables and the construction of phonology. In C. Ferguson, L. Menn and C. Stoel-Gammon (eds) *Phonological Development: Models, Research, Implications* (pp. 393–422). Timonium, MD: York Press.

Vihman, M.M. (1993) The construction of a phonological system. In B. de Boysson-Bardies, S. de Schonen, P. Jusczyk, P. McNeilage and J. Morton (eds) *Developmental Neurocognition: Speech and Face Processing in the First Year of Life* (pp. 411–419). New York: Springer.

Walker, E.A. and Bass-Ringdahl, S. (2008) Babbling complexity and its relationship to speech and language outcomes in children with cochlear implants. *Otology & Neurotology* 29 (2), 225–229; doi:10.1097/mao.0b013e31815f6673.

Warlaumont, A.S., Richards, J.A., Gilkerson, J. and Oller, D.K. (2014) A social feedback loop for speech development and its reduction in autism. *Psychological Science* 25 (7), 1314–1324; doi:10.1177/0956797614531023.

Whitehurst, G.J., Smith, M., Fischel, J.E., Arnold, D.S. and Lonigan, C.J. (1991) The continuity of babble and speech in children with specific expressive language delay. *Journal of Speech, Language, and Hearing Research* 34 (5), 1121–1129.

Zimmerman, F.J., Gilkerson, J., Richards, J.A., Christakis, D.A., Xu, D., Gray, S. and Yapanel, U. (2009) Teaching by listening: The importance of adult–child conversations to language development. *Pediatrics* 124 (1), 342–349; doi:10.1542/peds.2008-2267.

Part 2

Methods in Language Analysis and Assessment

3 On the Weight of Phones in Computing Phonological Word Proximity

Elena Babatsouli, David Ingram and Dimitrios Sotiropoulos

Introduction

Children's productions of target consonants have been the focus of research for a few decades. There are two main reasons why consonants have been studied more than vowels: (1) errors in vowels are more scarce; and (2) the pronunciation of vowels is generally more sensitive than that of consonants to dialectal differences. The proportion of consonants correct (PCC) (e.g. Shriberg *et al.*, 1997) has been widely used in the literature since the mid-1980s and also in practice for assessing children's consonants in typical and atypical language development. It was not until the early 2000s that a phonological measure was proposed to evaluate whole-word productions. Ingram and Ingram (2001) and Ingram (2002) introduced the phonological mean length of utterance (PMLU) as the arithmetic mean of the PMLU of individual words, which is defined as the sum of the produced vowels and the substituted consonants plus twice the correctly produced consonants. The same authors introduced the proportion of word proximity *per word*, referred to as *phonological word proximity* (PWP), as the proportion of the produced PMLU to the target PMLU, with the PWP for a number of words in a speech sample being the arithmetic average of the PWP of individual words.

Several researchers have applied PMLU and PWP to evaluate speech performance in monolingual and bilingual child speech. Taelman *et al.* (2005) discussed how to use CLAN (MacWhinney, 2000) to compute PMLU and PWP using large sets of speech data. Bunta *et al.* (2009) compared three-year old Spanish-English bilingual children to their monolingual peers to compute, among other quantities, PWP and PCC. They found that while PWP and PCC differ in general, bilinguals only differ on PCC from their monolingual peers in Spanish and that when comparing the Spanish and English of the bilingual participants, PCC was significantly different but PWP was similar. Burrows and Goldstein (2010) compared PWP and PCC accuracy in Spanish-English bilinguals with speech sound disorders (SSDs) to age-matched monolingual peers. MacLeod *et al.* (2011) compared the rate of change between PWP and PCC for two groups of 20 children each, at the ages of 18 months and 36 months. One of the groups involved monolingual English children while the other involved bilingual French-English children. Their results showed that the rate of change of PWP was larger than that of PCC for each group and that the bilingual children's performance in their stronger language was similar to that of the monolingual children.

Another look at the proportion of PWP was taken by Babatsouli *et al.* (2014). Instead of defining PWP *per word*, they defined it *cumulatively* for all the words in a speech sample. This enabled them to express PWP for the whole speech sample analytically in terms of the PCC, the proportion of consonants deleted (PCD) and the proportion of vowels (PV) in the target speech, and obtain upper and lower PWP bounds in general.

The present study takes yet another look at PWP in order to question whether the correctly produced consonants should be weighted twice as much as vowels and substituted consonants. This weighting factor, 2, was decided arbitrarily by Ingram and Ingram (2001) and Ingram (2002) and the effect of its choice on the sensitivity of PWP to changes in PCC and PCD has not been examined to date. The analytical expression derived by Babatsouli *et al.* (2014) provides the starting point for such an examination in the present study which is motivated by the need to provide a measure that is more sensitive to errors, in order to evaluate PWP in child speech. Ingram (2015) and Ingram *et al.* (January 2018) point out that, when comparing typically developing children to children with SSD, PCC changes are not uniform across categories of word complexity: monosyllabic words without consonant clusters, monosyllabic words with at least one consonant cluster, multisyllabic words without consonant clusters, multisyllabic words with at least one consonant cluster. Their preliminary results on typically developing children show that both syllabicity and clusters add to word complexity, as measured by PCC. However, 'it was found that one group of children with SSD showed a similar pattern to the typically developing children in that they showed a correlation between word complexity and PCC. These children were considered to be having a phonological delay' (Ingram, 2015: 100). A second group of children with SSD did not show a significant correlation between word complexity and PCC. These children were considered to have an articulatory problem; there were consonants that they could not produce regardless of a word's complexity.

Such cases as well as others will be examined here, in light of how to compute PWP with respect to the value of the relative weight between correct consonants on the one hand and vowels and substituted consonants on the other. Therefore, the analysis in the present study will provide an insight on how to assess PWP in child speech samples, not only for all the words in the samples but also for different categories of word complexity in them.

Phonological Word Proximity for any Relative Weight between Phones

Relative weight of 2 between correct consonants and substituted consonants (and vowels)

Ingram and Ingram (2001) and Ingram (2002) introduced the PWP *per word* as follows:

$$\mathrm{PWP} = (2\mathrm{CC} + \mathrm{CS} + \mathrm{V})/(2\mathrm{TC} + \mathrm{TV}) \tag{1}$$

where CC is the number of consonants in the word correctly produced, CS is the number of consonants substituted, V is the number of produced vowels, TC is the number of target consonants in the word, and TV is the number of target vowels in the word. Therefore, in computing PWP per word using Equation (1), correctly produced consonants (CC) are weighted *twice* as heavily as substituted consonants and produced vowels. PWP for a number of words in a speech sample was subsequently obtained as the arithmetic average of the PWPs per word. However, the effect of different relative weights between correctly produced and substituted consonants cannot be calculated on such a cumulative PWP, but only on the PWP of individual words. For this reason, the analysis in the present study will be performed on a cumulative PWP which is calculated as the weighted average of the PWPs per word.

Babatsouli *et al.* (2014) expressed the PWP of Equation (1) in terms of the PCC, the proportion of phonemes deleted (PPD), and the proportion of vowel phonemes (PV) to all phonemes, as follows:

$$\mathrm{PWP} = p\mathrm{PCC} + (1 - p)\,(1 - \mathrm{PPD}), \quad p = (1 - \mathrm{PV})/(2 - \mathrm{PV}) \tag{2}$$

Then, by taking the weighted average of the PWPs per word given by Equation (2), Babatsouli *et al.* (2014) obtained a cumulative PWP for all the words in exactly the same form as Equation (2), with the three phonological parameter components, PCC, PPD and PV now computed as the weighted averages of their corresponding values per word. For example, the cumulative PCC is now the proportion of correctly produced consonants in the whole speech sample to the target consonants in the whole speech sample as well. The cumulative PWP as expressed by Equation (2) made it possible to obtain, in general, its upper and lower bounds.

Any relative weight between correct consonants and substituted consonants (and vowels)

In order to analyze the effect of the weighting factor for correctly produced consonants on the cumulative PWP, a general weight equal to $n + 1$ is considered, where n is any real number greater than zero, as correctly produced consonants should be weighted more than substituted consonants. The weight which was taken by Ingram and Ingram (2001) and Ingram (2002) and adopted by Babatsouli *et al.* (2014) as equal to 2 ($n = 1$), is a special case of the general $n > 0$ considered here. Following a similar derivation to that in Babatsouli *et al.* (2014), the cumulative PWP for a general $n > 0$ now becomes

$$\text{PWP} = p\text{PCC} + (1 - p)\,(1 - \text{PPD}), \quad p = n\text{PC}/(1 + n\text{PC}) \qquad (3)$$

where PC = 1 – PV is the proportion of consonant phonemes in targeted speech. It is seen that when $n = 1$, Equation (3) reduces to Equation (2). Further, the weight of PCC, p, is an increasing function of nPC while the weight of PPD, $1 - p$, is a decreasing function of nPC.

The numerical values of the two weights are depicted in Figure 3.1 for different values of nPC. It is seen that the weight of PCC is smaller than the weight of PPD for nPC values smaller than 1, the two weights are equal for nPC equal to 1, while the weight of PCC is larger than the weight of PPD for nPC values larger than 1. In Ingram's proposition, n is equal to 1 and, therefore, the weight of PCC is always smaller than the weight of PPD,

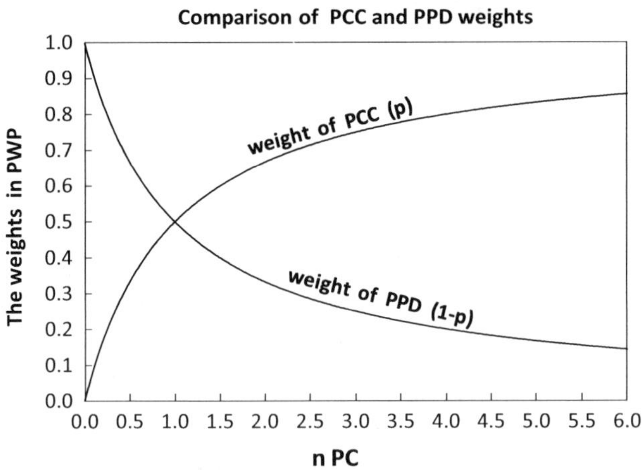

Figure 3.1 The weights of the proportion of consonants correct (PCC) and the proportion of phonemes deleted (PPD) versus nPC; $n + 1$ is the relative weight between correctly produced consonants and all other phones, and PC is the proportion of consonant phonemes

independent of the speech sample, as the proportion of consonant phonemes, PC, is smaller than 1.

The weight of PCC, p, will now be compared to the weight of the proportion of consonants deleted to the target consonants, for different values of n. To do this, PPD is written in terms of its two components, the proportion of consonants deleted to the target consonants, PCD, and the proportion of vowels deleted to the target vowels, PVD, as the sum of the following two products:

$$\text{PPD} = \text{PCD (PC)} + \text{PVD (PV)} \quad (4)$$

The weights of PCD and PCC in computing PWP of Equation (3) can now be compared by their ratio which, using Equation (4), becomes:

$$(1 - p)\text{PC}/p = 1/n \quad (5)$$

It may be seen that for any n larger than 1, the weight of PCD is smaller than the weight of PCC; for n equal to 1 (Ingram's proposal), the weight of PCD is equal to the weight of PCC; and for any n smaller than 1, the weight of PCD is larger than the weight of PCC. Therefore, the effect of different values of the relative weight between phones on the relative contributions of PCC and PCD in PWP is given quantitatively by Equation (5).

Differentiating Phonological Word Proximity across Productions of the Same or Different Speech Samples

We will now examine the effect of the relative weight of phones on differentiating PWP across different productions of the same or different speech samples. Depending on the relative change in PCC and PPD across speech productions, we seek a relative weight of phones which would better differentiate the PWP.

Uniform *p*

First, the proportion of consonant phonemes is taken to be the same between different speech samples. This includes the case in which different productions of the same speech sample are considered. Under these circumstances, the weights of PCC and PPD in PWP, which are p and $1 - p$ respectively, are uniform across the different productions.

Using Equation (3) for the PWP of each speech production and then subtracting the two PWPs gives the magnitude of the change of PWP, ΔPWP, as:

$$|\Delta\text{PWP}| = |p\,\Delta\text{PCC} - (1 - p)\,\Delta\text{PPD}| \quad (6)$$

where ΔPCC denotes the change in PCC across the two productions and ΔPPD represents the change in PPD. To calculate the magnitude of ΔPWP using Equation (6), the relative change between ΔPCC and ΔPPD needs to be known. In general, there are four possible scenarios for the relative change of the PCC and the PPD between two speech productions. These scenarios are:

$$\text{(i)}\quad \Delta PPD = -\kappa\,\Delta PCC, \quad 0 \le \kappa \le 1 \tag{7}$$

$$\text{(ii)}\quad \Delta PPD = \kappa\,\Delta PCC, \quad 0 \le \kappa \le 1 \tag{8}$$

$$\text{(iii)}\quad \Delta PCC = -\lambda\,\Delta PPD, \quad 0 \le \lambda \le 1 \tag{9}$$

$$\text{(iv)}\quad \Delta PCC = \lambda\,\Delta PPD, \quad 0 \le \lambda \le 1 \tag{10}$$

Scenarios (i) and (iii) are more likely to occur as more correct consonant productions are usually accompanied by fewer deletions and more deletions are usually accompanied by fewer correct consonant productions. Although Scenarios (ii) and (iv) are less likely, they may also occur when PCC and PPD are both either increasing or decreasing. These four scenarios have implications for the change in consonants substituted across the two productions. These implications are discussed next.

Since the sum of the consonants correct, the consonants substituted, and the consonants deleted is equal to the target consonants, that is, CC + CS + CD = TC, dividing both sides of this equation by TC and considering two productions yields the following relationship between the changes in correct consonants (CC), consonants substituted (CS) and consonants deleted (CD) across the two productions:

$$\Delta PCC + \Delta CD = -\Delta PCS \tag{11}$$

Assuming no change in vowel deletions across the productions, the change in consonants substituted would be of the opposite sign of the change in consonants correct in Scenarios (i) and (ii) and of the opposite sign of the change in consonants deleted in Scenarios (iii) and (iv).

For an arbitrary value of n, the change in PWP between two speech productions will now be calculated for each of the aforementioned four scenarios.

Scenario (i)

Substitution of Equation (7) in Equation (6) gives the following magnitude of the change in PWP across the two productions:

$$|\Delta PWP| = |\Delta PCC|[\kappa + (1 - \kappa)\,p] \tag{12}$$

Using the definition of p in (3), the quantity in the bracket of (12) becomes equal to $(\kappa + n\text{PC})/(1 + n\text{PC})$ and, therefore, it is linearly dependent on κ. It is smaller than 1 and its upper limit is equal to 1, when $\kappa = 1$. Thus, the magnitude of the change in PWP is smaller than the magnitude of the change in PCC, with the two magnitudes getting closer to each other as nPC increases. But, more importantly, the bracket of (12) is larger than κ and, therefore, the PWP is more sensitive than PPD to changes in PCC. This is illustrated in Figure 3.2 where the ratio $|\Delta\text{PWP}|/|\Delta\text{PCC}|$ is plotted against nPC for $\kappa = 0.1, 0.4, 0.7$. When $\kappa = 1$, the ratio is equal to 1 independent of nPC, meaning that PWP is as sensitive as PPD to changes in PCC. When $\kappa = 0$, meaning that there is no change in the deleted phonemes between the two productions, the ratio is equal to p and is thus given by the p line in Figure 3.1. It is concluded that larger nPC and κ result in a more sensitive PWP to changes in PCC when changes in PCC and PPD are of opposite sign across productions.

Scenario (ii)

Substitution of Equation (8) in Equation (6) results in

$$|\Delta\text{PWP}| = |\Delta\text{PCC}|\,|-\kappa + (1 + \kappa)\,p| \tag{13}$$

when there is no change in the deleted phonemes between the two productions, $\kappa = 0$, and the ratio $|\Delta\text{PWP}|/|\Delta\text{PCC}|$ becomes equal to p, the same as in Scenario (i). When nPC is large, the ratio approaches 1. More importantly, the ratio is smaller or equal to κ for $n\text{PC} \leq 2\kappa/(1 - \kappa)$, meaning that when changes in PCC and PPD across productions are of the same sign, PWP is less sensitive than PPD to changes in PCC for these values of κ. For all other values of PWP, the ratio is more sensitive as in Scenario (i). This is shown in

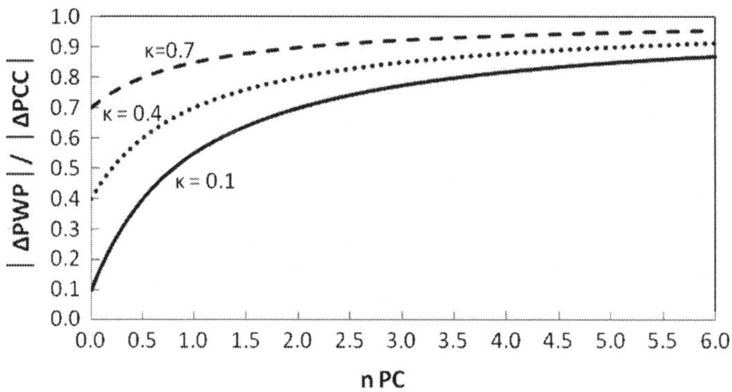

Figure 3.2 The sensitivity of proportion of word proximity (PWP) to changes in proportion of consonants correct (PCC) versus nPC for different values of κ when $\Delta\text{PPD} = -\kappa\,\Delta\text{PCC}$

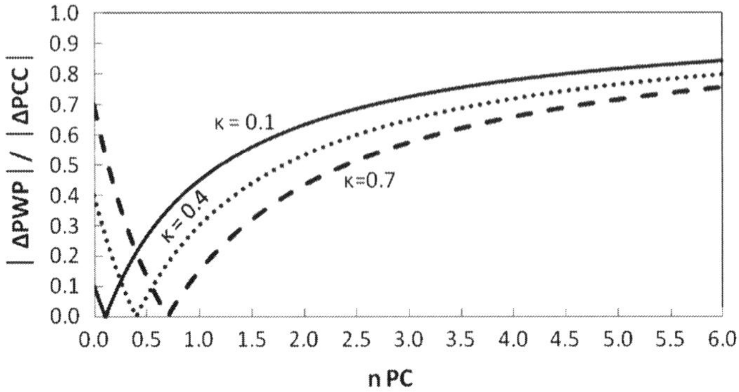

Figure 3.3 The sensitivity of proportion of word proximity (PWP) to changes in proportion of consonants correct (PCC) versus *n*PC for different values of κ when ΔPPD = κ ΔPCC

Figure 3.3 where the ratio is plotted against *n*PC for κ = 0.1, 0.4, 0.7. It is observed that there is a range of values of *n*PC, which is smaller for smaller κ, inside which increasing *n*PC and κ make PWP less sensitive than PPD to changes in PCC. When κ = 1, the ratio is 1 for *n*PC equal to 0, it diminishes for *n*PC equal to 1, and then it rises below κ = 0.7.

Scenario (iii)

Substitution of Equation (9) in Equation (6) gives

$$|\Delta\text{PWP}| = |\Delta\text{PPD}|[1 - (1 - \lambda)\, p] \tag{14}$$

when there is no change in the correctly produced phones, λ = 0, and the ratio |ΔPWP|/|ΔPPD| becomes $1 - p$ which is shown in Figure 3.1 against *n*PC. In this case, the smaller *n*PC, the more sensitive PWP is to changes in PPD. When the magnitudes of the change in PPD and PPC are equal, λ = 1, PWP changes as much as PPD across productions, attaining its maximum change, independent of *n*PC. It is noted that the bracket of Equation (14) is equal to $(1 + \lambda n\text{PC})/(1 + n\text{PC})$. Thus, the ratio is 1 for *n*PC equal to 0 and decreases as *n*PC increases approaching λ, while it increases for increasing λ. As a result, PWP is more sensitive than PCC to changes in PPD across productions. This is illustrated quantitatively in Figure 3.4, where the sensitivity of PWP to changes in PPD is plotted against *n*PC for λ = 0.1, 0.4, 0.7.

Scenario (iv)

Substitution of Equation (10) in Equation (6) yields

$$|\Delta\text{PWP}| = |\Delta\text{PPD}||(1 + \lambda)\, p - 1| \tag{15}$$

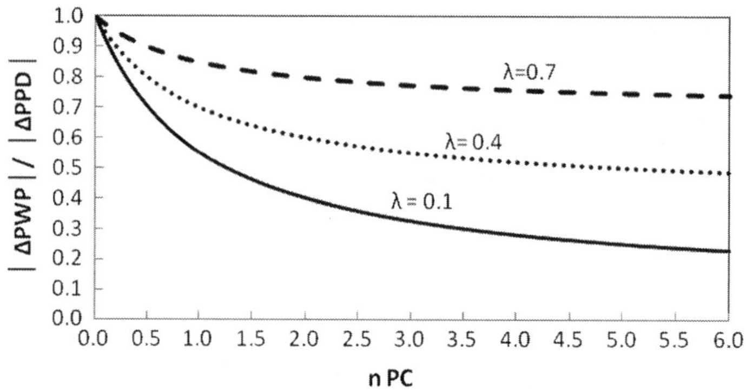

Figure 3.4 The sensitivity of proportion of word proximity (PWP) to changes in proportion of phonemes deleted (PPD) versus proportion of consonant phonemes (nPC) for different values of λ when $\Delta PCC = -\lambda\ \Delta PPD$

when $\lambda = 0$, the ratio $|\Delta PWP|/|\Delta PPD|$ becomes $1 - p$ as in Scenario (iii). Using the definition of p from (3), the ratio becomes $|\lambda n PC - 1|/|(nPC + 1)$. It is noted that for nPC equal to 0 the ratio is 1 independent of λ, it becomes zero when $\lambda n PC = 1$, and it approaches λ from below when nPC is large. These remarks may be observed in Figure 3.5 where the sensitivity of PWP to changes in PPD versus nPC for $\lambda = 0.1$, 0.4, 0.7 is shown quantitatively. There is a range of values of nPC, which is smaller for larger λ, inside which increasing nPC and λ make PWP less sensitive than PPD to changes in PCC. When $\lambda = 1$, the ratio diminishes for nPC equal to 1, and then it rises approaching 1 from below.

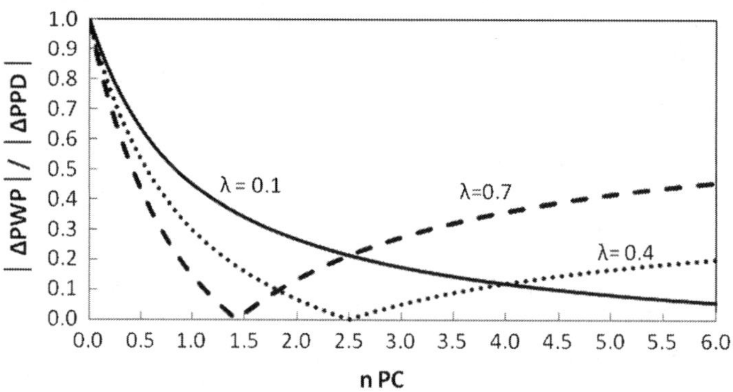

Figure 3.5 The sensitivity of proportion of word proximity (PWP) to changes in proportion of phonemes deleted (PPD) versus proportion of consonant phonemes (nPC) for different values of λ when $\Delta PCC = \lambda\ \Delta PPD$

Non-uniform p

Here, the sensitivity of PWP to changes in PCC or PPD across productions for different speech samples will be examined in view of an arbitrary relative weight between phones. The proportion of consonant phonemes across productions is in general considered different and, therefore, p is non-uniform. This case includes comparisons of a child's performance across speech samples that differ in the categories of word complexity in that they include, for example, monosyllabic words without consonant clusters, monosyllabic words with at least one consonant cluster, multisyllabic words without a consonant cluster, and multisyllabic words with at least one consonant cluster.

The pertinent question at hand is by how much the change in PC together with the changes in PCC and PPD would affect the value of the computed PWP. To answer this question in an exact mathematical manner will be more complicated than the uniform p case analyzed above and is outside the scope of the present chapter. Instead, two different approaches will be taken.

In the first approach, the PWP of one of the speech samples will be computed using the true values of PCC and PPD but not the true value of p. Instead, the p-value of the other speech sample will be used. How different would this approximate PWP be from the exact PWP calculated from the true p? If the difference is small, then the results for a uniform p presented above can be used.

Using Equation (3) to compute PWP for each one of the two ps, and then subtracting the two PWPs gives

$$\Delta \mathrm{PWP} = -\Delta p \; (1 - \mathrm{PCC} - \mathrm{PPD}) \qquad (16)$$

where $\Delta\mathrm{PWP} = \mathrm{PWP} - \mathrm{PWP}_1$ and $\Delta p = p - p_1$, where the quantities without subscript correspond to one of the speech samples and its production and with a subscript to the other. It is noted that the quantity in the parenthesis in Equation (16) is always smaller than 1, so that the change of PWP is smaller than the change of p. For a given n, Δp is obtained from the definition of p in (3) as

$$\Delta p = n\Delta\mathrm{PC}/[(1 + n\mathrm{PC} - n\Delta p)(1 + n\mathrm{PC})] \qquad (17)$$

where $\Delta\mathrm{PC} = \mathrm{PC} - \mathrm{PC}_1$. The dependence of Δp on $n\mathrm{PC}$ and $\Delta\mathrm{PC}$ will now be demonstrated quantitatively. The proportion of consonant phonemes in one of the speech samples is taken to be smaller than that of the other speech sample, that is, $\mathrm{PC}_1 = \alpha\mathrm{PC}$, $\alpha < 1$. Then, $\Delta\mathrm{PC} = (1 - \alpha)\mathrm{PC}$. Figure 3.6 depicts Δp versus $n\mathrm{PC}$ for $\alpha = 0.7, 0.8, 0.9$.

At first, we observe that Δp is quite small, less than 9% for all the cases shown in Figure 3.6. Secondly, it is observed that when $n = 1$ which gives

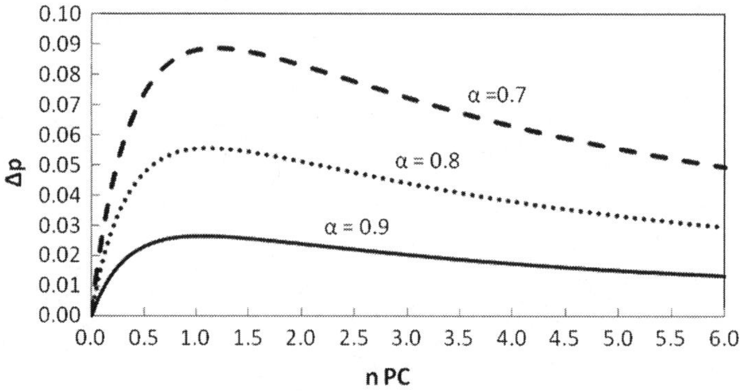

Figure 3.6 The dependence of the change in PCC weight, Δp, on the product of the relative weight of phones and the proportion of consonant phonemes, nPC, across speech samples whose ratio of consonant phonemes is α

Ingram's relative weight, Δp remains effectively constant for PC greater than 50% (or even lower). For $\alpha = 0.9$ the change in Δp is less than 0.5%, for $\alpha = 0.8$ it is less than 1%, and for $\alpha = 0.7$ it is less than 1.5%. This also holds true for an arbitrary n as long as nPC is greater than 50%. This means that an increasing relative weight of phones results in a larger range of PC values for which Δp remains effectively constant.

It is known (Nespor *et al.*, 2003) that the PC in adult speech is about 55% for stress-timed languages, like English, and about 50% for syllable-timed languages, like Spanish and Greek. Typical PC values for speech targeted by children during phonological development or for speech samples designed for assessment purposes usually exceed these values, as evidenced in the examples included in the following section. Therefore, in view of Equation (16), it is concluded that the PWP for a speech sample may be computed using the proportion of consonant phonemes of another speech sample, if the ratio of consonant phonemes is between 0.7 and 1.43.

Children's Speech Illustrating the Mathematical Analysis

Speech samples from two children will be considered here to illustrate the mathematical analysis presented above. The first child is a typically developing Greek-English bilingual child whose naturalistic word productions at the age of three years are examined. The second child is a monolingual English child diagnosed with SSD whose speech data were elicited at the age of five years and 11 months. In the two examples, two issues will be dealt with in view of the analytical results obtained above: (a) examining the effect of the relative weight of phones, $n + 1$, on computing the change in

PWP between words of different categories of word complexity. Specifically, the two word categories that will be examined are monosyllabic words containing only singleton consonants and monosyllabic words containing at least one consonant cluster, and (b) examining how well the approximation of Equation (16) holds for different relative weights of phones in computing the PWP of one word category using the proportion of consonants of the other word category.

A bilingual child's English at age three years

A Greek-English bilingual child's speech in English was elicited at the age of three years during routine interaction with an adult interlocutor (the mother). The child, a female, was born and raised in Greece, where Greek is the language of the ambient environment. She was exposed to English from the age of one year onwards exclusively through her mother's fluent second language (L2) English, which is close to the Standard American rhotic variety. From age one until age three, when the data presented here were elicited, the child's input in Greek came from her father and from the ambient Greek environment, while from age two onwards, the child's input in Greek also came from interactions at a day care school. The child is otherwise a typically developing bilingual; recent literature on bilingual acquisition accounts for increasing diversity in bilingual exposure and use (e.g. Babatsouli & Ingram, 2015; Kehoe, 2015).

A hand-held Olympus WS11-311M was used by the first author to digitally record the child's utterances. She also transcribed the data in IPA and entered them in a CLAN (MacWhinney, 2000) database. The child's speech was recorded on seven different days during the first 16 days following her third birthday. There is a total of four hours of recording at an average of 34 minutes per day. The total number of utterances in English is 514, containing 1590 word tokens, resulting in an average length of sentence (ALS) of 3.1 words. The mother addressed the child only in English, but the child sometimes code-switched, replying in Greek. During the aforementioned period of speech elicitation, the total number of child utterances in Greek is 734, containing 3871 word tokens, at an ALS equal to 5.3 words. ALS in terms of words was proposed by Nice (1925) as a measure of progress in child speech, and was shown by Parker and Brorson (2005) to be correlated to mean length of utterance (MLU) in terms of morphemes, as proposed by Brown (1973). We see that this child's ALS in English at age three is considerably lower than in Greek. This is attributed to the fact that the child's amount of input in Greek was larger than that in English, and that the child's speech development was ongoing. However, it ought to be mentioned that the child's ALS became comparable in the two languages by the age of three years and nine months.

The 45 monosyllabic words with singleton consonants which were targeted by the child, together with her typical productions in brackets, are as follows: *back* [bæt], *beach* [bi:ʦ], *bed* [bet], *bit* [vɪt], *car* [tæl], *case* [ʦeɪs], *cat* [tæt], *cows* [taʊs], *day* [deɪ], *dog* [dɒt], *door* [dɔ:l], *fish* [fɪʃ], *five* [faɪf], *food* [fu:t], *four* [fɔ:l], *full* [fʊɫ], *hair* [heəl], *have* [sæf], *head* [hed], *here* [sɪə], *hide* [ʃaɪt], *juice* [ʤu:s], *kiss* [tɪs], *leave* [li:f], *lick* [lɪt], *look* [lʊt], *loose* [lu:s], *moon* [mu:n], *more* [mɔ:l], *mouse* [maʊs], *nice* [naɪs], *nose* [noʊz], *now* [naʊ], *pull* [pʊɫ], *put* [pʊt], *rain* [veɪn], *red* [ve:t], *right* [vaɪt], *sea* [si:], *sit* [sɪt], *teeth* [ti:s], *wash* [voʧ], *what* [vɒt], *where* [veəl], *yes* [jes].

Further, the 38 monosyllabic words with at least one consonant cluster which were targeted by the child, together with her typical productions in brackets, are as follows: *block* [bɒt], *boots* [bu:ts], *box* [bɒts, pɒ], *bread* [be:t], *bridge* [bi:ʤ], *bring* [bin], *brush* [bʌʃ], *cold* [tɔ:d], *clean* [ti:n], *clear* [tɪəl], *clock* [tɒt], *doesn't* [tʌzən], *dream* [di:m], *farm* [sa:m], *flat* [fæt], *floor* [fɔ:l], *found* [faʊn], *grab* [dæb], *help* [seəp], *left* [le:], *lost* [lɒst], *milk* [mɪət], *once* [vʌts], *place* [peɪs], *seeds* [si:ds], *slide* [sa:ɪt], *small* [smɔ:], *spoon* [spu:n], *stopped* [stɒpt], *street* [sti:t], *things* [si:nts], *throw* [ʃoʊ], *toast* [toʊst], *train* [teɪn], *trash* [tæʃ], *trouble* [tʌbl̩], *try* [taɪ], *washed* [vɒst].

As expected, there were variations in the child's productions of some words because her phonological development was ongoing. Examples of such variations in the words with singleton consonants are: *loose* [lu:s, du:s] and *have* [sæf, hæf]. We note that [d] as a substitute of target *l* does not occur frequently at age three because the lateral was acquired in CV and CVC contexts several months before. The child is stopping the coronal lateral to [d], as stopping is a common simplification process in phonological development (e.g. Bernhardt & Stemberger, 1998). As opposed to the targeted lateral, the child's English glottal fricative was acquired much later, several months after age three. Although in monolingual English development *h* is usually deleted (e.g. Smit, 1993), this bilingual child's English *h* is produced as [s, ʃ], possibly due to the interference of the targeted Greek voiceless velar fricative, *x*, also substituted by [s, ʃ] in her speech.

Examples of variations in the production of the words with a consonant cluster are: *toast* [toʊst (2), toʊs, toʊt, stoʊst], *stopped* [stɒpt (2), spɒ], *place* [peɪs, ble], *spoon* [spu:n (4), pu:n, smu:n], and *flat* [fæt, flæt, sfæt]. We note that most variability observed in these productions was a result of repetition in the same utterance or in consecutive utterances. For instance, production of *spoon* varied when the child repeated the utterance *bring me another spoon* → [spu:n, pu:n], and on another day the utterance *I don't have another spoon* → [spu:n, smu:n]. Variable productions involve common phonological processes in child developmental speech (e.g. Bernhardt & Stemberger, 1998). Consonant cluster reduction occurs word finally in *st* which is reduced to either [s] or [t] in *toast*, and word initially in *pl*, *fl* which are reduced to [p] and [f] in *place* and *flat*, respectively, in accordance with sonority considerations where the more sonorant second member in the cluster gets deleted (e.g. Ohala, 1999). Voicing of the labial stop occurs by assimilation to the adjacent lateral in *place* [ble]. Also, [place] metathesis of labial to coronal occurs in *stopped* [spɒ]. Lastly, added syllable complexity, also referred to as *consonant clusters by excrescence* (CCEs) (Babatsouli, 2016) is also found in these examples. CCEs, whereby a non-targeted consonant, e.g. [s], is epenthesized next to a targeted consonant, e.g. [t] or [f], occur in *toast* [**s**toʊst] and *flat* [**s**fæt]. The pattern is argued to be an articulatory as well as a phonological mechanism that enables children to practice non-acquired consonant singletons and clusters. This pattern has been observed in both typical and atypical child speech development (Babatsouli, 2016, and references therein), though also evidenced in adult progressive speech degeneration (Ball *et al.*, 2004), where it may be an attempt to implement repair.

The child's variations in productions of words were included in calculating PCC and PCD. The results are:

Monosyllabic words with singleton consonants:	PC = 0.59, PCC = 0.64, PCD = 0.0
Monosyllabic words with consonant *clusters*:	PC = 0.71, PCC = 0.51, PCD = 0.19

The child's monosyllabic words with only singleton consonants have a PC equal to 59%, above the average PC for adult English speech which is 55% (Nespor *et al.*, 2003), while the monosyllabic words with a consonant cluster have an even larger PC equal to 71%, as expected. The corresponding p-values with $n = 1$ for the two word categories are 0.37 and 0.415, respectively. For $n = 2$, they are 0.541 and 0.587. The true PWP values are computed using Equation (3). For $n = 1$, the PWP values of the two word categories are 0.87 and 0.69, respectively, and for $n = 2$, they are 0.81 and 0.66. Since Δp is very small between the two word samples for both $n = 1$ and $n = 2$, the change in PWP for the two cases may be viewed in terms of the analytical results presented above for a uniform p between speech samples.

Even though the child did not produce vowels accurately, these pronunciation errors are not taken into account in PWP computations because the focus is on whether vowels are produced and whether they are produced in the target word position and not whether they are accurate, following Ingram (2002). Given that Δ(PCC) = 0.13 and Δ(PPD) = Δ(PCD PC) = −0.135, this child's performances between the two word categories belong to Scenario (iii) above described by Equation (9), since Δ(PCC) = −0.96 Δ(PPD). Therefore, as concluded from the analysis of Scenario (iii) above and the quantitative results of Figure 3.4, the ratio $|\Delta\text{PWP}|/|\Delta\text{PPD}|$ will become smaller as nPC increases. Furthermore, the ratio is expected to be larger than $\lambda = 0.96$, which is the ratio $|\Delta\text{PCC}|/|\Delta\text{PPD}|$. Indeed, for $n = 2$ the ratio $|\Delta\text{PWP}|/|\Delta\text{PPD}|$ is equal to 1.11, smaller than 1.33, its value for $n = 1$. The ratio being larger than 1 falling outside the scale of Figure 3.4 is attributed to assuming a null Δp in drawing Figure 3.4, which is not exactly the case between the child's word categories.

Now, suppose the PWP of one word category is computed from the PC of the other word category. How far off is this approximate PWP expected to be from the true PWP for the two *n*s, $n = 1$ and $n = 2$, in view of the analytical results of the previous section? Since Δp is very small, 0.045 and 0.046, respectively, for $n = 1$ and $n = 2$, the approximate PWP is expected to be near the true PWP. Indeed, when approximating either the words with singleton consonants or the words with consonant clusters, Equation (16) gives $\Delta\text{PWP} = 0.02$, a very small number. This shows quantitatively the practical application of computing PWP using the proportion of consonants of another speech sample, if Δp between the two samples is small.

A child with speech sound disorder

The child considered in the second example is a monolingual American English-speaking male child at age five years and 11 months diagnosed with SSD. His speech was recorded during his responses to pictures representing single words shown to him and was subsequently IPA transcribed. There were 18 target monosyllabic words with singleton consonants and 16 target monosyllabic words with at least one consonant cluster.

The CV and CVC monosyllabic words are: *bed, chair, doll, fish, gun, leaf, mouth, nose, page, rouge, rug, shoe, soap, that, thumb, tub, vase, watch*. The monosyllabic words with consonant clusters are: *black, green, fork, glove, horse, mask, sled, smooth, snake, spoon, spring, squirrel, star, string, three, truck*.

Transcription and analysis of the male child's realizations resulted in the following:

Singleton consonant words: PC = 0.64, PCC = 0.18, PCD = 0.28
Consonant *cluster* words: PC = 0.76, PCC = 0.18, PCD = 0.47

There were no vowel errors. It is interesting that the child's PCC is the same whether the words contain clusters or not; the inability to produce certain sounds regardless of a word's complexity may be interpreted as an articulatory effect (Ingram *et al.*, 2018). Since there is no change in PCC across the two word categories, $\Delta(\text{PCC}) = 0$. The corresponding *p*-values computed from (3) with $n = 1$ are 0.39 and 0.43, respectively, for singleton consonants and consonant cluster words. Therefore, if PWP for the consonant cluster words is approximated by Equation (16) using the *p* corresponding to the words with only singleton consonants, it will only differ from the true PWP by less than 4%. If $n = 2$ instead of $n = 1$ is used in computing *p*, then its values for the words with only consonant singletons and the words with a consonant cluster are respectively 0.56 and 0.60, resulting again in a very small error for PWP when using the *p* of the other word category.

Lastly, the case of a uniform PCC between speech samples just seen above warrants further analysis, the results of which can be used in practice for arbitrary Δ(PPD) as well as a Δp that is not negligible. It will be useful to see which relative weight of phones, $n + 1$, would differentiate better PWP between word categories whose PCC is invariable. Without going through the algebraic details, the use of Equation (3) four times, twice for each n to compute the PWP for each word category, results in

$$\Delta\text{PWP}_1 - \Delta\text{PWP}_2 = -(p_2 - p_1)\ \Delta\text{PPD} \tag{18}$$

where Δ is the change of the quantity of interest (PWP or PPD) across word categories and the subscript refers to the first or second n used in computing p and PWP. In (18), p may be computed for either category as it will yield the same result. This is because the difference $(p_2 - p_1)$ changes negligibly for any changes in PC values larger than about 50%, independent of n. This was observed in Figure 3.6. Comparing $(p_2 - p_1)$ values with subscript 2 referring to $n = 2$ and subscript 1 referring to $n = 1$ at different PC values larger than about 50%, it is seen that they are practically the same. For example, for PC = 50%, $p_1 = 0.333$ and $p_2 = 0.5$ and, thus, $p_2 - p_1 = 0.167$. For PC = 75%, $p_1 = 0.429$ and $p_2 = 0.6$ and, thus, $p_2 - p_1 = 0.171$. The change in the difference $(p_2 - p_1)$ is indeed negligible. Derivation of Equation (18) is based on this observation.

What does Equation (18) imply for practical applications? To answer this, first let the subscript 1 refer to the smaller of the two n-values chosen. Then $p_2 - p_1$ is positive and for negative ΔPPD (for example PPD for monosyllabic words with only singleton consonants minus PPD for words with a consonant cluster), the left-hand side becomes positive. For negative ΔPPD, ΔPWP is positive independent of the n chosen as ΔPCC = 0, giving that ΔPWP is larger for the smaller n. Distinguishing PWP between categories of word complexity is useful in practice and, therefore, it is better in such cases, as the one considered here, to use as small an n as possible. Ingram's proposition of $n = 1$ is the smallest integer n that can used for optimal results. Furthermore, Equation (18) gives the difference in the change of PWP for two arbitrary values of n, for a given ΔPPD. To get a feeling for the amount that this difference changes for different values of n, it is now computed for PC = 60% and $n = 0.5$, $n = 1$, and $n = 2$. ΔPWP for $n = 0.5$ is larger than ΔPWP for $n = 1$ by the amount 0.14 times the absolute value of ΔPPD. In turn, ΔPWP for $n = 1$ is larger than ΔPWP for $n = 2$ by the amount 0.17 times the absolute value of ΔPPD.

Summary and Recommendations for Practical Use

The purpose of the mathematical analysis and of the examples presented above is to provide a guide for practical use. That is, given a speech sample, one ought to be able to select the relative weight of phones in such a way as to make a better assessment using the measure of PWP. We briefly summarize our results in non-mathematical terms as follows.

(a) When the proportion of consonants correct is similar between different children's productions of the same speech sample, it is recommended that correct consonants are weighted by the lower limiting value 1 ($n = 0$), if the largest change of phonological word proximity across the speech productions is desired. In such a case, the change of phonological word proximity is equal to the change of the proportion of phonemes deleted, which can then be used instead since it is simpler to compute. The larger the weight of correct consonants used, the smaller the change of phonological word proximity across the speech productions. Lastly, the proportion of consonant phonemes in the speech sample affects the change of phonological word proximity in exactly the same way as the weight of correct consonants; the larger the proportion of consonant phonemes, the smaller the change of phonological word proximity.

(b) When the proportion of phonemes deleted is similar between different speech productions of the same sample, it is recommended that correct consonants are weighted as much as possible, if the largest change of phonological word proximity across the speech productions is desired. The largest possible change of phonological word proximity is equal to the change of the proportion of consonants correct, which can then be used instead because it is easier to calculate. Finally, the weight of correct consonants affects the change of phonological word proximity in exactly the same way as the proportion of consonant phonemes in the speech sample; the larger the proportion of consonant phonemes, the larger the change of phonological word proximity.

(c) When the change of the proportion of consonants correct is similar in magnitude to the change of phonemes deleted between two speech productions of the same sample, the change of phonological word proximity is similar to the change of the proportion of consonants correct, which can then be used instead for assessing phonological word level.

(d) When the change of the proportion of consonants correct is smaller and of the opposite sign than the change of the proportion of phonemes deleted between two speech productions of the same sample, a small weight of correct consonants is recommended to be used if a large change of phonological word proximity is desirable, as in case (a). Also, as in case (a), the smaller proportion of consonant phonemes results in a larger change of phonological word proximity. Independently of the weight used for correct consonants, the change of phonological word proximity is larger than the change of the proportion of consonants correct and, therefore, it is preferable to use if a larger change of phonological proximity across the speech productions is desired.

(e) When the change of the proportion of phonemes deleted is smaller and of the opposite sign to the change of the proportion of consonants correct between two speech productions of the same sample, a large weight of correct consonants is recommended to be used if a large change of phonological word proximity is desirable, as in case (b). Also, as in case (b), the larger proportion of consonant phonemes results in a larger change of phonological word proximity. The change of phonological word proximity is larger than the change of the proportion of phonemes deleted and, thus, it is better to use when a larger change of phonological word proximity is sought across the speech productions.

(f) Further, when phonological word proximity is compared between speech productions of different samples, as is the case of different categories of word complexity such as words with consonant singletons and words with consonant clusters, the results and recommendations in (a), (b), (c), (d) and (e) above are applicable when the change of the proportion of phonemes between the speech samples is between 0.7 and 1.43, independent of the weight used for correct consonants in computing phonological word proximity. This range of values increases as the weight used for correct consonants is closer to 1 than 2.

It is emphasized that the *limiting* cases included in the discussion above are not intended to undermine the importance of using PWP but to shed light on its proper use (relative weight of phones) depending on the relative change of its components between speech performances. Lastly, it is noted that when PWP is to be used in establishing norms for large populations, *smaller* differentiations of PWP between performances will result in smaller data scattering and, therefore, the relative weight of phones must be picked *inversely* to the cases where larger differentiations of PWP are desirable.

Conclusion

The effects of the relative weight of phones and of the proportion of consonant phonemes on differentiating phonological word proximity across speech productions were examined analytically. The mathematical analysis was illustrated in the examples of two children's speech samples, one typically developing, and the other with SSD. Of particular interest may be the natural speech production of the three-year old typically developing child whose variability in consonant errors during development also occurred in the repetition of sentences. Further, the mathematical results were summarized in simple terms in order to provide a guide for practical use. However, in the formulae suggested for computing phonological word proximity, vowel errors were ignored when they did not involve deletions. Therefore, if one is interested in focusing on vowel errors in child speech or in assessing second language speech where vowel mispronunciation occurs even in advanced L2 learners, the results of the present study cannot be used directly. They need to be extended to include inaccurate vowels in an analogous manner as when substituted consonants were included in computing phonological word proximity.

Acknowledgements

Preliminary results of this study were presented at the *International Symposium on Monolingual and Bilingual Speech 2015*, which took place on 7–10 September 2015 in Chania, Crete, Greece.

References

Babatsouli, E. (2016) Added syllable complexity in a child's developmental speech and clinical implications. *Clinical Linguistics & Phonetics* 30 (8), 628–648.

Babatsouli, E. and Ingram, D. (2015) What bilingualism tells us about phonological acquisition. In R.H. Bahr and E.R. Silliman (eds) *Routledge Handbook of Communication Disorders* (pp. 173–182). Routledge: Taylor & Francis.

Babatsouli, E., Ingram, D. and Sotiropoulos, D. (2014) Phonological word proximity in child speech development. *Chaotic Modeling and Simulation* 4 (3), 295–313.

Ball, M.J., Code, C., Tree, J., Dawe, K. and Kay, J. (2004) Phonetic and phonological analysis of progressive speech degeneration: A case study. *Clinical Linguistics & Phonetics* 18 (6–8), 447–462.

Bernhardt, B.M. and Stemberger, J.P. (1998) *Handbook of Phonological Development: From a Nonlinear Constraints-based Perspective*. San Diego, CA: Academic Press.

Brown, R. (1973) *A First Language: The Early Stages*. Cambridge, MA: Harvard University Press.

Bunta, F., Fabiano-Smith, L., Goldstein, B.A. and Ingram, D. (2009) Phonological whole-word measures in three-year-old bilingual children and their age-matched monolingual peers. *Clinical Linguistics & Phonetics* 23, 156–175.

Burrows, L. and Goldstein, B.A. (2010) Whole word measures in bilingual children with speech sound disorders. *Clinical Linguistics & Phonetics* 24, 357–368.

Ingram, D. (2002) The measurement of whole-word production. *Journal of Child Language* 29, 713–733.

Ingram, D. (2015) Whole-word measures: Using the pCC-PWP intersect to distinguish speech delay from speech disorder. In C. Bowen (ed.) *Children's Speech Sound Disorders* (2nd edn) (pp. 100–104). Oxford: John Wiley.

Ingram, D. and Ingram, K. (2001) A whole-word approach to phonological analysis and intervention. *Language, Speech, and Hearing Services in Schools* 32, 271–283.

Ingram, D., Williams, L. and Scherer, N.J. (2018, January) Are speech sound disorders phonological or articulatory? A spectrum approach. In E. Babatsouli and D. Ingram (eds) *Phonology in Protolanguage and Interlanguage* (pp. 27–48). Sheffield: Equinox.

Kehoe, M. (2015) When place does not fall into place: A case study of a child with diverse linguistic input. In M. Yavaş (ed.) *Unusual Productions in Phonology: Universals and Language Specific Considerations* (pp. 159–182). New York: Psychology Press.

MacLeod, A.A., Laukys, K. and Rvachew, S. (2011) The impact of bilingual language learning on whole-word complexity and segmental accuracy among children aged 18 and 36 months. *International Journal of Speech and Language Pathology* 13, 490–499.

MacWhinney, B. (2000) *The CHILDES Project: Tools for Analyzing Talk* (3rd edn). Mahwah, NJ: Lawrence Erlbaum.

Nespor, M., Peña, M. and Mehler, J. (2003) On the different roles of vowels and consonants in speech processing and language acquisition. *Lingue e Linguaggio* 2, 203–229.

Nice, M.M. (1925) Length of sentences as a criterion of a child's progress in speech. *Journal of Educational Psychology* 16, 370–379.

Ohala, D. (1999) The influence of sonority on children's cluster reductions. *Journal of Communication Disorders* 32, 397–421.

Parker, M.D. and Brorson, K. (2005) A comparative study between mean length of utterance in morphemes (MLUm) and mean length of utterance in words (MLUw). *First Language* 25, 365–376.

Shriberg, L., Austin, D., Lewis, B., McSweeney, J. and Wilson, D. (1997) The percentage of consonants correct (PCC) metric: Extensions and reliability data. *Journal of Speech, Language, and Hearing Research* 3, 708–722.

Smit, A.B. (1993) Phonologic error distributions in the Iowa-Nebraska articulation norms project: Consonant singletons. *Journal of Speech and Hearing Research* 36, 533–547.

Taelman, H., Durieux, G. and Gillis, S. (2005) Notes on Ingram's whole-word measures for phonological development. *Journal of Child Language* 32, 391–400.

4 Investigating Typical and Protracted Phonological Development across Languages

Barbara May Bernhardt and
Joseph Paul Stemberger

Introduction

Over the past century, researchers have examined data from diverse languages in order to discover and potentially explain similarities and differences in language systems. One primary goal has been to discover characteristics that occur across languages ('universals') versus those that pertain specifically to a given language (e.g. Bybee, 2006; Chomsky & Halle, 1968). The major area of focus has been adult language, but with some attention to children's language development, both typical and protracted. Because children's early language has reduced complexity compared with the adult language, acquisition researchers suggest that developmental data may highlight basic universal limitations (constraints) on language, with protracted development further affording opportunities to observe a greater variety of constraints operating over an extended period (Ingram, 1989; Jakobson, 1968). Some researchers suggest that such constraints are innate (e.g. Chomsky & Halle, 1968; Jakobson, 1968), but others argue that the constraints derive from limitations in cognition, brain and body (e.g. Bates & MacWhinney, 1982; Bernhardt & Stemberger, 1998; Hayes, 1999; Pierrehumbert, 2001). Regardless of the source of constraints, crosslinguistic developmental data may reveal both frequent patterns across languages and language-unique patterns, the former suggestive of universal tendencies (Locke, 1983) and the latter of language-specific influences (e.g. Ingram, 2012; Pye *et al.*, 1987). Pye *et al.* (1987) observed that acquisition of a relatively complex phonological element, the affricate /t͡ʃ/, was generally earlier in Quiché Mayan than in English. In Quiché Mayan, the affricate is very frequent (one of the five most frequent consonants in the language) and has a high functional load in the language, whereas in English it is infrequent (one of the five least frequent phonemes). Thus, universal tendencies can be tempered by frequency and functionality.

Such data emphasize the crucial importance of crosslinguistic studies for addressing issues of universality in language, yet very few studies have been conducted using equivalent methodology across languages. The crosslinguistic study discussed in this chapter describes phonological acquisition in monolingual children with typical development (TD) or protracted phonological development (PPD), with a similar methodology for each language. Congruent with the discussion above, the overarching objective of the large study is to inform theories on the broad questions of universality versus diversity in phonological development.

The theoretical orientation for this crosslinguistic study is constraint-based nonlinear phonology (Bernhardt & Stemberger, 1998), which describes phonological elements and their interactions and patterns from the level of the phonological phrase to the features that make up a segment. Figure 4.1 shows the prosodic section of the hierarchy. The phonological phrase contains prosodic words with different levels of prominence (stress) within the phrase. The prosodic word is composed of feet – groupings of syllables with different levels of prominence. Syllables have several major components (Hooper, 1976; Prince & Smolensky, 2004): (a) the onset, which includes consonants or glides preceding (b) the nucleus (stress-bearing unit), (c) the coda, and (d) the rime (a grouping of the nucleus and coda). Across languages, a syllable nucleus (and therefore, rime) is obligatory, whereas the onset is often obligatory and the coda optional. The rime timing units (elements) that attract stress to the syllable are considered 'weight-bearing' or 'moraic'. In some languages, the coda consonant is moraic if the vowel is lax or short, e.g. in English, which prefers minimally bimoraic syllables.

Figure 4.2 displays feature system (geometry) below the level of the prosodic hierarchy (Figure 4.1). The features and relationships are presented according to Bernhardt and Stemberger (1998), an extension of Sagey (1986) and McCarthy (1988). The bolded elements refer to the /b/ of the example in Figure 4.1. Each segment is composed of features reflecting manner of articulation (organized around the Root node), laryngeal status and place of articulation. The Root node defines the group of features for a particular segment, and represents the link between the segment and the higher level prosodic structure. Proposed systems differ in the features included in the hierarchy and their definition, in the assignment of binary values and in the structure of the geometry, just as there are discussions about the structure of the prosodic hierarchy. For the crosslinguistic study, we are adopting the basic framework as shown in Figures 4.1 and 4.2, but other frameworks could also be used to account for the phenomena observed.

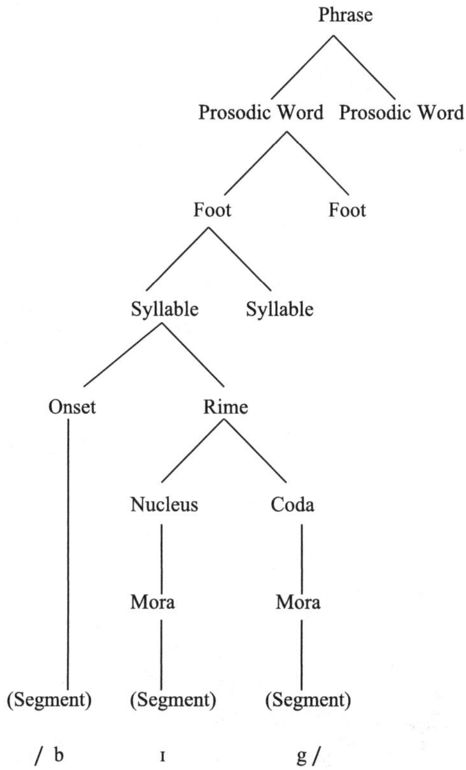

Figure 4.1 Phonological hierarchy from the phrase to the segment

For 'adult' phonology, researchers have investigated both the prosodic structures and segment/feature systems of languages (e.g. de Lacy, 2007). However, a comprehensive crosslinguistic comparison of word structure, segments and their interactions remains to be done for developing phonological systems, specifically taking into account the relative levels of complexity within each language. Within-language analyses in the project have revealed interactions between the stress and structure of the syllable and the accuracy of the segments, unstressed initial syllables showing many more and different mismatch (error) patterns than stressed syllables (Chávez-Peón *et al.*, 2012; Schretlen, 2013, both for Spanish). However, to address the main question of the proposed study concerning universality, many additional within- and between-language comparisons need to be done that can take into account language type and relative complexities.

A number of methodological variables need to be considered, however, before deriving conclusions about universal or non-universal patterns in development. The optimal study would have identical or at least near-identical methodology across languages: (a) matched groups of children in

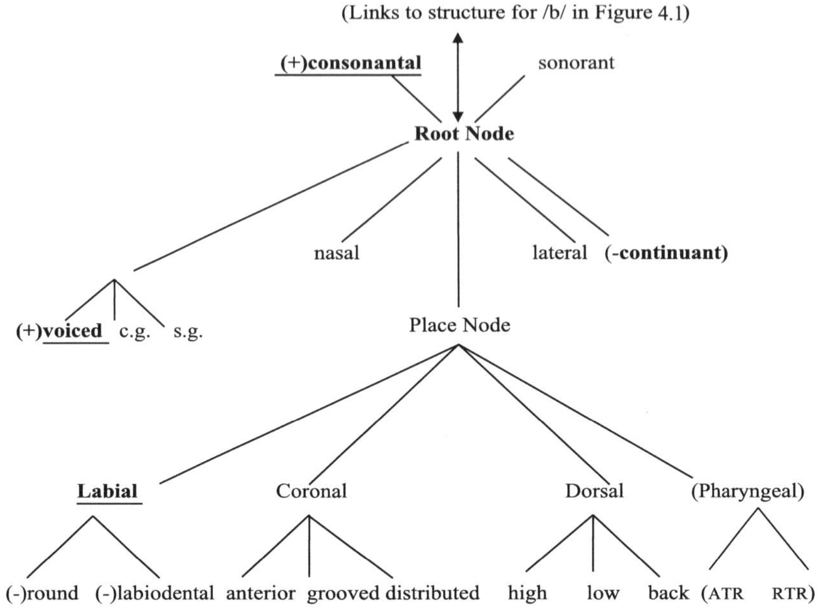

Figure 4.2 Feature hierarchy from the segment to the terminal features

terms of participant number, ages, gender, socio-economic status, birth order, general language skills, hearing status and other developmental factors; (b) sufficient participants in each group to have statistical power; (c) similar elicitation, recording, transcription and analysis procedures; and (d) equivalent levels of training and knowledge in the research teams to be able to collect and analyze the data in a similar fashion. Because the crosslinguistic study includes participants with PPD, the crosslinguistic and cross-cultural definitions of PPD are also relevant. In a language with simpler phonology (e.g. no clusters, few long words, minimal use of codas), the overall accuracy might be higher in both TD and PPD groups. Given a child with a particular level of phonological development, the child might be included in the TD group in a language with a simpler phonological system, but in the PPD group in a language with a more complex phonological system. Accounting for imbalances caused by differences in the adult system is a particular challenge for crosslinguistic comparison. However, such between-language differences can be partially mitigated through consideration of a number of methodological variables.

This chapter first describes the general methodology for the crosslinguistic project, describing solutions to challenges in diversity of sampling and transcription. The subsequent section addresses the need to account for potential variability in within-language data, focusing on dialectal influence (Mandarin; Granada Spanish) on children's pronunciations, and the interaction of word structure and features in interpreting variable developmental patterns (French). The third section outlines whole-word comparisons across several languages, with a further discussion about TD and PPD samples. Specific comparisons follow that illustrate some of the methodological considerations in crosslinguistic comparison and provide insights into universal versus language-specific phenomena: i.e. for Mandarin and Spanish diphthongs, and for German, English and Icelandic word-initial fricatives. A final section returns to the overarching objective about universality and explores implications of the current study for future research. Links are provided to project resources for clinical and research purposes. (In addition to the theoretical objective, the study has clinical objectives: to develop materials for phonological elicitation and analysis and intervention, and to provide training opportunities for academics and speech-language pathologists across a number of countries and regions.)

Methodology

The following section describes the general methodology for the crosslinguistic study in terms of data collection and analysis. Subsequent sections outline two of the common ways in which that methodology diverges across languages: sampling differences and transcription conventions. Finally, the project's solutions to those differences are presented and discussed.

General methods

The objective across languages is to collect data from 20–30 monolingual children aged three to six years, designated locally as having PPD, plus, where funding permits, from age- and dialect-matched TD peers. Exclusion criteria for both TD and PPD samples include sensorineural hearing loss, severe chronic otitis media, major language comprehension or cognitive delays, and major orofacial anomalies. Limited sentence production is not an exclusionary criterion. A native speaker tests the children in a quiet room, usually in a pre-school centre, in a 45–60 minute session. The data are digitally recorded with a high-quality audio-recording device (most often with a M-Audio Microtrack II digital recorder and a Sennheiser remote system, i.e. transmitter EK 100 G2 and receiver SK 100 G2, with Countryman remote lapel microphones). Where feasible, video-recordings are also made. For each language, a word list of approximately 100 words is developed for picture-/photo-naming. Project leaders and local investigators choose words familiar to children that cover all segments of the language (both consonants and vowels, at least twice in all word positions) and the major word structures (stress patterns,

CV sequences, word lengths). Ten words are elicited twice or three times each using either pictures or objects as a warm-up activity and to examine within-word variability later. Additional testing includes a hearing screening and a language comprehension test (when one exists), a short spontaneous language sample, and a parental questionnaire about the child's development and language use. A transcription-conventions document is developed in conjunction with the local team and project leaders. A native speaker of the dialect area then transcribes the sample, with reliability of transcription confirmed with a second native speaker or project leader experienced with transcription. (Further discussion of transcription follows below.) Data are then entered into Phon, a free phonological program for entry and analysis of phonological development data (https://www.phon.ca/), either locally or in the first author's laboratory at the University of British Columbia. Data are double-checked for accuracy of adult targets and alignment. Export of the data into spreadsheets allows further data analysis including statistical comparisons where feasible.

As can be seen above, the objective is to provide a common methodology across languages with similar (1) sample characteristics, (2) word list types, (3) data collection procedures, (4) transcription conventions and (5) data entry and analysis procedures. While the objective is generally achieved for items (2), (3) and (5), items (1) and (4) are more challenging. They are addressed in more detail below.

Sampling characteristics

Research is constrained by the availability of participants and the time and financial resources available. Many, but not all, language teams are able to find the target number of participants in the designated age range, including matched control groups of TD children. There are small variations in the size of the age groups, reflecting recruitment challenges. Developmental levels are generally the same because of the criteria for inclusion, with the possible exception of the degree of PPD. We return to the discussion of the PPD designation in our crosslinguistic comparison below.

Transcription conventions

As is well documented, achieving transcription agreement is difficult even for transcribers who speak the same language and have the same amount and type of training. This is particularly true for child speech or more 'disordered' speech, and if the transcribers use narrower transcription (Shriberg & Lof, 1991). Consensus-building activities and practice can enhance reliability, as can acoustic analysis, e.g. examining VOT, frication, formants, nasality or duration (Bernhardt & Stemberger, 2012). For the project, the teams from both the host region (British Columbia, Canada) and the other regions or countries work together from the outset to develop a set of transcription conventions that can be relatively equivalent across languages but respect the traditions within the various regions/countries. The following discussion outlines differences among transcribers and the project solutions for broad transcription.

(1) *Word-initial (WI) glottal stops.* Transcribers differ on whether they want to include or exclude a WI glottal stop, when the glottal stop is not phonemic in the adult language, and so is predictable (for adults). For the project, the convention of the local transcription team is followed. For analysis, transcribed WI glottal stops are counted as deletions if there is a different target consonant, but identified as glottal stops in detailed mismatch analyses. Because the data for the project come primarily from single-word elicitation, words starting with vowels are post-pausal and can have an initiating glottal stop (in adult speech). Thus, even when the child is not using many or any WI consonants, it is difficult to know whether the glottal stop is replacing the consonant or is an artefact of the single-word production (where the child has acquired the adult pattern that words cannot start with a vowel post-pausally).
(2) *Word-final (WF) glottal stops.* Transcribers also differ as to whether they want to include or exclude an unpredictable WF glottal stop, whether or not the target has a WF consonant. For the project, the convention of the local transcription team is followed. For analysis, transcribed WF glottal stops are counted as deletions if a target consonant is missing, but identified as glottal stops for future considerations and in detailed mismatch analyses. If a child uses very audible WF glottal stops in connected speech for target consonant codas (and perhaps also uses them word medially), there is a higher probability that the glottal stop is a type of place-holder for the timing unit of the target consonant.
(3) *Standard local transcription preferences.* Research teams in the various countries tend to have their own interpretation of at least some aspects of the International Phonetic Alphabet (IPA, 2015). The project accepts the local conventions, but acknowledges any differences in crosslinguistic comparisons. The three examples we relate here come from Spanish, Icelandic and Swedish. In Spanish, what is transcribed as palatoalveolar [t͡ʃ] (implying retracted, post-alveolar tongue tip) is actually alveopalatal [t͡ɕ] (with advanced tongue tip and maintaining grooving; Kochetov & Colantoni, 2011), but it is nevertheless transcribed as [t͡ʃ]. In contrast, for languages where /t͡ʃ/ has a more posterior place of articulation, the alveopalatal may be transcribed as alveopalatal and considered a mismatch (often with an ungrooved tongue shape). Another example concerns Icelandic: what is transcribed as the palatal stop [c] is in fact a fronted velar [k̟] (Árnason, 2011), but it is traditionally transcribed as [c]. For Swedish, consonant length in adult speech is predictable from vowel length (short after a stressed long vowel, and long after a stressed short vowel; Schaeffler & Wretling, 2003), and native speakers prefer to transcribe only the vowel length.

Regarding narrow transcription, there can be greater disagreement (Shriberg & Lof, 1991). In the project, differences have been resolved as described below.

(1) *Allophonic variation*. Examples here concern Granada Spanish and Icelandic. For Spanish, voiced stops show lenition in adult speech intervocalically (e.g. /b/ as [β]); the fricative/approximant is not *phonemically* different from a stop that the child might use instead, and native speaker transcribers do not always distinguish between the stops and fricative/approximants in the transcriptions. For all the data, a non-native transcriber verifies stop versus continuant allophones spectrographically, and adjusts the adult target to match the child production. No mismatch is indicated for the child in *agreement* with the initial transcription (i.e. the adult target is adjusted to match the child production). If development and use of the voiced 'stops' is the objective of analysis, the adult targets can be re-adjusted to match what they would typically be in that context. For both Granada Spanish and Icelandic, voiced 'fricatives' are generally more approximant-like than fricative-like (Árnason, 2011; Martínez Celdrán & Fernández Planas, 2007). They are transcribed using fricative symbols, in accordance with local transcription conventions, but interpretation of the results takes into account their approximant characteristics. Another allophonic pattern relates to the Granada Spanish dialect. When coda /s/ lenites in adult Granada Spanish, a short [h]-like element (highly variable in duration, if present at all) can replace it (Martínez Celdrán & Fernández Planas, 2007), and the vowel laxes. In the project, a second transcriber verifies presence of aspiration on the spectrogram, and includes the [h] in both the adult and child forms, but the native speaker transcribers consider only the laxness of the vowel (and not the presence of an optional [h]-like element) to be clinically relevant and so do not generally transcribe the [h].

(2) *Transitional versus actual epenthesis*. Word initially, consonant sequences can be challenging to articulate. Sometimes children epenthesize a small vocalic element either after a coda consonant or between consonants in a cluster. Adult native speakers may also produce non-phonemic vowel-like elements in certain clusters; these are generally regarded as transitional elements and so tend not be transcribed. For the study, audible epenthetic 'vowels' shorter than 40 msec are written as superscripts (e.g. [ˈgᵊris]), while vowels of 60 msec or longer are perceived as full vowels and written on the main line (e.g. [gəˈris]). This convention implies that there are two sources to these vowel-like elements (a 'loose juncture' where a very short gap appears between two consonants but is not actually a vowel; and a true vowel with its own articulatory targets, inserted to allow a child to produce both consonants in a cluster). Two predictions can be made: (a) there is a bimodal distribution of duration, with

little or no overlap; and (b) the elements transcribed as vowels should be within the duration range of target unstressed vowels in the child's speech. These predictions are being verified in an ongoing study of clusters.

(3) *Children's vocal tracts.* A child's vocal tract anatomy generally includes a high flattish tongue body in a proportionally small oral cavity (by adult standards). Thus, sibilants such as /s/ are often de-grooved or flattened, and the tongue body is high enough to cause frication along a longer front-back axis than in adult speech. For the study, an attempt was made to distinguish such productions from [s]/[z] by transcribing them as [sᶿ]/[zᶞ] (if dentalized with a flattish (but not fully flat) tongue and a low-enough tongue body), or alveolopalatal [ɕ]/[ʑ] (if ungrooved with a too-high tongue body).

Although full agreement is unlikely across languages, the reliability of transcription has been enhanced by these methods. For Granada Spanish, after consensus building, agreement for segments was high: 96% for TD samples and 93.6% for PPD samples. What has become clear during the consensus-building process is that transcribers often hear and agree on most aspects of the child's pronunciation, when those characteristics are brought to their attention. One difference across languages is that different things are considered irrelevant for transcription, because of differing local conventions or assumptions about importance for adult or clinical populations. The team learns together how to agree on what matters, which symbols to use, and how to interpret the symbols.

As a final note on methodology, the development of transcription conventions includes identification of multiple acceptable adult targets in the dialect area, so that children are not penalized for 'non-standard' pronunciations learned from adult input. Finding out what the adult target might be has proven to be relatively challenging for all of the languages. Even well-trained native speakers can be unaware of how their idiolect reflects or does not reflect the local dialect versus the 'standard'. For the study, speech samples have been collected from at least one adult from the dialect area, but with too few speakers to adequately reflect adult variation. In addition, the teams have consulted literature on the dialect. Through meetings with the local teams, time is spent in determining the range of possibilities for the adult targets.

As an example, Granada Spanish, an Andalusian dialect of Spanish, has a number of specific characteristics, some of which include: (1) use of [s] for 'z' and 'c' before front nonlow vowels (*seseo*) or [θ] (*ceceo*, most common in Northern Peninsular Spanish, i.e. Madrid); (2) presence, deletion or reduction of coda consonants as noted above, i.e. coda [s] may be deleted, or replaced by [h]/[ʰ], with a general laxing of the vowel, e.g. *dos* [dos] ~ [dɔh] ~ [dɔʰ] ~ [dɔ] 'two'; (3) interchange of coda [l] and [r] or, in the case of the medial consonant, deletion of the liquid, with gemination of the following consonant: e.g.

alma 'soul' [alma/aɾma/amːa] or *sarten* 'frying pan' [saɾˈten/salˈtẽ̞/sat͜ˈtẽ̞] (note also /n/ deletion with vowel nasalization). For the Granada Spanish study, data were collected from three adults, who varied from one another on these characteristics and in terms of seseo/ceceo, sometimes within speaker. When setting up the adult targets for the child, then, the range of variation in the adult pronunciations needs to be taken into account. The child's particular pronunciation will be based on one particular adult variant, and all acceptable adult variants must be noted in the adult target set.

Within-language Analysis

When interpreting within-language results, one of the challenges is finding ways to ensure that observed patterns, particularly 'inconsistent' patterns, are attributable to a given participant's developmental performance rather than transcription or dialectal factors. In this section we discuss two results from within-language analysis in our study, one that follows from the discussion in the last section about adult targets (dialect variation) and one that reflects word-position effects on apparently variable phonemes. In the dialect case, the interpretation of data remains inconclusive, whereas in the second case, the word-position analyses bring clarity to the interpretation.

Dialect and Data Interpretation

We saw above that in a relatively small city such as Granada there can be considerable variation, even in adult speech. Such variation increases notably when the language in question is spread over a huge geographic area and is a second related language or dialect for speakers in the area of study. This is the case for Mandarin (also known as Putonghua), the most widespread language in China. The majority of children in China start learning Mandarin at pre-school around age three, if they are not already speaking it natively. The consonant inventory of standard Beijing Mandarin is presented in Table 4.1.

As Table 4.1 shows, coronal fricatives and affricates are a major component of the standard inventory; there are contrasts in tongue-tip placement and height of the tongue body: dentals (with advanced tongue tip and low tongue body); alveopalatals (with advanced tongue tip and high tongue body); and retroflexes (with retracted tongue tip). The laryngeal contrast is between voiceless unaspirated and voiceless aspirated stops and affricates.

In the first Mandarin analysis for the study, it was assumed that children were learning standard Mandarin. A consonant accuracy analysis was done for 30 TD four-year-olds living in Shanghai. On examining the children's pronunciations, a number of differences from the standard targets appeared

Table 4.1 Standard Beijing Mandarin consonant inventory

	Labial	*Dental*	*Retroflex*	*Alveopalatal*	*Palatal*	*Dorsal*
Stops	p pʰ	t tʰ				k kʰ
Affricates		ts tsʰ	tʂ tʂʰ	tɕ tɕʰ		
Fricatives	f	s	ʂ	ɕ		x
Nasals	m	n				(ŋ)
Approximants	w	l	ɻ		j	

(see Table 4.2), especially concerning the retroflexed consonants and rhotics, where some children did not produce retroflexes where they were targets, and others produced retroflexes where they were not targets. Because retroflexes and rhotics are often later developing across languages (e.g. English, Smit *et al.*, 1990), it was tempting to label these productions mismatches. However, Shanghainese, typically the children's home language/dialect, does not have retroflex sibilants; thus, Shanghainese-influenced *Mandarin* may also lack retroflexes, accounting for cases where children did not use retroflexes. For those children who used retroflexes where they did not appear in the standard, a recent study of Shanghainese Mandarin suggests some interesting sociodialectal changes which might be influencing that pattern. Starr and Juraksy (2004) observed that some young adult women (potentially mothers of the children in this study) were showing a hyper-correction phenomenon, using retroflexes where they were not present in adult Mandarin. Children may be exposed to such adult pronunciations, another factor that needs to be considered when accounting for the data. A further wrinkle in this analysis is that Duanmu (2000) suggests that the retroflex 'liquid /r/' is actually a fricative /ʐ/, making it part of the coronal fricative group instead of an approximant/liquid. Duanmu notes further that the alveopalatals may be pronounced as palatalized alveolars (e.g. [t͡sʲ]). Thus, when interpreting Table 4.2, the mismatches seen for the sibilants and the rhotics may actually be acceptable variants in adult speech.

Table 4.2 Numbers of typically developing Mandarin-speaking four-year-olds showing one or more mismatches by category ($n = 30$)

Vowels	*Tones*	*[–] > [+] retroflex*	*[+] >[–] retroflex*	*ɻ ɚ > various*	*t͡ɕ <> ɕ t͡ɕ, ɕ <> s*	*Dorsal <> coronal*	*Other*
4	13	13	20	19	8	3	11

Notes: Dorsal = velar. <> means that the consonants on either side of the arrows can replace each other.

Further to dialect, Table 4.2 shows that some TD children had tone and vowel mismatches, even at age four. Acoustic analysis of the tone trajectories for the children's Shanghainese Mandarin shows a smaller pitch range for the tones in comparison with the Beijing standard (Lai *et al.*, 2011). However, adult Shanghainese also has less extreme pitch changes in tones than Mandarin. Additionally, the Shanghainese adult vowel space is smaller than that of adult Beijing Mandarin; the children's vowel space is smaller yet. The children's Mandarin vowel system may also be Shanghainese influenced. Much more information is needed on the variants of Mandarin in the various regions of China, both from adults and children. For any language, it is vitally important to have sufficient information from adults of the dialect area, especially of the ages, genders and occupations that tend to have close contact with pre-school children.

Word Structure–Segment Interactions and Data Interpretation

Another source of variability for a specific phoneme in child productions is the position of the phoneme within a particular word. Previous reports suggest that segments may be less accurate in weak prosodic positions (Bernhardt & Stemberger, 1998; Rose, 2002). Weak prosodic positions include unstressed syllables, codas and cluster elements. Inconsistent production of a phoneme, then, is sometimes because of variable accuracy across word positions or stress contexts. In data collected for eight children with PPD speaking Canadian (Manitoba) French, there were significant effects of stress on a number of segment types (Figures 4.3 and 4.4; see also Bérubé *et al.*, 2012).

In multisyllabic words, for example, obstruents and /l/ were significantly more accurate in stressed than unstressed syllables (Figure 4.3) according to a Wilcoxon Rank Sum Test: for stops and fricatives: $z = 2.52$, $n = 8$, $df = 1$, $p = 0.01$, $r = 0.63$; for /l/, $z = 2.38$, $p = 0.01$. Rhotic clusters also showed an effect of syllable prominence ($z = 2.53$, $df = 1$, $n = 8$, $p = 0.01$, $r = 0.63$, Figure 4.4), unlike glide clusters ($z = 0.68$, $df = 1$, $n = 8$, $p = 0.50$, $r = 0.17$). Similarly, children matched a greater proportion of nasal vowels in stressed syllables ($Md = 0.96$) than in unstressed syllables ($Md = 0.56$), $z = 2.52$, $p = 0.01$, $r = 0.63$. The data underscore the relevance of nonlinear phonology in that higher level prosodic structure can affect the realization of lower level segments.

Within-language results are the first step in a crosslinguistic comparison. In this section we have shown two important considerations in data interpretation: (1) the importance of determining the adult targets; and (2) the necessity of evaluating the data to determine potential reasons for inconsistencies. 'Random' inconsistency can occur in both adult and child speech, but the analyst needs to rule out principled accounts for variability across diverse tokens before suggesting that a particular phoneme, word structure

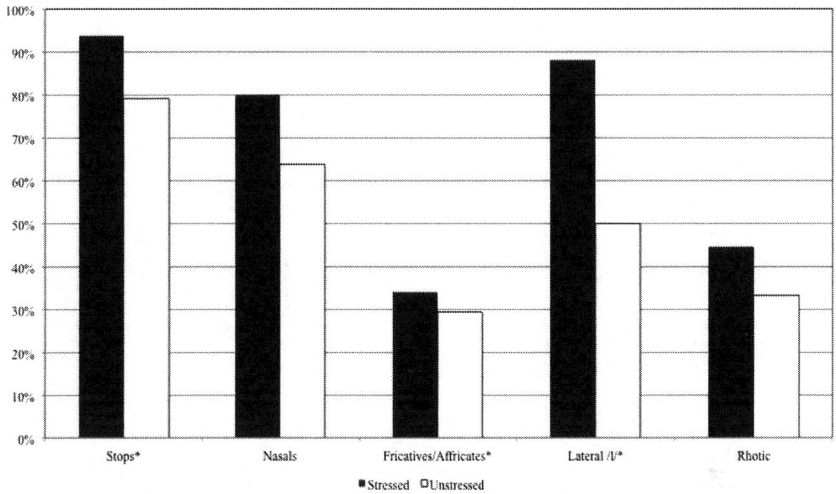

Figure 4.3 Sound class match (accuracy) data in stressed and unstressed syllables in multisyllabic words for eight Canadian French-speaking children with protracted phonological development

or lexical item is simply unstable at a certain point in development, no matter what the context. In addition to the prosodic effects noted above, inconsistency may also arise because of constraints on segmental sequences. A consonant or vowel may match the adult target in certain sequences, but not in others, e.g. *down* (with two coronal consonants) matching the adult target, but *dog*, with a coronal and dorsal (velar) showing assimilation ([gag]). The coronal is possible when there are two of them in the word, but vulnerable

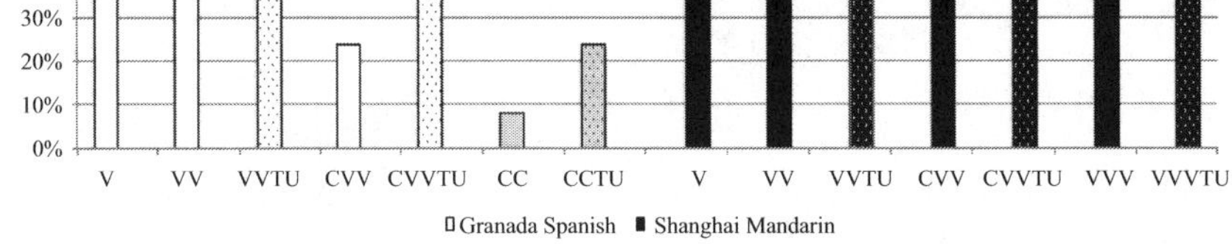

Figure 4.4 Match data for diphthongs, triphthongs (Mandarin) and word-initial clusters (Spanish) in two groups of eight children matched for age and level of protracted phonological development

when in sequence with a dorsal. By investigating the sources of variability in various individual samples, and comparing them first within a language group, and then across groups, we may reach a better understanding of universal constraints on the interaction of segments and word structures or sequences, something that has been insufficiently studied crosslinguistically. (See the chapters in Yavaş, 2014, for some attention to these topics.)

Between-language Results: Unity in Diversity

Moving from within-language analysis to between-language analysis brings a new set of challenges. Assuming that methodological and analysis procedures are consistent across languages, the first thing to consider is whether (a) the languages are similar enough to be compared (for the particular characteristics being focused on), and (b) the participant and elicitation samples are sufficiently matched between languages. Because the current project includes children labelled as having PPD, we also need to consider how the designation of PPD arises in the various languages and cultures.

Protracted Phonological Development across the Language Groups

Relative to designation of PPD, preliminary data analysis showed some inequivalences across languages. A whole word match (WWM) was calculated for the various samples (Table 4.3), showing ranges from less than 12% average WWM across the cohort with PPD (English, Icelandic) to about 40% (Mandarin and Granada Spanish), for word lists of about equivalent numbers. The mean age for all groups with PPD was in the four-year-old range, with some closer to 4;0 (English, Icelandic) and the remainder closer to 4;6 (and overall, the older children had higher scores as would be expected).[1]

The source of the differences in WWM across languages is unclear. Do languages with less complex phonology have higher WWM scores simply because they are phonologically 'easier' to learn? Were the word elicitation samples sufficiently similar in complexity, notwithstanding differences among languages in complexity? Or were there just simply differences among the specific children in the small samples in terms of degree of PPD? In terms of the languages, Icelandic and English have a more complex word structure than Mandarin and Spanish, even for words familiar to children (e.g. more cluster types, more different codas), suggesting that children with a tendency for PPD might have lower scores for those two languages, all else being equal (see the Appendix for the lists of words used at the time of data collection for Mandarin, Granada Spanish, Icelandic and Slovene). However, Slovene also has complex phonology with long words and clusters, and the WWM was more akin to that of

Table 4.3 Whole word match across languages, ages and participant groups

TD[a]	*PPD*	*Age group in years*	*Whole word match*
Mandarin		4	80%
Arabic			80%
Slovene			80%
Spanish			85.4%
	Mandarin	3–5 (Mean 4;2)	41.5%
	Granada Spanish	3–5 (Mean 4;6)	39.1%
	Slovene[b]	3–6 (Mean 4;7)	34.1%
	French	3;1–4;6[c]	25.6%
	German	3–5 (Mean 4;5)	18.9%
	English	3–5 (Mean 4;0)	12.7%
	Icelandic	3–5 (Mean 4;1)	11.6%

Notes: Whole word match means the child pronunciation matches the adult exactly, with the exception of slight deviations in place or voicing. See the Appendix for comparison of word list complexity in Mandarin, Spanish, Icelandic and Slovene. TD = typically developing; PPD = with protracted phonological development.

[a]Schmitt *et al.* (1983) showed a similar WWM score for English TD four-year-olds in a connected speech task.

[b]Only 4/54 children aged three years, which possibly inflates the WWM score.

[c]8 participants, compared with 29–30 for the other PPD groups; thus, mean is not reported.

Mandarin and Spanish. In part, this reflected the fact that the Slovene children were in the 4;6 range (mean age), but in addition, the data were collected in a typical pre-school setting. Thus, at least some of the children who were lagging behind their peers may in fact have been at the low end of typical. That is, the recruitment method for the participants in Slovenia did not specifically request children with PPD; rather, everyone who wanted to be tested was tested, and it is unlikely that in a sample of 54 children, there would have been more than 10 with notable PPD. That language is not always relevant shows up in the WWM scores for TD four-year-olds in the study: the scores were 80–85% not just for Mandarin and Spanish, with their simpler phonology, but also for Kuwaiti Arabic, which has a large consonant inventory (albeit few WI or WF clusters). Thus, complexity of language may be not as strong a factor as individual participant selection relative to degree of PPD. For the researcher, the question is how to resolve discrepancies among samples relative to PPD designation. The discrepancy is not particularly important for within-language analyses, except when comparing experimental and control groups. For example, the WWM scores did provide a cross-check on the PPD classification when there were matched groups of controls. In fact, in the Granada Spanish cohort, one child originally designated as PPD had a WWM similar to the age-matched controls, and thus was re-assigned to that cohort. Overall, however, the original classification as TD versus PPD has been consistent with the WWM scores.

Crosslinguistic comparisons are difficult to do if there are large discrepancies between groups; samples need to be evaluated for similarity. If global phonological variables match, then validity of more specific between-language comparison is enhanced. If the samples differ significantly in age or WWM, smaller sub-groups can be created, matching for age, gender (where possible) and various global phonological measures, e.g. WWM or percent consonants correct (PCC) scores. Participant matching reduces the sample sizes and therewith the potential for statistical power, but it does provide reassurance that interpretation is based on phonological differences rather than sampling differences. In general, the definition of PPD within and across languages remains an open question.

Between-language Comparisons for Specific Sound Classes

Keeping the cautionary notes discussed above in mind, the following discussion provides two crosslinguistic comparisons, one for WI fricatives in the same language family (Germanic), and one for diphthongs in two unrelated languages, Mandarin and Granada Spanish. In both cases, the major objective was to determine potentially 'universal' versus language-specific patterns.

Word-initial fricatives in three Germanic languages

In the early days of the crosslinguistic study, informal perusal of data from German-speaking children (Ullrich, 2004) showed differences from accounts of English development (as reported, for example, in Bernhardt & Stemberger, 1998); the phonetic inventory of each language and the relative frequency of phonemes appeared relevant both for the timeline of phoneme acquisition and for mismatch patterns that occurred.

The German PPD data for our crosslinguistic study were gathered in Cologne over a two-year period, allowing a relatively close match to the English sample relative to gender, size of age groups and, to a certain extent, severity of PPD (English mean WWM = 12%, German mean WWM = 19%). Thus, comparisons between the whole German and English samples of children with PPD (30 children each) have been possible (as in the comparison of fricative development, Bernhardt *et al.*, 2014). In contrast, for Icelandic–English comparisons, small variations in the size of the PPD age groups and severity levels have required minor reduction of the sample size. In a fricative comparison, adjusted sample sizes resulted in groups of 13 three-year-olds and 10 four-year-olds per language (Bernhardt *et al.*, 2015). The following comparison draws together findings from the two studies mentioned here, in order to further examine commonalities and differences.

The original motivation for studying fricatives was the observation that pre-schoolers with PPD often show low match proportions for the articulatorily complex fricatives and liquids (Bernhardt & Stemberger, 1998). The three languages do not have identical fricative inventories, and thus the two original studies compared only those fricatives that the languages have in common, matched for position in the word, and only in stress-initial words (avoiding any effects of word prominence, as noted in the previous section, and taking into account that all words in Icelandic are stress-initial). For this three-way comparison, we focus only on WI fricatives, because for each language, fricatives showed an overall match level of 38% in that position across participants. Fricatives in the comparison were: for English /f, v, s, z, θ, ʃ/; for German /f, v, z, ʃ/; and for Icelandic /f, s, θ/.

Both similarities and differences were expected across languages, based on the literature and assumptions about complexity and frequency. Expected similarities in terms of match (accuracy) levels were: (1) an overall low match for fricatives; (2) highest match levels for the voiceless labiodental /f/, probably because visual information provides support for acquisition that is minimally available for coronal fricatives (Fox & Dodd, 1999, German; Másdóttir, 2008, Icelandic; Smit *et al.*, 1990, English); (3) higher match levels for voiceless compared with voiced fricatives for German and English, because of the additional complexity of adjusting intraoral and subglottal pressures for the voiced fricatives (Bernhardt & Stemberger, 1998) (the voicing comparison was not relevant for Icelandic, which has voiced approximants rather than voiced fricatives as the 'cognates' to the voiceless fricatives; see Árnason, 2011); (4) lowest match levels for grooved sibilants ([+grooved], alternately designated as [+strident], Chomsky & Halle, 1968); and (5) low match levels for the infrequent (more marked) [–grooved] target /θ/ in Icelandic and English (Másdóttir, 2008; Smit *et al.*, 1990). In terms of mismatches, frequently expected patterns were: (1) a high frequency of manner mismatches, with the less complex obstruents, stops, appearing most commonly as substitutions (Bernhardt & Stemberger, 1998); and (2) ungrooved segments substituting for the [+grooved] coronal sibilants (Fox & Dodd, 1999; Smit *et al.*, 1990). Differences among the languages were predicted to reflect differences in phonetic frequency and inventory. Relative to frequency, some expectations were: (a) higher match levels for German voiced fricatives and /ʃ/ compared with English, where they are less frequent; and (b) higher proportions of substitutions with the [+spread glottis] feature for Icelandic than for German and English, because of Icelandic's higher frequency of [+spread glottis] segments ([h], pre-aspirated stops, post-aspirated stops, voiceless fricatives, voiceless sonorants). Relative to inventory, additional expectations were a higher frequency of: (a) palatal substitutions in German and Icelandic compared with English, because they have /ç/ in their adult inventories, while English does not; (b) [θ] substitutions in English and

Table 4.4 Match levels for word-initial fricatives in German, English and Icelandic preschoolers with protracted phonological development

Percent Match Range	*50–65%*	*35–49%*	*20–34%*	*11–19%*	*6–10%*
German	f v		z ʃ		
English		f z	v	θ	ʃ s
Icelandic		f s	θ		

Icelandic, because German lacks /θ/; and (c) affricate substitutions in German and English, because Icelandic lacks affricates.

Table 4.4 displays the relative match levels for the various fricatives across languages. The results supported some but not all of the predictions about relative match levels. The highest match was shown for /f/ across languages, but the sibilants varied more than expected. As predicted, the more frequent German /ʃ/ was more advanced than its English counterpart. Contrary to expectation, English /z/ had a higher match level than the more frequent German /z/, and Icelandic /s/ had a match level equivalent to that of /f/. The interdental was less advanced than /s/ in Icelandic (as predicted) but this was not true for the English sample. Voiceless fricatives fared better than voiced fricatives in German as expected, but not in English. Thus, simplicity and transparency (visibility) were relevant for /f/. Frequency appeared to enhance earlier acquisition of /v/ and /ʃ/ in German, but not /z/.

In terms of mismatch patterns, manner substitutions were relatively common, as predicted, but place substitutions were also common in German (which showed more other-fricative substitutions than in English). Other confirmed similarities were the use of ungrooved coronal fricatives for grooved ones, with the German children showing a relatively high proportion of lateralized fricatives (one solution to the 'grooving' challenge for tongue control, but appearing less often in the English and Icelandic samples). Expected inventory effects were noted: (1) palatal fricatives appeared more frequently in Icelandic and German than in English and both have higher proportions of palatals; (2) affricates substitutions were more frequent in English and German than Icelandic, reflecting the higher proportion of affricates in German and English; (3) as predicted, there was a higher proportion of [+spread glottis] substitutions in Icelandic, primarily [h], but also the more marked preaspirated stops and voiceless sonorants, substitutions which did not appear at all in German and English. Unexpectedly, [θ] often appeared as a substitution for /f/ in Icelandic, which is quite rare in English, but [f] appeared as a common substitution for /θ/ in Icelandic just as in English (where it has often been reported; e.g. Bernhardt & Stemberger, 1998). For the three languages, substitutions came primarily from other consonants in the adult inventory in Icelandic (80%) and English (71%) although less so in German (58%), due to the high frequency of lateralized fricatives, which are not in the inventory but are a pattern sometimes seen in children with PPD as a solution to the [+grooved] challenge (Bernhardt & Stemberger, 1998, Chapter 8; Smit *et al.*, 1990).

In summary, the results provide further insight into the question of universal versus within-language patterns. As previous research has shown, fricatives showed low match levels, reflecting their complexity and markedness (Bernhardt & Stemberger, 1998). The earlier acquisition of /f/ in comparison with the lingual fricatives diverges from crosslinguistic frequency of fricative types; /s/ is in fact a more frequent fricative across languages and is often considered the unmarked fricative (Maddieson, 1984). However, articulatory complexity also affects acquisition; in the case of /f/, its visibility and simpler articulation than lingual fricatives probably results in its earlier mastery. If the most frequent, unmarked, fricative for adult languages (/s/) is not the earliest acquired fricative of child language, child and adult universals diverge, even if children show some 'universal' tendencies across languages. The principle of universality applies, but for different targets. Further to the question about universal versus language-specific phenomena, a number of language-specific influences were observed, not just for segments, but also for features (supporting the notion that segments are not indivisible units, but are made up of components such as features). In German, /v/ was earlier acquired than in English; the high frequency of the *feature* [+labiodental] possibly promoted earlier acquisition of both segments with that feature, compared with English where /v/ is infrequent, reducing the overall frequency of [+labiodental] and the mastery level for both /v/ and /f/. The higher frequency of [+spread glottis] segments in Icelandic probably influenced the higher proportion of mismatches with that feature. Finally, if a language has particular segments in its inventory, a child appears to be more likely to use those in substitution patterns; solutions to negative constraints can usually be found within the language, because of overlaps between segments in their featural composition. Even if one feature is impossible to produce, other features of the target segment may be achievable. In replacing an impossible target with another one that matches some features, the child shows partial mastery of the combination needed for the full expression of the target. This can of course differ between children speaking one language, because there are options at every point, but it is more likely to differ across languages because of the differences in inventories across languages. What is universal is the drive to match the adult target, until such time as all the negative constraints can be overcome. How that plays out reflects the child's capacity for realization of syllable structure, features and their combinations and, most of the time, the options provided in the language.

Mandarin and Spanish diphthongs

The previous section discussed fricatives, a challenging sound class for acquisition. Compared with consonants, vowels are examined much less often, probably because they tend to be acquired relatively early (Bernhardt & Stemberger, 1998). However, this is more true of singleton vowels than vowel sequences, i.e. diphthongs or triphthongs, which are more challenging because they are more complex. Liu (2015) noted that a sample of 29 Mandarin-speaking children with PPD had notable mismatches for diphthongs and triphthongs, and an overview of the Granada Spanish PPD data showed similar patterns. In order to add to the vowel literature and to address the universality question with targets other than consonants, a preliminary comparison was therefore undertaken for these two languages. Although from different language families, they have two similarities that make a diphthong comparison intriguing: they both have rimes with few codas but nuclei that include 11 diphthong types, and equivalent numbers of rising and falling diphthongs (see Table 4.5[2]). The diphthong inventories overlap with each other, Spanish uniquely including /ui/, /oi/, and /ei/ and Mandarin uniquely including /uo/, /ye/, /ou/ and /ao/ (with the latter sometimes transcribed /au/).

Although there is similarity in terms of diphthongs, the languages also differ in several ways, in terms of:

(1) *Word structure*. Mandarin has a large proportion of monosyllabic words, with multisyllabic words being multimorphemic. There are no WI (or WF) clusters, although there are some word-medial (WM) consonant sequences across morpheme boundaries. Spanish has relatively few monosyllables but has monomorphemic disyllabic and multisyllabic words and both WI and WM consonant sequences.
(2) *Consonant inventory*. Mandarin has a larger inventory than Spanish (especially as it concerns coronal fricatives and affricates) and an aspiration rather than voicing contrast.
(3) *Monophthong inventory size*. Mandarin has nine, whereas Spanish has five.
(4) *Vowel sequence types*. Mandarin has four triphthongs (sometimes referred to as glide plus diphthongs, Duanmu, 2000), and Spanish, none.
(5) *Suprasegmental characteristics*. Mandarin is a tone language with five tones (one being the predictable neutral tone: Duanmu, 2000), whereas Spanish is a language with a variety of stress patterns, i.e. left-prominent, centre-prominent and right-prominent feet. Whether the similarities in the two languages would result in similar patterns for diphthong development, irrespective of the other differences, was the question. Expectations across the two languages were a lower match for diphthongs than for monophthongs and in terms of mismatch patterns, diphthong reduction, with the least sonorous element deleting most frequently within each diphthong.

Table 4.5 Diphthongs (and triphthongs[a]) in Mandarin and Granada Spanish elicitations

Language	*VV/VVV*[b]	*No. in test*	*Stress, Spanish*	*Words*[c]
Granada Spanish	Rising VV: <u>ui</u> ue ua ia io ie	17	12 stressed 5 unstressed (WF)	ruido llueve fuego hueso cuadro cuatro suave guante *agua (2)* *zanahoria gracias dinosaurio* pierna nieve hirviendo abierta
	Falling VV: ai au <u>oi</u> ei <u>eu</u>	10	9 stressed 1 unstressed (WI)	aire *bailando* jaula Paula (2) dinosaurio, hoy oigo (peine/penne; euro)[d]
Mandarin	Rising VV: <u>uo</u> ue ua ia io ie <u>ye</u>	20		ɚ^{MLM}tuo^{0} t͡sʰuo^{HL} suo^{MLM} t͡suo^{H}tsi(ə)^{0} pʰiŋ^{MH}kuo^{MLM} xua^{H} ʂua^{H}ja^{MH} ɕiaŋ^{H}tɕiao^{H} tian^{HL}ʂi^{H} tian^{HL}ʂi^{HL}tɕi^{H} tɕian^{H}paŋ^{MLM} ɕi^{MH}lian^{MLM} jye^{HL}liaŋ^{0} tsai^{HL}tɕian^{HL} ʂua^{H}ja^{MH} ɕie^{HL}ɕie^{0} ɕie^{MH}(tsi(ə)^{0}) xu^{MH}tie^{MH} kʰoŋ^{MLM}tɕʰye^{HL}
	Falling VV: ai <u>ao</u> (au)d <u>ou</u> ei	17		ai^{HL} tsʰai^{HL} niou^{MH}nai^{MLM} tsai^{HL}tɕian^{HL} tʰai^{HL}jaŋ^{0} ɕioŋ^{MH}mao^{H} pao^{H} pʰao^{MLM}pu^{HL} tsʰao^{MLM} pʰu^{MH}tʰao^{0} ou^{HL} ʂou^{MLM} lou^{MH}tʰi^{H} tʰou^{MH}fa^{0} ɕiao^{MLM}pʰɤŋ^{MH}jou^{0} fei^{H}tɕi^{H} pei^{H}tsi(ə)^{0}
	Triphthongs <u>uai uei</u> <u>iou iao</u>	4		tsuei^{MLM}(pa^{0}) ɕiao^{MLM}pʰɤŋ^{MH} jou^{0} jye^{HL}liaŋ^{0} ɕiaŋ^{H}tɕiao^{H}

Notes:
[a]Only Mandarin has triphthongs.
[b]Underlining indicates vowel sequences not in the other language.
[c]Italics indicates unstressed diphthongs in Spanish.
[d]Alternate pronunciations.

The procedures for the comparison followed the general procedures for data collection in the crosslinguistic study (see Methodology). The PPD samples for each language included 29 children, divided into three age groups from three to five years. In order to best equate the samples, two sub-groups of eight children each were selected with a similar age and degree of PPD: a mean age of 44 months for Spanish and 43 months for Mandarin, with percent consonant match (PCM) of 57.3% and 50.9%, respectively. Vowels being the target of interest, PCM was used to match samples, in order to exclude vowels from the matching procedures.

The single-word elicitation for Spanish included 103 words, with nine words repeated once; the Mandarin task included 80 words, the smaller list being sufficient to capture the major facets of Mandarin phonology (no WI consonant clusters, for example). Regarding diphthong word targets, Table 4.4 shows that the Spanish diphthongs occurred primarily in stressed syllables (21 in stressed syllables versus six in unstressed syllables), in this way being equivalent to Mandarin, which has relatively equal stress across syllables. There were more word types with diphthongs in the Mandarin word sample (37, versus 27 for Spanish), although there was an equivalent number of words with rising diphthongs (20 for Mandarin, 17 for Spanish). The overall difference in types thus primarily reflected a lower proportion of Spanish falling diphthongs in the sample. Word sample sizes were reduced further in the Spanish sample because of dialectal variation that allows [e] as a variant of /ei/, [u] as a variant of /eu/, or in certain slower speech contexts, diphthongs pronounced as two vowels with hiatus. Lack of familiarity with the Mandarin variants for diphthongs precluded data reduction for the Mandarin words. Because of the difference in word sample sizes, these data can be considered preliminary only, but do raise questions for future investigation.

Figure 4.4 and Table 4.6 show results from the descriptive analysis. (Statistical analyses were not done, because of the preliminary nature of the data from a small set of children.) As expected, the match level was higher for monophthongs than for diphthongs in both languages. Overall, the Mandarin diphthongs had higher match scores in spite of the lower PCM score for Mandarin. For both languages, timing unit match was uniformly higher than full segmental match, suggesting that at least some of the mismatch patterns did not involve diphthong reduction. The Spanish children had the same match level for diphthongs as the Mandarin children had for triphthongs (around 45–55%), even though the Spanish singleton vowels were 10% higher in match levels. Turning to rising versus falling diphthongs, there was minimal difference for the Mandarin data set, but the falling diphthongs fared

Table 4.6 Match comparisons for rising versus falling diphthongs in Mandarin and Spanish

	Rising VV full match	*Rising VV TU match*	*Falling VV full match*	*Falling VV TU match*
Granada Spanish	57.7%	65.9%	38.6%	51.4%
Shanghai Mandarin	67.5%	79.0%	80.5%	85.9%

somewhat worse than rising diphthongs for the Spanish children. The word *bailando* was partially responsible for the lower score, the only word where the diphthong was in an unstressed syllable. Even with exclusion of *dinosaurio* (the longest word), the falling diphthongs had overall lower match scores.

Regarding mismatches, the predominant pattern was deletion of the least sonorous element as predicted. But this was not uniform. The most sonorous of the two elements did delete in both languages some of the time. There were also other infrequent patterns, including metathesis, coalescence or deletion of the preceding consonant and maintenance of the diphthong.

Overall, two aspects of the preliminary comparison are intriguing: (a) the higher match proportion for Mandarin diphthongs than for Spanish, even though Mandarin data showed a lower PCM; and (b) equivalent match levels for the triphthongs in Mandarin and the diphthongs in Spanish. Any interpretation remains speculative; however, the question is whether diphthongs may have higher token frequency in Mandarin (they were more frequent in the sample of words for the full test in comparison with Spanish), and thus be more highly practised. Another question is whether having triphthongs also means that the less complex diphthongs may be more accurate, because there is something even more complex to learn. In terms of universal expectations, the major pattern of diphthong reduction, i.e. the least sonorous element deleting, was as would be expected by universal principles of phonology. However, as with many aspects of phonology, this was only probabilistic because in fact the most sonorous could delete, or other patterns could occur. Further study of diphthong development (vowels!) across languages is certainly warranted.

Conclusion

The overarching goal of the current crosslinguistic study is to determine universal versus language-specific aspects of phonological development. This chapter demonstrates some of the challenges facing any crosslinguistic project in children's phonological development and the set of solutions taken for the current study, given the complexities of international collaborations and differences among children, cultures, methods and languages. The examples of both within-language and between-language studies show the potential impact of crosslinguistic data: the greater the number of languages and countries, the richer and more diverse the data. However, the challenges of methodology need to be tempered by discussion, consensus-building, adult dialect definition and sample matching. Even the early results of the project speak to the complex interaction of articulatory complexity and language frequency as influences in phonological development. Some expectations about phonological universals are met, e.g. that unstressed syllables are weak prosodic domains where features may fail to surface, that the bulk of substitutions come from within the language's phonetic inventory, and that /f/ is an early fricative across at least the Germanic languages. But the data also show that language- and child-specific solutions can be found to resolve negative constraints. If the tongue cannot be grooved, a variety of phones might provide at least a partial match with the target.

When comparing across languages, the question is what can be compared. Currently, a set of papers is underway examining WI rhotic and lateral clusters with languages that have apical taps and/or trills. The unifying factors for the study are the focus on one particular topic and the processes of data collection. A long-term project is the analysis of word-structure development across the languages, because such data are relatively rare. Group study data are useful for examining larger questions statistically. However, individual child data are also informative about what is possible in language. A volume of case profiles is planned which will include all of the languages in the project. Some the data will be shared with Phonbank, so that other researchers can ask their own questions about phonological development, using the same data. As a final note, another major objective of the project has been to provide materials for speech-language therapists and researchers. The website phonodevelopment.sites.olt.ubc.ca has free assessment materials in the various languages, tutorials about transcription, phonology and scan analysis (in English, French and Spanish) for intervention planning and a set of fun-ological activities for clinical intervention (to date in Cantonese, English, French, Mandarin, Slovenian and Spanish).

Notes

(1) Whole word match means that the child's pronunciation of a specific word matches the adult target, or is considered 'close enough' by adult native speakers, with slight deviations in place or voicing ignored (see, for example, Schmitt *et al.*, 1983, where speech samples also showed an 80% WWM for four-year-olds for English).

(2) Rising diphthongs are those with rising sonority, in which the second element is more sonorous than the first, as in /ju/ (/iu/) or /wi/ (/ui/). Falling diphthongs are those with falling sonority in which the second element is less sonorous than the first, as in /au/ (/aw/) or /oi/ (/oj/).

(3) The word list for the English sample in the study is from the commercial Photo Articulation Test-3 and thus cannot be shared here (Lippke *et al.*, 1997). Updated lists for Mandarin, Granada Spanish and Slovene are on the website at phonodevelopment.sites.olt.ubc.ca.

(4) All Icelandic words are stress-initial (with the exception of some loan words not included here).

Acknowledgements

The authors would like to thank all the participants in the studies and the collaborators in the various countries for their enthusiastic engagement with us in this enterprise. They also gratefully acknowledge the Social Sciences and Humanities Research Council of Canada for the funding: Grants 410-2009-0348 and 611-2012-0164. The authors have no conflicts of interest regarding this research or chapter.

References

Árnason, K. (2011) *The Phonology of Icelandic and Faroese*. Oxford: Oxford University Press.

Bates, E. and MacWhinney, B. (1982) Functionalist approaches to grammar. In E. Wanner and L. Gleitman (eds) *Language Acquisition: The State of the Art* (pp. 173–218). New York: Cambridge University Press.

Bernhardt, B.H. and Stemberger, J.P. (1998) *Handbook of Phonological Development: From the Perspective of Constraint-based Nonlinear Phonology*. San Diego, CA: Academic Press.

Bernhardt, B.M. and Stemberger, J.P. (2012) Translation to practice: Transcription of the speech of multilingual children. In B. Goldstein and S. McLeod (eds) *Multilingual Aspects of Speech Sound Disorders in Children* (pp. 182–190). Bristol: Multilingual Matters.

Bernhardt, B.M., Romonath, R. and Stemberger, J.P. (2014) A comparison of fricative acquisition in German and Canadian English-speaking children with protracted phonological development. In M. Yavaş (ed.) *Unusual Productions in Phonology: Universals and Language-specific Considerations* (pp. 102–127). New York: Psychology Press.

Bernhardt, B.M., Másdóttir, T., Stemberger, J.P., Leonhardt, L. and Hansson, G.Ó. (2015) Fricative acquisition in English- and Icelandic-speaking preschoolers with protracted phonological development. *Clinical Linguistics & Phonetics* 29, 642–665.

Bérubé, D., Bernhardt, B.M., Stemberger, J.P. and Bacsfalvi, P. (2012) Nonlinear phonological analysis of the speech of Manitoba French-speaking preschoolers with protracted phonological development. Paper presented at the *International Conference of Clinical Phonetics and Linguistics*, 27–30 June, Cork, Ireland.

Bybee, J. (2006) *Frequency of Use and the Organization of Language*. Oxford: Oxford University Press.

Chávez-Peón, M.E., Bernhardt, B.M., Adler-Bock, M. *et al.* (2012) A Spanish pilot investigation for a crosslinguistic study in protracted phonological development. *Clinical Linguistics & Phonetics* 26, 255–272.

Chomsky, N. and Halle, M. (1968) *The Sound Pattern of English*. New York: Harper & Row.

de Lacy, P. (2007) *The Cambridge Handbook of Phonology*. Cambridge: Cambridge University Press.

Duanmu, S. (2000) *The Phonology of Standard Chinese*. Oxford: Oxford University Press.

Fox, A.V. and Dodd, B.J. (1999) Der Erwerb des phonologischen Systems in der deutschen Sprache. [Development of the phonological system in German]. *Sprache, Stimme und Gehör* 23, 183–191.

Hayes, B. (1999) Phonetically-driven phonology: The role of optimality theory and inductive grounding. In M. Darnell, E. Moravscik, M. Noonan, F. Newmeyer and K. Wheatly (eds) *Functionalism and Formalism in Linguistics, Vol. 1* (pp. 243–285). Amsterdam: John Benjamins.

Hooper, J.B. (1976) *An Introduction to Natural Generative Phonology*. New York: Academic Press.

Ingram, D. (1989) *Child Language Acquisition: Method, Description, and Explanation*. Cambridge: Cambridge University Press

Ingram, D. (2012) Prologue: Cross-linguistic and multilingual aspects of speech sound disorders in children. In S. McLeod and B. Goldstein (eds) *Multilingual Aspects of Speech Sound Disorders in Children* (pp. 3–12). Bristol: Multilingual Matters.

IPA (International Phonetic Alphabet) (2015) *Full IPA Chart*. See https://www.internationalphoneticassociation.org/content/full-ipa-chart.

Jakobson, R. (1968) *Child Language, Phonological Universals and Aphasia* (trans. A. Keiler). The Hague: Mouton. (Original work published 1941 as *Kindersprache, aphasie und allgemeine Lautgesetze*.)

Kochetov, A. and Colantoni, L. (2011) Coronal place contrasts in Argentine and Cuban Spanish: An electropalatographic study. *Journal of the International Phonetic Association* 41, 313–342.

Lai, Y., Bernhardt, B.M., Zhao, J. and Stemberger, J.P. (2011) Acoustic analysis of Mandarin tone in 4-year-old typically developing children in Shanghai. Poster presented at the *York Child Phonology Conference*, 15–17 June, York.

Locke, J.L. (1983) *Phonological Acquisition and Change*. New York: Academic Press.

Lippke, B.A., Dickey, S.E., Selmar, J.W. and Soder, A.L. (1997) *Photo Articulation Test – 3 (Revised)*. Austin, TX: Pro-Ed.

Liu, C. (2015) A Survey of Developmental Patterns in Mandarin Diphthong and Triphthong Acquisition by Preschoolers with Protracted Phonological Development. Unpublished graduating paper, University of British Columbia.

Maddieson, I. (1984) *Patterns of Sounds*. Cambridge: Cambridge University Press.

Martínez Celdrán, E. and Fernández Planas, A.M. (2007) *Manual de Fonética Española: Articulaciones y Sonidos del Español*. Barcelona: Ariel.

Másdóttir, T. (2008) Phonological Development and Disorders in Icelandic-speaking Children (PhD dissertation). Newcastle University, Newcastle. Printed in Reykjavík, 2008: Háskólaprent. ISBN: 978-9979-70-628-1.

McCarthy, J.J. (1988) Feature geometry and dependency. *Phonetica* 43, 84–108.

Pierrehumbert, J. (2001) Exemplar dynamics: Word frequency, lenition, and contrast. In J. Bybee and P. Hopper (eds) *Frequency Effects and the Emergence of Lexical Structure* (pp. 137–157). Amsterdam: John Benjamins.

Prince, A. and Smolensky, P. (2004) *Optimality Theory: Constraint Interaction in Generative Grammar*. Oxford: Blackwell.

Pye, C., Ingram, D. and List, H. (1987) A comparison of initial consonant acquisition in English and Quiché. In K. Nelson and A. van Kleeck (eds) *Children's Language, Vol. 6* (pp. 175–190). Hillsdale, NJ: Lawrence Erlbaum.

Rose, Y. (2002) Relations between segmental and prosodic structure in first language acquisition. In L. Santelmann, M. Verrips and F. Wijnen (eds) *The Annual Review of Language Acquisition* (vol. 2 , pp. 117–155). Amsterdam: John Benjamins.

Sagey, E.C. (1986) The representation of features and relations in non-linear phonology. Unpublished doctoral dissertation, Massachusetts Institute of Technology.

Schaeffler, F. and Wretling, P. (2003) Towards a typology of phonological quantity in the dialects of Modern Swedish. In D. Recasens (ed.) *Proceedings of the 15th International Congress of Phonetic Sciences (ICPhS)* (pp. 2697–2700). Barcelona: Universita autònoma de Barcelona.

Schmitt, L.S., Howard, B.H. and Schmitt, J.F. (1983) Conversational speech sampling in the assessment of articulation proficiency. *Language, Speech, and Hearing Services in Schools* 14, 210–214.

Schretlen, C. (2013) Prosodic structure patterns in multisyllabic word productions of Granada Spanish-speaking children with typical versus protracted phonological development. Unpublished master's thesis, University of British Columbia.

Shriberg, L.D. and Lof, G.L. (1991) Reliability studies in broad and narrow phonetic transcription. *Clinical Linguistics & Phonetics* 5, 225–279.

Smit, A.B., Hand, L., Freilinger, J.J., Bernthal, J.E. and Bird, A. (1990) *Journal of Speech and Hearing Disorders* 34, 779–798.

Starr, R. and Jurafsky, D. (2004) Phonological variation in Shanghai Mandarin. Paper presented at the *New Ways of Evaluating Variation* (NWAV)-33 Conference, 3 October, Ann Arbor, MI.

Ullrich, A. (2004) Nichtlineare Phonologische Analyse Deutschsprachiger Kinder [Nonlinear phonological analysis of German-speaking children]. Unpublished master's thesis, Julius Maximilians Universität.

Yavaş, M. (2014) *Unusual Productions in Phonology: Universals and Language-specific Considerations*. New York: Psychology Press.

Appendix: Word Lists for Mandarin, Granada Spanish, Icelandic and Slovene[3]

Mandarin

Pinyin	*CV Sequence*	*IPA*
bao1	CVV	pao^{H}
er3duo0	{V/VC}CVV	{ɚ/ɑɻ}^{MLM}tuo^{0}
zui3(ba)0	CVVV(CV)	tsuei^{MLM}(pa^{0})
shou3	CVV	ʂou^{MLM}
tou2fa0	CVVCV	tʰou^{MH}fa^{0}
jiao3	CVVV	tɕiao^{MLM}
xie2(zi0)	CVV(CV(V))	ɕie^{MH}(tsɨ(ə)^{0})
qun2zi0	CVCCV(V)	tɕʰyn^{MH}tsɨ(ə)^{0}
ping2guo3	CVCCVV	pʰiŋ^{MH}kuo^{MLM}
xi1gua{0/1}	CVCVV	ɕi^{H}kua{$^{0/H}$}
xiang1jiao1	CVVCCVVV	ɕiaŋ^{H}tɕiao^{H}
rou4	CVV	ɹou^{HL}
cai4	CVV	tsʰai^{HL}
wan3	CVC	wan^{MLM}
kuai4zi0	CVVVCV(V)	kʰuai^{HL}tsɨ(ə)^{0}
huai4le0	CVVVCV	xuai^{HL}lə^{0}
zhuo1zi0	CVVCV(V)	tʂuo^{H}tsɨ(ə)^{0}
shui3	CVVV	ʂuei^{MLM}
xi2lian3	CVCVVC	ɕi^{MH}lian^{MLM}
shua1ya2	CVVCV	ʂua^{H}ja^{MH}
chuang2	CVVC	tʂʰuaŋ^{MH}
men2	CVC	mɤn^{MH}
deng1	CVC	tɤŋ^{H}
ü2san3	VCVC	y^{MH}san^{MLM}
tai4yang0	CVVCVC	tʰai^{HL}jaŋ^{0}
yue4liang0	CVVCVVC	jye^{HL}liaŋ^{0}
xing1xing0	CVCCVC	ɕiŋ^{H}ɕiŋ^{0}
hua1	CVV	xua^{H}
niao3	CVVV	niao^{MLM}
gou3	CVV	kou^{MLM}
xiong2mao1	CVVCCVV	ɕioŋ^{MH}mao^{H}
fei1ji1	CVVCV	fei^{H}tɕi^{H}

(*Continued*)

Pinyin	*CV Sequence*	*IPA*
qi4che1	CVCV	tɕʰi^{HL}tʂʰɤ^{H}
qiu2	CVVV	tɕʰiou^{MH}
wa4zi0	CVCV(V)	wa^{HL}tsi(ə)^{0}
yu2	V	y^{MH}
niu2nai3	CVVVCVV	niou^{MH}nai^{MLM}
bei1zi0	CVVCV(V)	pei^{H}tsɨ((ə)^{0}
hong2de0	CVCCV	xoŋ^{MH}tə^{0}
tang2	CVC	tʰaŋ^{MH}
xie4xie0	CVVCVV	ɕie^{HL}ɕie^{0}
zai4jian4	CVVCVVC	tsai^{HL}tɕian^{HL}
shu1	CV	ʂu^{H}
dian4shi4ji1	CVVCCVCV	tian^{HL}ʂi^{HL}tɕi^{H}
sao3di4	CVVCV	sao^{MLM}ti^{HL}
ke2sou0	CVCVV	kʰɤ^{MH}sou^{0}
ma3	CV	ma^{MLM}
jian1bang3	CVVCCVC	tɕian^{H}paŋ^{MLM}
ba{1/4}ba0	CVCV	pa{$^{H/HL\}}$}pa^{0}
ai4	VV	ai^{HL}
bing3gan1	CVCCVC	piŋ^{MLM}kan^{H}
an4/en4	VC	{an^{HL}/ ɤn^{HL}}
kong3long2	CVCCVC	kʰoŋ^{MLM}loŋ^{MH}
diao4ü2	CVVV.V	tiao^{HL}y^{MH}
tiao4u3	CVVV.V	tʰiao^{HL}u^{MLM}
hu2die2	CVCVV	xu^{MH}tie^{MH}
re4	CV	ɹɤ^{HL}
pao3bu4	CVVCV	pʰao^{MLM}pu^{HL}
cao3	CVV	tsʰao^{MLM}
zhan4	CVC	tʂan^{HL}
reng1	CVC	ɹɤŋ^{H}
zhi1zhu1	CVCV	tʂɨ^{H}tʂu^{H}
chang4ge1	CVCCV	tʂʰaŋ^{HL}kɤ^{H}
chi1	CV	tʂʰɨ^{H}
shan1	CVC	ʂan^{H}
she2	CV	ʂɤ^{MH}
cuo4	CVV	tsʰuo^{HL}
jiu3	CVVV	tɕiou^{MLM}
qian2	CVVC	tɕʰian^{MH}
kong3que4	CVCCVV	kʰoŋ^{MLM}tɕʰye^{HL}

(*Continued*)

Pinyin	*CV Sequence*	*IPA*
er4	V	ɚ^{HL}
suo3	CVV	suo^{MLM}
liu4	CVVV	liou^{HL}
pu2tao0	CVCVV	pʰu^{MH}tʰao^{0}
di4di0	CVCV	ti^{HL}ti^{0}
bi3	CV	pi^{MLM}
lou2ti1	CVVCV	lou^{MH}tʰi^{H}
mi4feng1	CVCVC	mi^{HL}fɤn^{H}
xiao3peng2you0	CVVVCVCCVV	ɕiao^{MLM}pʰɤŋ^{MH}jou^{0}
gong1gong4qi4che1	CVCCVCCVCV	koŋ^{H}koŋ^{HL}tɕʰi^{HL}tʂʰɤ^{H}

Granada Spanish 2010 Word List

Word	*CV Sequence*	*IPA*
Object elicitation		
agua	'VCVV	'aɣ{wa/ua}
muñeca	CV'CVCV	mũ'ɲeka
Paula	'CVVCV	'paula
pescado/pez	CV'(C)CV(C)V	pe{s/θ/ʰ/ø}'ka{ð/ø}o
pez	'CV(C)	(pe{s/θ/ʰ/ø})
baño/bañera	'CVCV	'{b/β}aɲo
(bañera)	CV'CVCV	('{b/β}aɲera)
blanco	'CCVCCV	'blaŋko
flor	'CCV(C)	'flo{r/l/ø}
zapato	CV'CVCV	{s/θ}a'pato
reloj	CV'CV(C)	re'l{o/ɔ}{x/ʰ/ø)
Photo elicitation		
abierta	V'CVVCCV	a{b/β}{'je/ie}(ɾ/t)ta
agua	'VCVV	'aɣ{wa/ua}
azul	V'CV(C)	a'(s/θ}u{l/ɾ/ø}
elefante	VCV'CVCCV	ele'fan̪te
escalera	V(C)'CVCVCV	{e/ɛ}{s/ʰ/ø}ka'leɾa
estanque	V(C)'CVCCV	{e/ɛ}{s/ʰ/ø}'taŋke
hermano	VC'CVCV	eɾ'maãno
hipopótamo	VCV'CVCVC	ipo'potamo
hirviendo	VC'CVVCCV	iɾ'{b/β}{je/ie}n̪do

(*Continued*)

Word	*CV Sequence*	*IPA*
hoyo	'VCV	'oʝo
uvas	'VCV(C)	'uβ{a/a̯}{s/ ^{h}/ø}
aire	'(V)VCV	'aiɾe
euro	'(V)VCV	'{e}uɾo
Europa	'VVCVCV	{e}u'ɾopa
hoy	'VV	'oi
oigo	'VVCV	'oiɣo
hueso	'VVCV	'{g}{we/ue}so
martillo	CVC'CVCV	ma{ɾ/t}'tiʝo
mesa	'CVCV	'mesa
muñeca	CV'CVCV	mũ'ɲeka
nariz	CV'CV(C)	na'ɾi{s/^{h}/θ/ø}
nieve	'CVVCV	'n{ʝe/ie}βe
noche	'CVCV	'no{t͡ʃ/ʃ}e
pájaro	'CVCVCV	'pa{x/h}aɾo
pan	'CVC	'pa{ŋ/n}
pantalón	CVC'CVCVC	'pan̪talo{n/ŋ}
papá	CV'CV	pa'pa
Paula	'CVVCV	'paula
peine	'CVVCV/CVCCV	'p{ein/enn}e
pelo	'CVCV	'pelo
perro	'CVCV	'pero
pescado	CVC'(C)V(C)V	pe{s/θ/^{h}/ø}'ka{ð/ø}o
pierna	'CVCCV	'p{ʝe/ie}{ɾ/n}na
playa	'CCVCV	'plaʝa
pluma	'CCVCV	'pluma
primavera	CCVCV'CVCV	pɾima'{β/b}eɾa
princesa	CCVC'CVCV	pɾin̪{'θ/s}esa
bailando	CVV'CVCCV	{b/β}a'ilan̪do
baño	'CVCV	'{b/β}aɲo
barco	'CVCCV	'{b/β}aɾko
veinte	'CVVCCV	'{b/β}ein̪te
boca/la boca	'CVCV	'{b/β}oka
blanco	'CCVCCV	'{b/β}laŋko
bloque(s)	'CCVCV(C)	'{b/β}lok{e(ɛ)}{ s/^{h}/ø}
brazo	'CCVCV	'{b/β}ɾa{s/θ}o
bruja	'CCVCV	'{b/β}ɾu{x/h}a

(*Continued*)

Word	*CV Sequence*	*IPA*
techo	'CVCV	'te{t͡ʃ/ʃ}o
teléfono	CV'CVCVCV	te'lefono
toca	'CVCV	'toka
tortuga	CVC'CVCV	to{ɾ't}tuɣa
tres	'CCV(C)	'tɾ{e(ɛ)}{ s/ʰ/ø}
triángulo	CCV.'VCVCV	tɾi'aŋ{gɣ/}ulo
día	'CV.V	'{d/ð}i.a
dinosaurio	CVCV'CVVCVV	{d/ð}ino'sauɾ{io/jo}
dos	'CV(C)	'{d/ð}{o(ɔ)}{s/ʰ/ø}
dragón	CCV'CVC	d/ð}ɾa'ɣo{ŋ/n}
caballo	CV'CVCV	ka' {β/b}aʝo
casa	'CVCV	'kasa
cocodrilo	CVCV'CCVCV	koko'{d/ð}ɾilo
conejo	CV'CVCV	ko'ne{x/h}o
cuadro	'CVVCCV	'k{wa/ua}{d/ð}ɾo
cuatro	'CVVCCV	'k{wa/ua}tɾo
cruz	'CCV(C)	'kɾu{θ/s/ʰ/ø}
gato	'CVCV	'{g/ɣ}ato
gorra	'CVCV	'{g/ɣ}ora
guante	'CVVCCV	'{g/ɣ}{wa/ua}n̪te
guitarra	CV'CVCV	{g/ɣ}i'tara
globo(s)	'CCVCV(C)	'{g/ɣ}oβ{o/ɔ}(s/ʰ)
gracias	'CCVCVV(C)	'{g/ɣ}ɾa{θ/s}{ja/ia}{s/ʰ/ø}
grande	'CCVCCV	'{g/ɣ}ɾan̪de
foto	'CVCV	'foto
fuego	'CVVCV	'f{we/ue}ɣo
fútbol	'CVCCV(C)	'fu{t.b/bb}{o/ɔ}{l/ɾ/ø}
flecha	'CCVCV	'fle{t͡ʃ/ʃ}a
flor	'CCV(C)	'flo{ɾ/l/ø}
fresa	'CCVCV	'fɾesa
fruta(s)	'CCVCV(C)	'fɾut{a/a̹}(s/ʰ/ø)
saltando	CVC'CVCCV	sa{l/t}'tan̪do
sed	'CV(C)	's{e/ɛ}{d/ð/ø}
silla	'CVCV	'siʝa
sombrero	CVC'CCVCV	'som'bɾeɾo
suave	'CVVCV	's{wa/ua}βe
zanahoria	CVCV.'VCVV	{s/θ}ana'oɾ{ia/ja}

(*Continued*)

Word	*CV Sequence*	*IPA*
zapato	CV'CVCV	{s/θ}a'pato
chimenea	CVCV'CV.V	t͡ʃimẽ'ne.a
chocando	CV'CVCCV	t͡ʃo'kan̪do
chocolate	CVCV'CVCV	t͡ʃoko'late
jirafa	CV'CVCV	{x/h}i'ɾafa
jamón	CV'CVC	{x/h}a'mõ{ŋ/n}
jaula	'CVVCV	'{x/h}aula
juguete	CV'CVVCV	{x/h}u'{ɣ/g}ete
llave	'CVCV	'{d͡ʒ/ʝ}aβe
llorando	CV'CVCCV	{d͡ʒ/ʝ}o'ran̪do
llueve	'CVVCV	'{d͡ʒ/ʝ}{we/ue}βe
lámpara	'CVCCVCV	'lampara
lápiz	'CVCV(C)	'lapi{s/θ/ʰ/ø}
leche	'CVCV	'le{t͡ʃ/ʃ}e
luz	'CV(C)	'lu({θ/s/ʰ/ø})
ratón	CV'CV(C)	ra'to{ŋ/(n)}
regalo	CV'CVCV	re'{ɣ/g} ɣalo
reloj	CV'CV(C)	re'l{o/ɔ}{x/ʰ/ø)
rojo	'CVCV	'roxo
ruido	'CVVCV	'r{ui/wi}{ð/d}o

Icelandic 2009 Word List[4]

Word	*CV Sequence*	*IPA*
afi	V:CV	a:ʋɪ
elda	VCCV	ɛlta
epli	VCCCV	ɛhplɪ
ofn	VCC	ɔpn̥
opna	VCCCV	ɔhpna
ungi	VCCV	uɲcɪ
bangsi	CVVCCV	pauŋsɪ
banka	CVVCCV	pauŋ̊ka
bók	CVV:C	pou:k
bolti	CVCCV	pɔl̥tɪ
peli	CV:CV	pʰɛ:lɪ
peysa	CVV:CV	pʰɛi:sa
blóm	CCVV:C	plou:m
blaðra	CCVCCV	plaðra

(*Continued*)

Word	*CV Sequence*	*IPA*
bleia	CCVV:CV	plɛi:ja
plástur	CCVVCCVC	pʰlaustʏr̥
brauð	CCVV:C	prœy:θ
prins	CCVCC	pʰrɪns
prinsessa	CCVCCVC:V	pʰrɪnsɛs:a
bjalla	CCVCCV	pjatla
dúkka	CVCCV	tuhka
datt	CVCC	taht
draugur	CCVV:CVC	trœy:{ɣ/ɰ}ʏr̥
tær	CVV:C	tʰai:r̥
tennur	CVC:VC	tʰɛn:ʏr̥
tromma	CCVC:V	tʰrɔm:a
tré	CCC:V:	tʰrj:ɛ:
tveir	CCVV:C	tʰʋɛi:r̥
geispa	CVVCCV	cɛispa
geit	CVV:C	cɛi:t
gíraffi	CV:CVC:V	ci:raf:ɪ
kjóll	CCVVCC	cʰjoutl̥
kíkja	CVVCV	cʰi:ca
kind	CVCC	cʰɪnt
kyssa	CVC:V	cʰɪs:a
gaffall	CVC:VCC	kaf:atl̥
gagga	CVC:V	kak:a
kanína	CV:CV:CV	ka:ni:na
kartafla	CVCCVCCV	kʰar̥t{a/ɛ}pla
koddi	CVC:V	kʰɔt:ɪ
kona	CV:CV	kʰɔ:na
kubbar	CVC:VC	kʰʏp:ar̥
glas	CCV:C	kla:s
gluggi	CCVC:V	klʏc:ɪ
klukka	CCVCCV	kʰlʏhka
greiða	CCVV:CV	krɛi:ða
grís	CCV:C	kri:s
krókódíll	CCVVCVCVCC	kʰroukɔtitl̥
krummi	CCVC:V	kʰrʏm:ɪ
mús	CV:C	mu:s
mjólk	CCVVCC	mjoul̥k
mjólka	CCVVCCV	mjoul̥ka

(*Continued*)

Word	*CV Sequence*	*IPA*
nagli	CVCCV	naklɪ
nef	CV:C	nɛ:f
hnerra	CVC:V	n̥ɛr:a
fiðrildi	CVCCVCCV	fɪðrɪltɪ
fugl	CVCC	fʏkl̥
fullt	CVCC	fʏl̥t
fjórir	CCVV:CVC	fjou:rɪr̥
flauta	CCVV:CV	flœy:ta
fluga	CCV:CV	flʏ:{ɣ/ɰ}a
frɔskur	CCVCCVC	frɔskʏr̥
þumall	CV:CVCC	θʏ:matl̥
þrír	CCV:C	θri:r̥
sippa	CVCCV	sɪhpa
sól	CVV:C	sou:l̥
sög	CV:C	sœ:x
spil	CCV:C	spɪ:l̥
stelpa	CCVCCV	stɛ̥lpa
stóll	CCVVCC	stoutl̥
skæri	CCVV:CV	scai:rɪ
skegg	CCVC:	scɛk:
skip	CCV:C	scɪ:p
skór	CCVV:C	skou:r̥
slanga	CCVVCCV	stlauŋka
slaufa	CCCVV:CV	stlœy:fa
smekkur	C(C)CVCCVC	s(p)mɛhkʏr̥
springa	CCCVCCV	spriŋka
snuð	CCCV:C	stnʏ:{θ/ð̥}
strætó	CCCVV:CVV	strai:tou
strákur	CCCVV:CVC	strau:kʏr̥
skríða	CCCV:CV	skri:ða
svín	CCV:C	sʋi:n
sjó(num)	CCVV:	sjou:
sjóræningi	CCVV:CVVCVCCV	sjou:rainiɲcɪ
hjarta	CVCCV	çar̥ta
hjóla	CVV:CV	çou:la
vagn	CVCC	ʋakn̥
vasi	CV:CV	ʋa:sɪ
vatn	CVCCC	ʋahtn̥
jólasveinn	CVV:CVCCVVCC	jou:lasʋɛitn̥
jakki	CVCCV	jahcɪ
lamb	CVCC	lamp

(*Continued*)

Word	*CV Sequence*	*IPA*
lampi	CVCCV	lam̥pɪ
lesa	CV:CV	lɛ:sa
lita	CV:CV	lɪ:ta
lögga	CVC:V	lœk:a
lyfta	CVCCV	lɪfta
lykta	CVCCV	lɪxta
hlaupa	CVV:CV	l̥œy:pa
ljón	CCVV:C	ljou:n
rautt	CVVCC	rœyht
renna	CVC:V	rɛn:a
rigning	CVCCVCC	rɪknɪŋk
risaeðla	CVCV.VCCV	rɪsa.ɛðla
rúlla	CVC:V	rul:a
hringur	CVCCVC	r̥iŋkʏr̥
hægt	CVVCC	haixt
hattur	CVCCVC	hahtʏr̥
hundur	CVCCVC	hʏntʏr̥

Slovene 2009 Word List

Word	*CV Sequence*	*IPA*
lev	'CVC	'lɛu̯
dolg	'CVC	'dok
dim	'CVC	'dim
koš	'CVC	'kɔʃ
noč	'CVC	'no͡tʃ
nos	'CVC	'nos
sok	'CVC	'sok
suh	'CVC	'sux
šal	'CVC	'ʃal
zob	'CVC	'zob̥
dež	'CVC	'dəʃ
črn	'CCC/CVCVC	'͡tʃ(ə)r(ə)n
voz	'CVC	'vos
tiger	'CVCVC	'tigər
buča	'CVCV	'bu͡tʃa

(*Continued*)

Word	*CV Sequence*	*IPA*
hiša	'CVCV	'xiʃa
juha	'CVCV	'juxa
miza	'CVCV	'miza
okno	VC'CV	ok'no
riba	'CVCV	'riba
roka	'CVCV	'rɔka
šola	'CVCV	'ʃola
taca	'CVCV	'ta͡tsa
vaza	'CVCV	vaza
žaba	'CVCV	'ʒaba
žoga	'CVCV	'ʒoga
fižol	CV'CVV	fi'ʒou̯
nebo	CV'CV	nɛ'bo
jezik	'CVCVC	'jɛzik
zadaj	'CVCVC	'zadai̯
velik	'CVCVC/CV'CVC	{'vɛlik/vɛ'lik}
balon	CV'CVC	ba'lon
rumen	'CV'CVC	ru'mɛn
banana	CV'CVCV	ba'nana
čebela	CV'CVCV	t͡ʃɛ'bela
darilo	CV'CVCV	da'rilɔ
lisica	CV'CVCV	li'si͡tsa
žirafa	CV'CVCV	ʒi'rafa
jagoda	'CVCVCV	'jagɔda
veverica	'CVCVCVCV/CVCV'CVCV	{'vevɛri͡tsa/vevɛ'ri͡tsa}
čokolada	CVCV'CVCV	t͡ʃɔkɔ'lada
nogavica	CVCV'CVCV	nɔga'vi͡tsa
avto	'VVCV	'au̯tɔ
ura	'VCV	'ura
očala	V'CVCV	ɔ't͡ʃala
gnezdo	CCVC'CV	'gnezdɔ
zvezda	'CCVCCV	'zvezda
krompir	CCVC'CVC	k{r/r̩}{ɔ/ə}m'pir
špageti	CCV'CVCV	ʃpa'geti
postelja	'CVCCVCCV/CV'CCVCCV	{'postelja/po'stelja}
helikopter	CVCV'CVCV	xɛli'koptər
steklenica	CCVCCV'CVCV	stɛklɛ'ni͡tsa
grad	'CCVC	'grad̥

(*Continued*)

Word	*CV Sequence*	*IPA*
ključ	'CC(C)VC	'kʎu t͡ʃ
kruh	'CCVC	'krux
slon	'CCVC	'slɔn
sneg	'CCVC	'sneg̊/'snek(ʰ)
vlak	'CCVC	'vlak
krof	'CCVC	krëf
prazen	'CCVCVC	'prazɛn
trebuh	'CCVCVC	'trebux
zvonec	'CCVCVC/'CCVCC	'zvɔnɛ t͡s
svinčnik	'CCVCCCVC	'svin t͡ʃnik
gumb	'CVCC	'gump(ʰ)/'gumb̥
list	'CVCC	'list
prst	'CVCCC	'pərst
cesta	'CVCCV	't͡sesta
metla	'CVCCV	'mɛtla
kocke	'CVCCV	kot͡ske
hrbet	'CVCCVC	'xərbətʰ
sonce	'CVCCV	'son t͡sɛ
medved	'CVCCVC	'mɛdvɛd
zajtrk	'CVCCVCC	'zai̯tərk
mleko	'CCVCV	'mleko
knjiga	'CC(C)VCV	{'kniga/'knʲiga/'kɲiga}
plava	'CCVCV	'plava
srajca	'CCVCCV	'srai̯ t͡sa
krava	'CCVCV	krava
drevo	CCV'CV	drɛ'vo
glava	'CCVCV	'glava
streha	'CCVCV	'strexa
vrata	'CCVCV	'vrata
zgoraj	'CCVCVC	'zgɔra{i̯/j}
dva	'CCV	'd{v/ʋ̞/ʋ}a
spi	'CCV	'spi
stol	'CCVC	'stou̯
tla	'CCV	'tla
škarje	'CCVCCV	'ʃkarjɛ
hruška	'CCVCCV	'xruʃka
mravlja	'CCVVC(C)V	'mrau̯ʎa
rdeč	VC'CVCC/'CCVC	{ər'de t͡ʃ/'rde t͡ʃ]

(*Continued*)

Word	*CV Sequence*	*IPA*
usta	ˈVCCV	ˈ(ʔ)usta
sladoled	CCVCVˈCVC	sladɔˈleḓ
blagajna	CCVˈCVCCV	blaˈgai̯na
klobasa	CCVˈCVCV	klɔˈbasa
zdravnica	CCCVVˈCVCV	zdrau̯ˈni t͡sa
brisača	CCVˈCVCV	briˈsa t͡ʃa
kmetija	CCVˈCVCV	kmɛˈtija
hladilnik	CCVˈCVCCVC	xlaˈdilnik
peskovnik	CVCˈCVCVC	pɛˈskou̯nik
igrišče	VˈCCVCCV	iˈgriʃt͡ʃɛ
zobna ščetka	ˌCVCCVˈCCVCCV	ˌzobnaˈʃ t͡ʃetka
pomaranča	CVCVˈCVCCV	pɔmaˈran t͡ʃa
kenguru	CVCCVˈCV	kɛnguˈru
mehurčki	CVCˈCVCCCV	mɛˈxur t͡ʃki
gugalnica	CVˈCVCCV/CV	guˈgalni t͡sa

5 Bilingual Speech Assessment for Maltese Children

Helen Grech, Barbara Dodd and Sue Franklin

Introduction

Published research on children's speech development is mainly related to studies of monolingual English-speaking children (Zhu & Dodd, 2006). More recently, there has been increased interest in children acquiring other languages (e.g. Ballard & Farao, 2008 for Samoan; Fox, 2000 for German; MacLeod *et al.*, 2011 for Québécois French; To *et al.*, 2012 for Hong Kong Cantonese). Research suggests that children acquiring different languages have some language-specific developmental phonological processes indicating that findings for one language are not applicable to other languages (e.g. Amayreh & Dyson, 1998 for Arabic; Grech, 1998 for Maltese; Macleod *et al.*, 2011 for Québécois French; So & Dodd, 1994 for Cantonese; Zhu & Dodd, 2000 for Putonghua). During the past couple of decades research on bilingual acquisition has become of more interest.

Studies on bilingual phonological acquisition include those for Spanish-English (Fabiano & Goldstein, 2005), Cantonese-English (Holm & Dodd, 2006), German (Lleó *et al.*, 2003), Welsh-English (Munro *et al.*, 2005), Arabic-Swedish (Salameh *et al.*, 2003) and French-English (Sundara *et al.*, 2006). There are indications that children exposed to early sequential bilingualism show different patterns of phonological acquisition from those of monolingual children of the respective languages (e.g. Grech & Dodd, 2008; Holm & Dodd, 1999c). Further, sequential bilingual children may exhibit differences in type and number of errors from simultaneous bilingual ones (De Houwer, 2009). When Wright and Gildersleeve-Neumann (2005) compared 11 monolingual English-speaking children with five Russian-English bilingual children (two of whom learned Russian and English simultaneously and three of whom acquired English once their Russian was established), they found that the sequentially bilingual participants made more consonant errors than the simultaneous bilingual children and that overall the bilingual participants made more errors than the monolingual subjects.

The finding that bilingual children's phonological acquisition differs from that of monolinguals of either of the languages spoken indicates that having two phonologies affects the course of acquisition. This is in line with the *Interactional Dual Systems Model* for the mental organization of more than one language. The model asserts that bilingual children have two separate phonological systems, but that those two systems can influence one another. Paradis (2001) reported such crosslinguistic features in the productions of bilingual children. The model fits with data from other studies of bilingual children (e.g. Holm & Dodd, 1999a, 1999b, 1999c for Cantonese-English, Italian-English and Punjabi-English, respectively; Johnson & Lancaster, 1998 for Norwegian-English; Keshavarz & Ingram, 2002 for Farsi-English; Salameh *et al.*, 2003 for Swedish-Arabic. On the other hand, Navarro *et al.* (1995) found no atypical phonological processes in the speech of 11 successive bilingual Hispanic-English pre-school children in the US. Other studies report that successive bilingual individuals tend to superimpose an unknown system on the more established one (e.g. Watson, 1991).

Zhu and Dodd (2006) reviewed the varying reports concerned with the phonological development of bilingual children (e.g. Johnson & Lancaster, 1998). They concluded that apparently conflicting findings may reflect differences between the different language pairs learned, or the comparative length of exposure to a child's two languages.

Research describing bilingual phonological acquisition is limited in terms of the language pairs studied and the language learning contexts investigated. Data are often reported from studies where the children's first language is that of their immigrant parents in a country where the dominant language is English (e.g. Goldstein & Washington, 2001 for Hispanic children in the US; Stow & Dodd, 2003 for Pakistani Heritage languages in the UK). They are in a community where one language is spoken apart from the home language. The child becomes bilingual as a result of the shift of linguistic environment. However, there also exist simultaneous bilingual individuals where acquisition of two or more languages occurs very early in their lives. De Houwer (2009) refers to two sub-groups of such children, i.e. those who have bilingual first language acquisition (BFLA) when there is no chronologic difference in the exposure of both languages, and those children who are early second language learners (ESLLs) and are exposed to a second language on a regular basis between 8 and 48 months of age. de Houwer also refers to formal second language acquisition whereby children are introduced to second language literacy at about 60 months of age. Second language acquisition (SLA) and English language learners (ELLs) or equivalent terms used in non-English contexts refer to learning the second language at school. Sequential acquisition can also refer to learning subsequent languages at any time during life.

Another important limitation of the available data on bilingual children's acquisition of speech is that, very often, the two languages studied come from the same language family and share similar phonological characteristics. There is evidence that research findings from two Indo-European languages (e.g. English-French, Spanish-English) differ from those for other language pairs even though one of the languages in the pair is the same (Zhu & Dodd, 2006). Further, the number of children involved in these studies has been extremely small (many are case studies), with the consequence that there are no normative data for many language pairs, limiting the assessment and diagnosis of speech disorders. Studies in English-speaking countries have established and standardized assessments to identify children with speech difficulties but no such protocols are available for the Maltese population. The authors attempted to address such a gap in the knowledge base concerned with speech acquisition in the Maltese context by developing a bilingual speech and language assessment and administering it on a large sample of Maltese children.

The work described in this chapter is solely related to the children's speech, although this forms part of a broader study related to Maltese speech and language acquisition (see Grech *et al.*, 2011b, for reference to the *Language Assessment for Maltese Children*). A summary of the findings relating to the speech development for monolingual and bilingual Maltese children aged between 24 and 72 months is provided. Some of the findings reported in Grech and Dodd (2008) are summarized in the Results section below. Standard scores for monolingual Maltese-speaking children and bilingual children are included as Appendices in this chapter. The reliability and validity measures of the speech data are also discussed.

The phonologies of Maltese and English have their origins in two different language families (Semitic and Indo-European). The consonant inventory of Maltese is similar to that of English (with /ʔ/ and /ts/ being *additional* Maltese phonemes while the English /θ/, /ʒ/ and /ð/ are not part of the Maltese inventory). The vowel systems are also very similar in relation to English received pronunciation (RP) and Standard Maltese. However, the two languages differ in their phonotactics. Maltese has a greater range of possible consonantal clusters and consonantal sequences and is characterized by multisyllabic lexemes (Borg & Azzopardi-Alexander, 1997). Further information relating to the phonology of Maltese can be found in Grech (1998). A speech test standardized on English-speaking children, such as the *Diagnostic Evaluation of Articulation and Phonology (DEAP)* (Dodd *et al.*, 2002), is therefore not applicable since it does not cater for Maltese phonotactics and should not be used to assess Maltese-speaking children. The use of English-only standardized tests when clinicians evaluate non-native English speakers has often been reported (e.g. Skahan & Lof, 2007), and should be avoided as it may lead to misdiagnosis of a speech disorder.

Clinicians need language-specific tools to identify children with speech and/or language difficulties, since it is well known that children with an early history of speech/language impairment may be at risk for continuing communication difficulties particularly related to written language development (Shriberg & Kwiatkowski, 1994). Educational achievement is also related to early speech and language abilities (Bickford-Smith *et al.*, 2005) as well as social, emotional or behavioural challenges (Rome-Flanders & Cronk, 1998). It was therefore considered crucial to develop a speech assessment that can identify children who have speech impairment in Malta. The objectives of this study were to construct and standardize a speech assessment battery appropriate for children acquiring language in the bilingual language learning context of Malta. Traditionally assessments for children in bilingual contexts have consisted of two separate tests, one for each language. This does not reflect the reality of the way in which bilingual children use language in terms of language mixing and word borrowing. Indeed, to respond appropriately in the required language may require an added degree of metalinguistic control. Uniquely, in this speech assessment children are able to use Maltese or English in response to each stimulus item. Scoring and analysis also cater for language mixing (for details see the test manual in Grech *et al.*, 2011a). This assessment is also meant to capture the crosslinguistic effects in case of bilingual language acquisition which Goldstein and Gildersleeve-Neumann (2015) report.

The Maltese sociolinguistic context

The Maltese Islands have a complex language learning context. There are two official languages (Maltese and English); most children are bilingual in that they have some knowledge of both languages but one of the languages may be dominant. Reports from parents indicate that in some homes one of the languages may be used exclusively while other families use both languages (Grech & Dodd, 2008) so that the child is exposed to two languages at home soon after birth (simultaneous acquisition). In comparison, some children are exposed to only Maltese or English at home, followed by exposure to their second language in the community usually by 36 months of age when they start attending pre-school (early sequential acquisition). There is a dearth of knowledge as to whether and how Maltese monolingual children differ from their bilingual peers in terms of crosslinguistic interaction. Given the Maltese scenario, bilingual children would be expected to cope better in the different *monolingual* contexts that they may encounter at school or elsewhere. For example, a typical Maltese bilingual child would be able to communicate effectively with Maltese monolingual grandparents or adults; yet if the child goes to an English-speaking school s/he will encounter no difficulties with communicating with his peers and educators.

In this study, data from children reported by the caregivers to be simultaneously bilingual (as defined above) were analyzed and reported separately from data of the children who were reported to be exposed to Maltese or English at home (referred to as monolingual in this study). The term *monolingual* in the Maltese context has to be treated with caution and refers in this chapter to home exposure. The language learning context of Malta, where most people have some knowledge of two languages, reflects emerging patterns of language use in the European Union, due to population shifts, where many people have some knowledge and functional use of at least two languages although one language may be dominant. Given the influx of migrants in Malta, particularly following its full membership as a European Member State in 2004, children living in Malta have become exposed to other languages, especially at school. The Italian television channels used to play a role in language exposure to children in Malta and, as a result, Italian was acquired as the third language, specifically by watching Italian films and shows. However, with the introduction of computers and the internet at home, Italian TV lost its popularity. What we have today in the Maltese Islands is mainly bilingual Maltese and English exposure to varying degrees. By 10–11 years of age children are taught the third language at school and sometimes even a fourth language, these usually being Italian, French or German. The Maltese National Curriculum is bilingual (Maltese and English), so even children of expatriates are bound to be introduced to Maltese and English once they attend school if their home language is different. The newly launched policy for bilingual education in the early years (Ministry of Education and Employment, 2016) will play a major role in exposing all children (from pre-school years) to both Maltese and English, with both languages given equal importance.

The Maltese Islands have a relatively small number of inhabitants (approximately 420,000). However, there are many Maltese residing in other countries, particularly in Australia, the UK, the United States and Canada. Maltese (which is one of the 23 official languages of Europe) is therefore spoken on other continents. For example, according to the Australia 2011 Census, residents whose country of birth is Malta totalled 116,195 (stat.data.abs.gov.au, accessed 19 February 2017). Estimates by the UK National Statistics Office of Maltese-born UK residents in 2015 were 22,000 (https://www.ons.gov.uk/peoplepopulationandcommunity/populationandmigration/internationalmigration/datasets/populationoftheunitedkingdombycountryofbirthandnationality, accessed 17 February 2017). More than 70,000 Maltese immigrants and descendants were estimated to be living in the US in the mid-1990s (http://www.everyculture.com/multi/Le-Pa/Maltese-Americans.html, accessed 11 January 2015). Slavik (2001) provides figures from the Canadian Census in 1996, indicating that one-third of the approximately 30,000 people of Maltese ethnic origin use Maltese as their home language. Slavik reported that around 75% of first-generation Maltese-Canadians speak Maltese or Maltese with some English to siblings, whereas 22% of second-generation Maltese-Canadians speak Maltese or Maltese with some English. It is estimated that close to 500,000 use spoken Maltese worldwide (https://www.ethnologue.com/language/mlt, accessed 28 July, 2017). Consequently, the research study reported here informs practitioners within and outside Maltese territory. It also adds value to the European Union's promotion of multilingualism among EU citizens which is believed to lead to the individual's self-improvement and as a means for more job opportunities and growth across the EU economy (European Commission, 2008).

Research Questions

The *Maltese-English Speech Assessment* (MESA) (Grech *et al.*, 2011a) was constructed and evaluated to address the following research questions:

- Does the MESA demonstrate that a single battery can effectively assess mono- and bilingual children?
- Do the speech acquisition patterns for these two populations differ?
- Is the MESA a reliable and valid test of speech development?
- Does the MESA distinguish between typically developing children and those with delayed or disordered speech, making the assessment a useful tool for clinicians working with Maltese-speaking children?

Method

The sample

The public registry of births for the Maltese Islands was accessed to draw a random sample of 1000 Maltese children aged 24–72 months. All children whose parents consented to participate in the project (a total of 241 children) were assessed on a picture-naming task to evaluate phone articulation, phonology and consistency of word production. The children were also assessed for oro-motor skills and the ability to repeat phonotactically complex words. The sample included a total of 134 girls and 107 boys. Twenty-two participants were aged 24–35 months, 35 were 36–41 months, 45 were 42–47 months and 40 were 48–53 months. Information was collected from the carers relating to whether the children had an underlying sensory, cognitive or anatomical/physiological condition, family history of communication difficulties and other factors such as socio-economic status that could reflect on their speech and language acquisition. However, this information did not result in exclusion of children from the study unless the assessment distressed them. The rationale for this decision was to avoid over-diagnosis of impairment, since data identifying typical performance must be based on a representative sample of the total population.

Other information related to the primary language of the child, and language/s used at home was collected. The children were allowed to use the language they chose (either Maltese or English). Ninety-two children (38.17%) were reported by parents to speak both Maltese and English at home, 138 (57.26%) were reported to speak Maltese and 11 (4.56%) only English at home (see Tables 5.1 and 5.2 for details of the sample).

The assessment battery (MESA)

Standardized speech assessments are based on one of three main approaches, i.e. the phonetic, linguistic and psycholinguistic approach. The latter focuses on how a speech impairment occurs and attempts to explain its cause by analyzing and not merely describing the individual's linguistic behaviour. In principle, the psycholinguistic approach supports the notion that a speech impairment results from a breakdown in the speech processing chain. This may occur at any level, such as peripheral hearing, auditory discrimination of phonemes, accurate storing of words, planning of speech output and/or execution of speech. Dodd *et al.* (2002) constructed the DEAP on the basis of this approach and claim that deficits at any level of the model reflect a specific sub-group of speech impairment. Hence, the DEAP is not only a robust clinical tool that leads to differential diagnosis of speech disorder but also taps into the respective deficits that can be directly addressed in intervention. The DEAP was therefore considered as the most robust assessment on which to base the MESA. The MESA (Grech *et al.*, 2011a) consists of four tests that assess articulation, phonology, consistency of production and oro-motor skills.

- *The Articulation Assessment* is meant to identify perceptually any phonemes that cannot be produced by the child. The assessment includes 42 pictures depicting all consonant and vowel sounds in English and

Table 5.1 Maltese sample by age and gender

Age in months	*Total no. of age cohort*	*No. of girls*	*No. of boys*
24–35	20	9	11
36–41	36	23	13
42–47	45	27	18
48–53	40	19	21
54–59	34	11	23
60–65	37	25	12
66–72	29	20	9
Total	241	134	107
% of sample	100%	56.6%	44.4%

Table 5.2 Maltese sample by language learning context

Age in months	*Maltese*	*English*	*Maltese-English*	*Total per cohort*
24–35	10	1	11	22
36–41	18	2	15	35
42–47	23	2	20	45
48–53	28	1	11	40
54–59	22	1	11	34
60–65	22	1	14	37
66–72	15	3	10	28
Total	138	11	92	241
% of sample	57.26	4.56	38.17	100

Maltese. If a picture is not named spontaneously by the child, the administrator attempts to elicit it through imitation in syllable context or in isolation. The pictures are different from those used in the DEAP and were selected on the basis of clarity, cultural familiarity and age appropriateness.

- *The Phonology Assessment* is meant to determine the use of developmental phonological processes (surface speech error patterns) that are produced by the child. These may include the language-specific ones (e.g. compensatory vowel lengthening; Grech, 1998) universal ones (e.g. fronting) and in some instances atypical patterns. Children are asked to name the same 42 pictures and in the same order as in the articulation subtest, although these have a different coloured background.
- *The Inconsistency Assessment* allows the administrator to evaluate the consistency of production (stability) of the child's contrastive phones. When considered as part of the test battery, this assessment enables the identification of those children whose speech is inconsistent but who have no oro-motor difficulties. Children are required to name 17 pictures on three separate trials within one session.
- *The Oro-motor Assessment* evaluates the child's oro-motor function in relation to his/her diadochokinetic (DDK) skills for sequencing and intelligibility. Imitation of isolated and sequenced movements involving speech musculature is also assessed via a separate subtest. Another subtest involves the repetition of a list of 11 words, some of which are multisyllabic; some include syllable-initial consonantal clusters. For this subtest the child is asked to repeat the word uttered by the administrator, three times consecutively. This word repetition test was included specifically because of the syllabic structure of Maltese and the wide range of multiple combinations of consonantal cluster possibilities as well as multisyllabic words. Examples of words in this subtest include: /tpɪnʤɪ/ 'colouring', /hwɛɪɛʧ/ 'clothes', and /sʊfɐrɪnɐ/ 'match'.

The MESA portfolio includes the *Manual*, which provides clear instructions for its administration. The *Stimulus Book* contains pictures that are culturally appropriate, age appropriate and colourful. This was checked by piloting the test on Maltese children of varying ages. Clinicians were also approached for feedback before confirming the list of pictures to be used. The pictures are visually attractive to children between 24 and 72 months, the target age group. The *Score Sheets* are colour coded for ease of reference and allow for entry of raw scores for each section. Different subtests can be carried out in separate sessions (but close in time), particularly if the test is being used for review purposes. The articulation test is easy and quick to score, whereby the clinician is only expected to circle any phones that the child does not produce in the adult form. Phonetic transcription according to the International Phonetic Alphabet (IPA) is required for the phonology test. This allows for the identification of error patterns and idiosyncratic phoneme production. Quantitative analysis is recommended to calculate percent consonants correct (PCC) and percent vowels correct (PVC) for the different language codes (e.g. Maltese, Maltese-English). PCC and PVC measures are used regularly to index the phonological skills of children. PCC measures are reported to be linguistically and psychometrically valid (Shriberg *et al.*, 1997).

The Inconsistency test score is calculated as a percentage of the number of words produced differently in three trials in relation to the total number of words produced three times. In case of the word repetition subtest the child is not penalized if s/he utters the word with the correct syllabic structure but uses 'systemic error patterns'. For example, if the word /hwɛɪɛʧ/ is replaced by [twɛɪɛʧ] this is considered correct for the sake of this subtest since it is meant to assess the production of the syllabic structure including the use of consonantal clusters. A percentage of correct word production is recorded for this subtest. The other subtests are easy to score, whereby accurate production is given a score and the total score per subtest is noted. Speech-language pathologists (SLPs) are expected to administer the test, score, analyze the data and compare them to typical data. Table 5.3 summarizes the MESA subtests and what they are meant to assess.

Procedure

Most of the children were assessed at home in one or two sessions. During each one-hour session short breaks were given as often as was considered necessary. A few children were assessed in the University Communication Therapy Teaching and Research Clinic following parental request. Pre-assessment criteria were set in relation to the test administrators' language use for instruction. Maltese was used to give assessment instructions unless the child was English speaking. If unsure, the examiner used the language chosen by the child. When caregivers reported that the child was bilingual, Maltese was used. A novel feature was that the children

Table 5.3 Summary of MESA subtests

Subtest	*Contents*	*Function*	*Analysis*	*Language version*
Articulation assessment	42 colourful pictures with identical plain-coloured background, compiled in a soft bound booklet	Assesses articulation skills	Mismatched/ omitted phones	Maltese and English
Phonology assessment	As above but with different colour-coded background	Assesses aspects of child's phonology	Qualitative and quantitative analyses; identification of child's use of phonological processes (error patterns); percent consonants correct (PCC) and percent vowels correct (PVC)	Maltese and English
Inconsistency assessment	17 target words represented in pictures with yellow background	Assesses consistency of production	Inconsistency score is calculated based on DEAP analysis	Maltese and English
Oro-motor skills assessment	Child asked to repeat after clinician string of sounds/ words or to make oral movements	• Diadochokinesis (DDK) assessment • Consonantal clusters and multisyllabic words assessment • Imitation of single oral and sequenced movements	Specific analytic criteria defined in manual	Instructions administered in child's preferred language

had the choice to respond in either language. Ideally, bilingual children should be tested in both languages. For the MESA study this was not done since data collection already involved considerable time commitment due to the administration of the MESA and a language assessment battery, which extended to two home visits for most children. This decision was also supported by there being only three additional English phonemes which do not exist in Maltese phonology; i.e. /θ, ð, ʒ/. It has been reported (e.g. Grech, 1998) that the Maltese use /t/ and /d/ for /θ, ð/, respectively, when speaking English (generalization of Maltese phonology). Meanwhile, /ʒ/ is the least frequently used phoneme of English (Ball & Müller, 2005). The MESA score sheets allow for code-switching, the data showing that most children produced some words in both languages (Grech & Dodd, 2008). If in the middle of a picture naming task the child shifts to name the picture in the other language, the administrator will record and transcribe the child's utterances accordingly. The child is encouraged to name the respective picture/s in the *other language*. However, if the child does not produce the translation equivalent, the administrator continues the testing.

Reliability of the Maltese-English Speech Assessment

The accuracy and consistency of the MESA was measured by test-retest reliability and inter-rater reliability. Test-retest reliability was estimated by testing 5% of the sample twice (mean age: 51.6 months). The between-test interval was less than five weeks. Inter-rater reliability was measured in relation to the degree of consistency between persons scoring, transcribing and analyzing the children's speech. The audio-recordings of 12 children (5% of Maltese normative sample; mean age: 46.3 months) were transcribed and analyzed by two independent examiners.

Validity

The content and concurrent validity of the MESA were established in different ways. The data from the typically developing children using MESA were compared with those in Azzopardi (1997) and Grech (1998). These studies presented data from typically developing children. Azzopardi's (1997) phonological study investigated the development of Maltese consonants and some consonant clusters in four-year-old Maltese-speaking children. A cross-sectional study of 10 children was carried out. Parents were interviewed and relevant screening measures were applied before including children in the study. A phonological sample was collected at each child's home using picture elicitation materials designed specifically for this study. The sample was transcribed and analyzed using the Phonological Assessment of Child Speech (PACS; Grunwell, 1985). The results indicated that: (a) fricatives and liquids were most likely to be misproduced; (b) only five developmental processes (error patterns) were observed, thus indicating that the children had eliminated most developmental phonological processes; and (c) many of the clusters were produced consistently.

Grech's (1998) exploratory study was related to the phonological development of 21 normally developing Maltese-speaking children. The children were recorded in their natural settings at four different stages between the ages of 24 and 42 months. The data collected were transcribed narrowly and analyzed. Each child's phonetic/phonological inventory was identified; various developmental phonological processes were also recorded throughout the period of study. A developmental profile was collated for the group, indicating trends of stages of phonological development. This profile was compared crosslinguistically. The data fit in with current theories highlighting universal phonological acquisition particularly in the early years. As predicted, some language-specific behaviour was also observed.

The usefulness of the MESA was also validated by data from a clinical population (not part of the larger cohort of the study). It was hypothesized that data from children who had been clinically identified with speech sound disorder would differ from that of the *normative* sample and from that of children with *other* communication impairments. Differential diagnosis of these children with impairments was made by a clinician using various speech and language assessment tools that are not *standardized* on the local population because standardized tests for Maltese children were unavailable. The same criteria as for the *normative* sample were applied with regard to the decision as to whether these children were considered monolingual or bilingual. The clinician administered the MESA to 17 children with speech impairment and 13 children with one or more of the following, but who did not exhibit a speech impairment: autistic spectrum disorder, attention deficit and hyperactivity disorder, learning difficulties, fluency, word finding, dysphonia and specific language impairment.

Results

The analyses completed on the speech data included the following quantitative measures: percent consonants correct (PCC), percent vowels correct (PVC), percent inconsistency score, diadochokinetic score (DDK), single and sequenced oral movements (SSM) scores and word repetition (WR) score. Z-scores, standard scores and percentiles were calculated for each age band, for monolingual and bilingual children aged between 36 and 72 months of age, allowing the detection of children performing below the typical range for this cohort. Data of the children who were younger than 36 months of age were not converted to standard scores and presented in the appendices because of the limited number of subjects. Standard scores are given in Appendices A–L, where it can be seen that for both monolingual and bilingual children, scores for PCC and word repetition follow a developmental trajectory (although this is less clear for the oromotor measures).

Analyses of the data for consonant accuracy (PCC) for the monolingual Maltese-speaking and the bilingual children indicated an increase in phonological competence over the age range and differences between children exposed to one as opposed to two languages at home are reported (see Table 5.4) in Grech and Dodd (2008). Other analysis of phonological processes (error patterns) and consistency of production are also reported in Grech and Dodd (2008). The authors indicated no significant difference in the number of phonological processes used between those exposed to one or two languages at home, for the younger cohort ($F_{1,91} = 1.99$, $p = 0.162$). For older children (46–72 months), however, children exposed to two languages at home had fewer phonological processes than children exposed to only one language ($F_{1,130} = 7.77$, $p < 0.01$). The children exposed to two languages at home had suppressed the developmental processes more rapidly than those exposed only to Maltese.

As for the consistency subtest, it is reported in Grech and Dodd (2008) that the bilingual children aged between 24 and 47 months had a mean inconsistency score of 7.78% (*SD* 9.7, Range 0–41%) on the 17 words in the consistency test, while older (48–72 month olds) bilingual speakers had a mean inconsistency score of 1.56% (*SD* 4.9, Range 0–21). The younger monolingual Maltese speakers (24–47 months of age) produced 15.09% (*SD* 21.5, Range 0–85%) of the 17 words in the consistency test inconsistently over three productions, while older children had a mean inconsistency score of 4.39% (*SD* 7.5, Range 0–41%). A one-way ANOVA (four groups: younger and older children exposed at home to Maltese and English or Maltese) was significant ($F_{1,207} = 11.328$, $p < 0.001$). Post hoc Bonferroni tests established that younger bilingual children were more consistent than younger children from homes where only Maltese was spoken (mean difference 7.3, $p < 0.05$). There was no difference in consistency between the older children from different

Table 5.4 Test-retest correlation for quantitative measures (within subjects)

Score type	*Intraclass correlation*	*95% confidence interval*		*F*			
		Lower bound	*Upper bound*	*Value*	*df1*	*df2*	*Sig*
PCC	0.705	0.131	0.925	5.774	8	8	0.011*
DDK	0.665	0.057	0.913	4.968	8	8	0.018*
Inconsistency	0.187	–0.504	0.733	1.462	8	8	0.302
Word repetition[a]	–	–	–	–	–	–	–
Oro-motor movements	0.458	–0.245	0.845	2.689	8	8	0.092

Notes: Since the test was only repeated once, the single measures result is reported. PCC = percentage consonant correct; DDK = diadochokinesis.

[a]Word repetition scale has zero variance items.

*$p < 0.05$.

language backgrounds. Younger children exposed only to Maltese at home were less consistent than older children (mean difference 10.7, $p < 0.001$), but this was not true for the bilingual group.

Reliability

Test-retest reliability. Since the tests were up to five weeks apart and since the younger children may be both somewhat inconsistent and developing fairly rapidly, one might predict that test-retest results will not demonstrate perfect agreement but should be highly correlated. The correlation between the scores is summarized in Table 5.4. The test scores between measures were all significantly correlated with the exception of inconsistency. The agreement percentage on the production of consonants and error patterns is summarized in Table 5.5. Consonant production is highly consistent across the two times of testing. Error patterns are also generally consistent but there are some exceptions, notably fronting. An error pattern was considered to be used by a child if this occurred at least five times. The same criterion was applied for acknowledging error patterns in the main study as reported in Grech and Dodd (2008) and in the DEAP (Dodd *et al.*, 2002).

Inter-rater reliability. The correlation between scores is summarized in Table 5.6. It can be seen that all measures correlate significantly. The agreement percentage on the production of consonants and error patterns is summarized in Table 5.7. Intriguingly there is low agreement for fronting, but other measures have high agreement.

Comparison with a clinical sample

Table 5.8 summarizes the clinical data. The two groups of the clinical sample were well matched. There was a trend for the speech impaired group to be younger, but this was not significant. Table 5.9 shows the quantitative severity measures of the clinical sample, indicating that the speech impaired group produced more consonant errors, are more inconsistent and do not produce more vowel errors than those with no speech difficulties. There is a trend towards significance for DDK scores. There was no significant difference for other oro-motor measures between the two clinical groups. There was no significant difference between the two groups for percentage correct word repetition. Tables 5.10 and 5.11 refer to the severity measures of the clinical sample for articulation skills and phonological processes, respectively. Most sounds were articulated by the children in both clinical groups except for the ones highlighted in Table 5.10. It can be seen that the speech impaired children have more sounds missing and a higher proportion of missing sounds. The mean usage of developmental processes for the clinical sub-groups expressed as whole numbers is indicated in Table 5.11; it can be seen that the developmental processes are more common in the speech impaired category for 11/12 processes.

Table 5.5 Test-retest agreement percentage on the production of consonants and error patterns

Items	*Agreement (%)*
Consonants	
z	100
d	100
v	100
g	100
s	100
f	100
k	100
ʃ	91.67
r	91.67
ts	100
ʤ	91.67
ʧ	100
Error patterns	
Cluster reduction	96.83
Weak syllable deletion	91.67
Consonant harmony	100
Syllable initial consonant deletion	91.67
Syllable final consonant deletion	91.67
Reduplication	100
Gemination	91.67
Compensatory vowel lengthening	100
Fronting	75.00
Fronting of fricatives	58.33
Gliding	68.42
Lateralization of /r/	91.67
Stopping	100
Deaffrication	100
Devoicing	91.67
Affrication	100
Voicing	100
Methatesis	100
Backing	91.67

Table 5.6 Inter-rater correlation for quantitative measures

Score type	*Intraclass correlation*	*95% Confidence interval*		*F*			
		Lower bound	*Upper bound*	*Value*	*df1*	*df2*	*Sig*
PCC	0.714	0.267	0.908	6.004	11	11	0.003**
DDK	0.544	−0.013	0.843	3.386	11	11	0.027*
Inconsistency	0.803	0.421	0.943	9.132	10	10	0.001**
Word repetition[a]	1.000	1.000	1.000	–	12	–	–
Oro-motor movements	0.651	0.121	0.893	4.737	10	10	0.011*

Notes: Since each rater took one measurement, the single measures result is reported.
PCC = percentage consonant correct; DDK = diadochokinesis.
[a]For Word repetition scale 100% agreement between raters was obtained.
$*p < 0.05$;
$**p < 0.01$.

Discussion

Does the Maltese-English Speech Assessment demonstrate that a single battery can effectively assess mono- and bilingual children?

The results from the MESA were consistent with a developmental trajectory and it was possible to develop standard scores for test administration since the population tested in this study represent 2% of the total population in question (see Appendices A–L). This applies to both monolingual and bilingual children. This calculation is based on the average number of annual births in Malta which is around 4000 (National Statistics Office and Public Registry; personal communication). The assessment battery worked particularly well with respect to the children's use of both languages, which was quite common. In an entirely monolingual test it is problematic to decide how to deal with items where another language is used; since in this test either English or Maltese was acceptable all responses could be used in the analysis.

Does the speech acquisition pattern for these two populations differ?

The data highlighted in Appendices A–L indicate that children reported to be monolingual differed from children reported to be bilingual in Maltese and English. The Appendices indicate a clear pattern of faster phonological acquisition for bilingual children as from 42 months of age when compared to the monolingual cohort. This 'positive transfer' is in line with other studies (e.g. Kehoe *et al.*, 2001; Lleó *et al.*, 2003). In this context positive transfer refers to when multilingual children exhibit speech sound skills that are more advanced than their monolingual peers.

Table 5.7 Inter-rater agreement percentage on the production of consonants and error patterns

Items	*Agreement (%)*
Consonants	
z	100
d	100
v	100
g	100
s	100
f	100
k	100
ʃ	100
r	91.67
ts	100
ʤ	100
ʧ	100
Error patterns	
Cluster reduction	97.53
Weak syllable deletion	83.33
Consonant harmony	100
Syllable initial consonant deletion	91.67
Syllable final consonant deletion	91.67
Reduplication	100
Gemination	91.67
Compensatory vowel lengthening	100
Fronting	58.33
Fronting of fricatives	33.33
Gliding	71.43
Lateralization of /r/	91.67
Stopping	91.67
Deaffrication	75.00
Devoicing	83.33
Affrication	100
Voicing	100
Methatesis	100
Backing	83.33

However, these findings are not in line with those reported by Fabiano-Smith and Goldstein (2010) for Spanish-English speaking children who did not exhibit acceleration (i.e. a faster rate of acquisition) when compared with monolingual peers on overall phonological accuracy, although these skills in the bilingual children were within the normal range of their monolingual counterparts in both English and Spanish. The data collected in this study

Table 5.8 Characteristics and statistical comparison of the clinical sample

	Speech impaired	*No speech difficulties*	*Statistical significance*
N	17	13	
Age (in months)	61 (13) 38–84	69 (11) 51–84	F (1,28) = 3.492; p = 0.072
Gender	5 girls, 12 boys	1 girl, 12 boys	
Language background	4 bilingual 13 monolingual	4 bilingual 9 monolingual	

indicate that early bilingual exposure might enhance phonological acquisition. The claim that children in a bilingual learning context may be at an advantage for spoken phonological acquisition is supported by other researchers who looked at children exposed to more than one language (e.g. Bialystok *et al.*, 2005 for English-Spanish or Hebrew; Yavaş & Goldstein, 2006 for Spanish-English). Children who are regularly exposed to more than one spoken language would need to discriminate between languages using phonological cues and consequently become aware of the constraints specific to each language's phonology and increase their phonological knowledge.

Is the Maltese-English Speech Assessment a reliable and valid test of speech development?

This study also addressed the question as to whether the MESA is a reliable and valid clinical tool which distinguishes between typically developing

Table 5.9 Quantitative severity measures of the clinical sample

	Speech impaired	*No speech difficulties*	*Statistical significance*
No. of subjects	17	13	F
PCC	78.5 (25) 12–100	93.4 (8.4) 73–100	F (1,28) = 4.388*
PVC	99.8 (0.3) 99–100	100 (0)	F (1,28) = 1.73; NS
Inconsistency	19.2 (21) (0–64)	6.5 (6.7) 0–18	F (1,28) = 4.429*
DDK	3.7 (2.8) 0–6	5.38 (1.7) 0–6	F (1,28) = 3.968; p = 0.056
Single/sequenced Oro-motor movements	4.9 (1.9) 0–6	5.4 (1.0) 3–6	F (1,28) = 0.735; NS
% Correct word repetition	60.5 (33.5) 0–100	80.9 (22.8) 39–100	F (1,28) = 3.57; p = 0.07; NS

Notes: Scores for speech impaired/no speech difficulties represent mean, standard deviation (in parenthesis) and range, respectively. PCC = percentage consonant correct; PVC = percentage vowels correct; DDK = diadochokinesis.
*$p < 0.05$; NS = not significant.

Table 5.10 Severity measures of the clinical sample (articulation skills)

Missing speech sound	*% of children with missing phone*	
	Speech impaired	*No speech difficulties*
Voiced alveolar fricative /z/	12	8
Voiced labiodental fricative /v/	12	0
Voiced velar plosive /g/	18	8
Voiceless labiodental fricative /f/	12	0
Voiceless velar plosive /k/	6	8
Voiceless postalveolar fricative /ʃ/	18	8
Alveolar approximant/tap/trill /r/	24	0
Voiceless alveolar affricate /ts/	29	0
Voiceless postalveolar affricate /tʃ/	24	0

children and those with delayed or disordered speech. Table 5.5 highlights a high correlation between test and retest for quantitative measures. Table 5.6 indicates that a high percentage test-retest agreement was reached in relation to the children's production of consonants and error patterns. The relatively low agreement for fronting of fricatives and gliding may be due to the fact that these developmental error patterns are often very unstable; in some instances there was a four to five week gap between test and retest which may have reflected on phonological developmental progress. Similarly, a high correlation was obtained for inter-rater quantitative measures. Table 5.7 shows a high percentage agreement for the children's production of

Table 5.11 The mean usage of phonological processes for the clinical sub-groups expressed as whole numbers

Phonological process	*Speech impaired*	*No speech difficulties*
Mean cluster reduction occurrence per child	13	10
Weak syllable deletion	10	2
Consonant harmony	10	10
Initial consonant deletion	17	2
Final consonant deletion	24	8
Syllable reduplication	4	0
Vowel lengthening	17	6
Fronting	32	11
Gliding	18	17
Stopping	8	1
Delinking affricates	28	8
Voicing errors	48	3

consonants and error patterns when rated by different assessors. The relatively low agreement for fronting and gliding may be due to the fact that gliding and fronting are difficult to perceive even in the case of a trained ear; transcription was supported by audio-recordings which were often affected by poor signal-to-background noise ratio. The MESA is therefore a reliable tool to measure aspects of speech of monolingual and bilingual Maltese children. The error patterns are consistent with those found in the DEAP (Dodd *et al.*, 2002) for children who chose to do the test mainly in English and with Azzopardi (1997) and Grech (1998) for Maltese-speaking children. This contributes to the validity of the MESA. Its validity is further supported by the clinical sample data.

Does the Maltese-English Speech Assessment distinguish between typically developing children and those with delayed or disordered speech (making the assessment a useful tool for clinicians working with Maltese-speaking children?)

The quantitative severity measures of the clinical sample summarized in Table 5.9 show that the children in the speech impaired group produced more consonant errors, were more inconsistent and did not produce more vowel errors than those with no speech difficulties. This points towards the validity of the MESA as a clinical tool for the diagnosis of speech impairment. There is a trend towards significance for DDK scores; the difference is probably due to fronting (/k/→[t]) rather than sequencing, fluency or precision of articulation. The fact that there is no significant difference for other oro-motor measures between the two clinical groups replicates other findings for speech disordered children and normally speaking controls. Only children with motor speech disorder do poorly on these tasks, as opposed to children with phonological disorder. Percentage correct word repetition just failed to reach significance ($p = 0.07$), but the mean scores were 60.5% versus 80.9% correct. Tables 5.10 and 5.11 indicate that the speech impaired group showed more missing phones and phonological processes. Therefore, the MESA proved to be a clinically discriminatory and a valid tool for the assessment of speech disorders, since the two groups differed on key measures specific to speech, but not, as could be predicted, on the oro-motor measures. The MESA will aid clinicians in differentiating between *typical* language development patterns and language disorder and in directing the most effective intervention to children who struggle with developing phonetic and phonological skills.

Conclusion

The MESA is an innovative protocol where the subtests devised are truly bilingual in nature. Hence, a child living in Malta would be tested in Maltese and/or English depending on which language/s (or language mix) s/he would be exposed to. This innovation is time-cost efficient in that bilingual children do not need to go through two different tests for checking proficiency of speech skills since, as indicated above, the Maltese use mainly Maltese phonemes when speaking English. However, if the clinician has time, it would be ideal to administer the test in both English and Maltese to the bilingual child.

It also reflects the reality of the way in which children use language in a bilingual situation. The MESA has been shown to be a clinically useful tool for assessing children differentiating between sub-types of speech disorder. Administration of the complete battery should enable the tester to differentiate between disorders of articulation (organic and functional), delayed phonological development, consistent and inconsistent phonological disorder and childhood apraxia of speech. Clinicians using the MESA will be able to reach a differential diagnosis that determines choice of evidence-based treatment approach. Therefore the MESA leads to the improvement of the quality of life of the communication disordered population. Moreover, as was hypothesized, the data collected clearly show that children reported to be monolingual by parents differ from children reported to speak both Maltese and English at home in terms of phonological acquisition patterns. From the point of view of the test battery itself, it is clear that the standard scores for bilingual and monolingual children need to be given separately.

The results have implications for education, speech language pathology, psychology and linguistics. For education, teachers of Maltese-speaking children currently have little information about the language competence of typically developing children at school entry, since 'test-book' knowledge is derived from studies of monolingual English speakers in the UK and US. The study's results will allow curriculum modification to better suit children's competence and improve learning outcomes. SLPs currently have no normative data on the rate and course of speech development in Maltese, making choice of intervention targets difficult. Educational psychologists' assessment of verbal cognitive ability is hampered by the dearth of information on Maltese speech and language development. It is hoped that other researchers would use the same framework to develop similar assessments for other bilingual groups in European Member States and elsewhere.

Appendix A: Standard Scores for Quantitative Measure: Monolingual Percent Consonants Correct

Standard scores	*Raw scores*					
	Group 2 36–41 months	*Group 3 42–47 months*	*Group 4 48–53 months*	*Group 5 54–59 months*	*Group 6 60–65 months*	*Group 7 66–72 months*
17						
16						
15						
14						
13						
12	99–100	100		100		
11	95–97	96–99	97–100	98–99		99–100
10	87–90	92–93	95–96	96	99–100	97
9	80–82	88	90–92	95	98	91–93
8	79	83–86	86–88	94		86–87
7	72	80	82	91–92		85
6			80			
5						
4					88	
3						
2						
1						

Appendix B: Standard Scores for Quantitative Measure: Bilingual Percent Consonants Correct

Standard scores	*Raw scores*					
	Group 2 36–41 months	*Group 3 42–47 months*	*Group 4 48–53 months*	*Group 5 54–59 months*	*Group 6 60–65 months*	*Group 7 66–72 months*
17						
16						
15						
14						
13						
12	100					
11	96–99	98–100		100		100
10	93–95	94–97	100		92–100	99
9	91	90		99		98
8	86–87	89		96		
7		89–90				96
6		87–88	91			
5		74				
4						
3						
2						
1						
0						

Appendix C: Standard Scores for Quantitative Measure: Monolingual Percent Vowels Correct

Standard scores	Raw scores					
	36–41 months	*42–47 months*	*48–53 months*	*54–59 months*	*60–65 months*	*66–72 months*
17					100% All groups	100% All groups
16						
15				100		
14						
13						
12						
11		100				
10	100		100			
9	87		99			
8						
7						
6						
5						
4						
3				99		
2						
1						
0						

Appendix D: Standard Scores for Quantitative Measure: Bilingual Percent Vowels Correct

Standard scores	*Raw scores*					
	Group 2 36–41 months	*Group 3 42–47 months*	*Group 4 48–53 months*	*Group 5 54–59 months*	*Group 6 60–65 months*	*Group 7 66–72 months*
17		100% All groups	100% All groups	100% All groups		
16						
15						
14						
13						
12						
11	100					
10					100	100
9						
8						
7						
6						97
5					99	
4						
3						
2						
1						

Appendix E: Standard Scores for Quantitative Measure: Inconsistency Monolingual Scores

Standard scores	*Raw scores*					
	36–41 months	*42–47 months*	*48–53 months*	*54–59 months*	*60–65 months*	*66–72 months*
17						
16			41	35		
15	71					24
14		46–53			12	
13						
12			18–19	12	6	12
11	29	18–24	12			6–7
10	12–20	6–12	6	6	0	
9	0	0	0	0		0
8						
7						
6						
5						
4						
3						
2						
1						
0						

Appendix F: Standard Scores for Quantitative Measure: Inconsistency Bilingual Scores

Standard scores	*Raw scores*					
	36–41 months	*42–47 months*	*48–53 months*	*54–59 months*	*60–65 months*	*66–72 months*
17						
16						
15					6	
14	21		21	12		
13		24				6
12	13	20		6		
11		12	6			
10	6	6			0	
9	0	0	0	0		0
8						
7						
6						
5						
4						
3						
2						
1						
0						

Appendix G: Standard Scores for Quantitative Measure: DDK Monolingual Scores

Standard scores	*Raw scores*					
	36–41 months	*42–47 months*	*48–53 months*	*54–59 months*	*60–65 months*	*66–72 months*
17						
16						
15						
14						
13						
12	6		6			
11	5	5–6	5	5–6	6	6
10	3–4	4	4	4	5	5
9	2	3	2–3	3	4	
8		2		2		4
7	0	0	0		2	
6				0		2
5					0	
4						
3						
2						
1						
0						

Appendix H: Standard Scores for Quantitative Measure: DDK Bilingual Scores

Standard scores	*Raw scores*					
	36–41 months	*42–47 months*	*48–53 months*	*54–59 months*	*60–65 months*	*66–72 months*
17						100% All groups
16						
15						
14						
13						
12	6					
11	5	6	6	6	6	
10	4	4–5	4–5			
9	2	3		5	4	
8		2	2			
7	0		0		2	
6		0		3		
5						
4						
3						
2						
1						
0						

Appendix I: Standard Scores for Quantitative Measure: SSM Monolingual Scores

Standard scores	Raw scores					
	36–41 months	42–47 months	48–53 months	54–59 months	60–65 months	66–72 months
17						
16						
15						
14						
13	6					
12						
11	5	6	6	6		
10	4	5	5		6	6
9	3					
8	2	2–3	4	5		
7	1	1				
6		0	2	4		
5						
4					3	5
3						
2						
1						
0						

Appendix J: Standard Scores for Quantitative Measure: SSM Bilingual Scores

Standard scores	*Raw scores*					
	36–41 months	*42–47 months*	*48–53 months*	*54–59 months*	*60–65 months*	*66–72 months*
17						100% All groups
16						
15						
14						
13						
12	6					
11	5		6	6		
10		6		5	6	
9	4					
8	3			4		
7				3		
6		5	5			
5					3	
4						
3						
2						
1						
0						

Appendix K: Standard Scores for Quantitative Measure: Word Repetition Monolingual Scores

Standard scores	*Raw scores*					
	36–41 months	*42–47 months*	*48–53 months*	*54–59 months*	*60–65 months*	*66–72 months*
17						
16						
15						
14						
13						
12	100					
11	90–94	100	100	100	100	100
10	67–79	91				96
9	64	82				91
8	33–34	50–73	82	91	82	80
7	27		72		72	
6				82		
5					64	64
4						
3						
2						
1						
0						

Appendix L: Standard Scores for Quantitative Measure: Word Repetition Bilingual Scores

Standard scores	*Raw scores*					
	36–41 months	*42–47 months*	*48–53 months*	*54–59 months*	*60–65 months*	*66–72 months*
17						
16						
15						
14						
13						
12						
11	100				100	100
10	82	91–100		100		
9	64				94	
8						
7	37					
6				67		97
5		27				
4						
3						
2						
1						
0						

References

Amayreh, A. and Dyson, A. (1998) The acquisition of Arabic consonants. *Journal of Speech, Language, and Hearing Research* 41, 642–653.

Azzopardi, S. (1997) Phonological development of consonants in 4-year-old Maltese children. Unpublished dissertation, University of Malta.

Ball, M. and Müller, N. (2005) *Phonetics for Communication Disorders.* Mahwah, NJ: Lawrence Erlbaum.

Ballard, E. and Farao, S. (2008) The phonological skills of Samoan speaking 4-year-olds. *International Journal of Speech-Language Pathology* 10 (6), 379–391.

Bialystok, E., Luk, G. and Kwan, E. (2005) Bilingualism, biliteracy, and learning to read: Interactions among languages and writing systems. *Scientific Studies of Reading* 9, 43–61.

Bickford-Smith, A., Wijayatilake, L. and Woods, G. (2005) Evaluating the effectiveness of an early years language intervention. *Educational Psychology in Practice* 21 (3), 161–173.

Borg, A.J. and Azzopardi-Alexander, M. (1997) *Maltese.* London: Routledge.

De Houwer, A. (2009) *Bilingual First Language Acquisition.* Bristol: Multilingual Matters.

Dodd, B., Crosbie, S., Zhu, H., Holm, A. and Ozanne, A. (2002) *The Diagnostic Evaluation of Articulation and Phonology.* London: Psychological Corporation.

European Commission (2008) *Speaking for Europe: Languages in the European Union.* Luxembourg: Office for Official Publications of the European Communities. See http://library.umac.mo/e_resources/org_publications/b11868156.pdf.

Fabiano, L. and Goldstein B. (2005) Phonological cross-linguistic effects in bilingual Spanish-English speaking children. *Attachment and Human Development* 3, 56–63.

Fabiano-Smith, L. and Goldstein, B. (2010) Phonological acquisition in bilingual Spanish-English speaking children. *Journal of Speech, Language, and Hearing Research* 53, 160–178.

Fox, A. (2000) The acquisition of phonology and the classification of speech disorders in German-speaking children. Unpublished PhD thesis, University of Newcastle-upon-Tyne.

Goldstein, B. and Gildersleeve-Neumann, C. (2015) Bilingualism and speech sound disorder. *Current Deventmental Disorders Reports* 2, 237–244; doi:10.1007/s40474-015-0049-3.

Goldstein, B. and Washington, P. (2001) An initial investigation of phonological patterns in 4-year-old typically developing Spanish-English bilingual children. *Language, Speech, and Hearing Services in Schools* 32, 153–164.

Grech, H. (1998) Phonological development of normal Maltese speaking children. Unpublished PhD thesis, University of Manchester.

Grech, H. and Dodd, B. (2008) Phonological acquisition in Malta: A bilingual learning context. *International Journal of Bilingualism* 12, 155–171.

Grech, H., Dodd, B. and Franklin, S. (2011a) *Maltese-English Speech Assessment (MESA).* Malta: University of Malta.

Grech, H., Franklin, S. and Dodd, B. (2011b) *Language Assessment for Maltese Children (LAMC).* Malta: University of Malta.

Grunwell, P. (1985) *Phonological Assessment of Child's Speech (PACS).* Windsor: NFER-Nelson.

Holm, A. and Dodd, B. (1999a) Differential diagnosis of phonological disorder in two bilingual children acquiring Italian and English. *Clinical Phonetics and Linguistics* 13, 113–129.

Holm, A. and Dodd, B. (1999b) An intervention case study of a bilingual child with phonological disorder. *Child Language Teaching and Therapy* 15, 139–158.

Holm, A. and Dodd, B. (1999c) A longitudinal study of the phonological development of two Cantonese-English bilingual children. *Applied Psycholinguistics* 20, 349–376.

Holm, A. and Dodd, B. (2006) Phonological development and disorder of bilingual children acquiring Cantonese and English. In H. Zhu and B. Dodd (eds) *Phonological*

Development and Disorders in Children: A Multilingual Perspective (pp. 86–325). Clevedon: Multilingual Matters.

Johnson, C. and Lancaster, P. (1998) The development of more than one phonology: A case-study of a Norwegian-English bilingual child. *International Journal of Bilingualism* 2, 265–300.

Kehoe, M., Trujillo, C. and Lleó, C. (2001) Bilingual phonological acquisition: An analysis of syllable structure and VOT. In K.F. Cantone and M.O. Hinzelin (eds) *Proceedings of the Colloquium on Structure, Acquisition and Change of Grammars: Phonological and Syntactic Aspects* (pp. 38–54). Hamburg: Universität Hamburg: Arbeiten zur Mehrsprachigkeit.

Kheshavarz, M. and Ingram, D. (2002) The early phonological development of a Farsi-English bilingual child. *International Journal of Bilingualism* 6, 265–300.

Lleó, C., Kuchenbrandt, I., Kehoe, M. and Trujillo, C. (2003) Syllable final consonants in Spanish and German monolingual and bilingual acquisition. In N. Müller (ed.) *(In)vulnerable Domains in Multilingualism* (pp. 191–220). Amsterdam: John Benjamins.

MacLeod, A.A.N., Sutton, A., Trudeau, N. and Thordardottir, E. (2011) The acquisition of consonants in Québécois French: A cross-sectional study of pre-school aged children. *International Journal of Speech-Language Pathology* 13 (2), 93–109; doi:10.3109/17549507.2011.487543.

Ministry of Education and Employment (2016) *A Language Policy for the Early Years in Malta and Gozo*. See https://education.gov.mt/en/Documents/A%20Language%20Policy%20for%20the%20Early%20Years%20Consultation%20Document.

Munro, S., Ball, M.J., Müller, N., Duckworth, M. and Lyddy, F. (2005) The acquisition of Welsh and English phonology in bilingual Welsh-English children. *Journal of Multilingual Communication Disorders* 3, 24–49.

Navarro, A., Pearson, B., Cobo-Lewis, A. and Oller, D. (1995) Early phonological development in young bilinguals: Comparison to monolinguals. Paper presented to the *American Speech, Language and Hearing Association Conference 1995*.

Paradis, J. (2001) Do bilingual two-year-olds have separate phonological systems? *International Journal of Bilingualism* 5, 19–38.

Rome-Flanders, T. and Cronk, C. (1998) Stability and usefulness of language test results under two years of age. *Journal of Speech and Language Pathology and Audiology* 2 (2), 74–80.

Salameh, E.-K., Nettlebladt, U. and Norlin, K. (2003) Assessing phonologies in bilingual Swedish-Arabic children with and without language impairment. *Child Language Teaching and Therapy* 19, 338–364.

Shriberg, L. and Kwiatkowski, J. (1994) Developmental phonological disorders I: A clinical profile. *Journal of Speech and Hearing Disorders* 51, 140–161.

Shriberg, D., Austin, D. and Lewis, B.A. (1997) The percentage of consonants correct (PCC) metric: Extensions and reliability data. *Journal of Speech, Language, and Hearing Research* 40, 708–722.

Skahan, S. and Lof, G. (2007) Speech-language pathologists' assessment practices for children with suspected speech sound disorders: Results of a national survey. *American Journal of Speech-Language Pathology* 16, 246–259.

Slavik, A. (2001) Language maintenance and language shift among Maltese migrants in Ontario. *International Journal of the Sociology of Language* 152, 131–152.

So, L. and Dodd, B. (1994) Phonologically disordered Cantonese-speaking children. *Journal of Clinical Linguistics & Phonetics* 8, 235–255.

Stow, C. and Dodd, B. (2003) Providing an equitable service to bilingual children in the UK. *International Journal of Language & Communication Disorders* 38 (4), 351–377.

Sundara, M., Polka, L. and Genesee, F. (2006) Language experience facilitates discrimination of /d/ in monolingual and bilingual acquisition of English. *Cognition* 100, 369–388.

To, C.K.S., Cheung, P.S.P. and McLeod, S. (2012) A population study of children's acquisition of Hong Kong Cantonese consonants, vowels, and tones. *Journal of Speech, Language, and Hearing Research* 56, 103–123; doi:10.1044/1092-4388(2012/11-0080).

Watson, I. (1991) Phonological processing in two languages. In E. Bialystock (ed.) *Language Processing in Bilingual Children* (pp. 25–48). Cambridge: Cambridge University Press.

Wright, K. and Gildersleeve-Neumann, C. (2005) Speech-sound development in preschoolers from bilingual Russian-English language environments. Poster presented at the *Oregon Speech-Language-Hearing Association Conference 2005*.

Yavaş, M. and Goldstein, B. (2006) Aspects of bilingual phonology: The case of Spanish-English bilingual children. In B. Dodd and H. Zhu (eds) *Phonological Development and Disorders: A Cross-linguistic Perspective* (pp. 265–285). Clevedon: Multilingual Matters.

Zhu, H. and Dodd, B. (2000) The phonological acquisition of Putonghua (Modern Standard Chinese). *Journal of Child Language* 27, 3–42.

Zhu, H. and Dodd, B. (2006) *Phonological Development and Disorders: A Multilingual Perspective.* Clevedon: Multilingual Matters.

6 Early Language Development in a Bilectal Context: The Cypriot Adaptation of the MacArthur-Bates CDI

Loukia Taxitari, Maria Kambanaros, Georgios Floros and Kleanthes K. Grohmann

Introduction

The investigation of language development over the past decades has mainly focused on monolingual development (e.g. Clark, 2004; Golinkoff *et al.*, 1999), although bilingual development has gained ground over the last 20 years, with researchers studying different aspects of it, from lexical and phonological development to the effects of bilingualism on cognitive function (e.g. Pearson & Fernández, 1994; Werker & Byers-Heinlein, 2008). Lexical and morphosyntactic development are both quite well described and different aspects of them are now well understood in monolingual populations; researchers have been tracing similarities and differences from bilingual populations.

A grey area between the two extremes, monolingualism and bilingualism, has recently received much-needed attention (Grohmann, 2014; Grohmann & Kambanaros, 2016): discretely *bilectal* populations (Rowe & Grohmann, 2013), that is, speakers in linguistic communities traditionally characterized as diglossic, where more than one variety of the same language co-exist. One such case is Cyprus, where the local dialect, Cypriot Greek (CG), co-exists with the standard variety, Standard Modern Greek (SMG); however, this approach can arguably be extended to countries in which distinct dialects co-exist with a higher standard, such as Germany, Great Britain, Italy, Norway or Switzerland.

Recent research on the development of Greek in Cyprus suggests that CG-speaking children acquire morphosyntax differently from their monolingual SMG-speaking peers in mainland Greece (Grohmann, 2011; Grohmann & Leivada, 2012; Kambanaros *et al.*, 2012). Also, Durrant *et al.* (2015) compared the phonological representations of familiar words between mono- and bidialectal 18-month-olds in British English and found that only monodialectal children could detect phonological mispronunciations of words, suggesting that multidialectalism may impact the degree of specificity of one's phonological representations in early infancy. The question then is whether children who are exposed to more than one language variety (that is, standard form, dialect, etc.) grow up more akin to monolinguals or to bilinguals, or whether there could be a third, intermediate, option between mono- and bilingualism with its own special characteristics (cf. Grohmann & Kambanaros, 2016; Kambanaros *et al.*, 2014).

One way to study language development is through the use of the MacArthur-Bates Communicative Development Inventory (CDI), a questionnaire addressed to parents of children who are asked to provide feedback on their child's language, mainly the lexicon and morphosyntax, through very specific targeted questions. The CDI has been adapted to over 63 languages and dialects, and more recently a growing number of bilingual CDIs are becoming available (for a full collection, see http://mb-cdi.stanford.edu). It has been widely used to describe children's language abilities at different ages, month by month: the number of words understood and produced, most popular words or semantic categories, word use, grammatical development, and more (Fenson *et al.*, 1994, 2000, 2007; Jørgensen *et al.*, 2010). Also, percentiles of collected samples can be produced and new data compared to available norms in order to help identify children at risk for language and communication difficulties. Data for various adaptations, both monolingual and bilingual, are now available online and can be used for comparisons between languages (see the Wordbank website at http://wordbank.stanford.edu).

Recently, Taxitari *et al.* (2015) used the CG adaptation of the MacArthur-Bates Communicative Development Inventory (CDI) to look at two- to three-year-olds' lexical development, through the study of translation equivalent (TE) pairs in a first pilot study with the tool. TE pairs refer to words with a different lexical form in two varieties with the same meaning. CG-speaking children were reported to produce many such TE pairs, that is, both a CG and an SMG word for the same concept. This behaviour is suggested to arise in contrast to mutual exclusivity, a well-known constraint in monolingual children's lexical development evidenced from around two years of age; mutual exclusivity refers to the tendency to attach a new label to a name-unknown object, as a way to avoid double labels for objects (Au & Glusman, 1990; Markman & Hutchinson, 1984; Markman *et al.*, 2003). CDI data from English- and French-speaking children, however, show that bilingual children actually make use of multiple labels for a single concept from very early in life, exhibiting a lack of, or overriding, mutual exclusivity from as young as 13 months of age (De Houwer *et al.*, 2006). Similarly, CG-speaking children use words from both varieties, CG and SMG, to refer to the same concept, departing from monolingual children's behaviour, who are rather reluctant to attach two labels to the same concept.

In the current study, we present data from the CG-CDI in children between 18 and 30 months, in three-month intervals. The CG-CDI has been adapted for Greek-speaking Cyprus and data from parents of young children have been collected in an effort to better understand early language development on the island. The aims of the study were twofold: to study early lexical and grammatical development, including the creation of a lexical-semantic as well as a morphosyntactic profile of bilectal children's language development, and to investigate specific aspects of bilectal children's early language development which could give us clues to the question as to how this group of children is best described linguistically. For the latter, we focus on TE pairs, which provide information on how flexibly concepts and words (acoustic forms) are treated by children in this bilectal population.

Method

Participants

Parents of children in five age groups (18, 21, 24, 27 and 30 months) participated in this study. Table 6.3 shows the mean age and standard deviation, as well as the gender distribution in each of the five groups. All children were recruited for the LexiKyp project (CG-CDI) through online outreach (Facebook, Cyprus Acquisition Team lab website, LexiKyp project website), other advertisements in the form of leaflets (nurseries, children's clinics, playgrounds), and recruiting events around Cyprus. Some parents were approached directly by the research team and others volunteered by contacting the project administrator themselves or signing up through an online registration system.

Along with the CG-CDI, parents were asked to answer a number of demographic questions which might relate to and affect language development, modelled after the Language and Background Development Questionnaire (Paradis *et al.*, 2010, 2011). These questions targeted information about different aspects of the child's development (premature birth, birth order in the family, frequent ear infections) and language environment (exposure to languages other than Greek, having a housemaid at home from a different country, or one of the parents not being Greek Cypriot), as well as parents' educational level and any history of language problems in the family (see section on Demographic Questions below for more details).

All children were exposed only to (Cypriot) Greek from birth, and on a daily basis. None of the children was systematically exposed to any other language; children were excluded if the parents reported that the child was exposed to another language for more than 10 hours per week. All children were full-term (not more than six weeks premature) and had no history of hearing problems, ear infections or any kind of language impairment/problem. The questionnaire was completed only by mothers.

Cypriot Greek and Standard Modern Greek

Over the past decades there has been considerable discussion in the literature regarding an exact definition of the linguistic situation in Greek-speaking Cyprus. Recently, Rowe and Grohmann (2013) suggested that the country is currently transitioning through a state of diglossia, and Tsiplakou (2014) argues for a partial convergence of a Cypriot *koiné* to SMG through innovative, structurally mixed forms together with systematic language alternation in the form of code-switching, code-mixing and register shifting. This Cypriot *koiné* is the variety used in urban centres on the island, retaining many of the characteristics of CG but also leaving behind many of the features of CG geographical sub-varieties and replacing them with more standard-like features. For the purposes of this paper, by CG we will refer to the CG *koiné*.

At all levels of linguistic description, there are similarities and differences between the two varieties, with some levels more closely related than others. Phonology and syntax seem to remain quite distinct in the two varieties, while morphological features tend to be more mixed in the *koiné*. There is still considerable debate in the literature as to whether CG and SMG form part of a continuum or not, and the question which arises is when exactly during language development these different features are acquired and when they become separated (or even merged). In the CG-CDI the focus is on lexical development, as well as on the development of different morphosyntactic features as explained in the next section, so we will not be concerned with phonology here.

Cypriot Greek-CDI: Words and sentences

The CG adaptation of the *MacArthur-Bates Communicative Development Inventory: Words and Sentences* (Fenson *et al.*, 1994) was used in this study. The *CDI: Words & Sentences* consists of two sections: Part I: *Words Children Use* and *Word Use*, and Part II: *Sentences & Grammar* and *Word Combinations*. Several demographic questions were given to parents before the questionnaire, which were based on an adaptation for Greek Cypriot parents of the *Developmental and Language Background Questionnaire* (Paradis *et al.*, 2010, 2011; Taxitari *et al.*, 2015).

Part I: Words children use and Word use

The first part of the CDI focuses on words and their use. The first section consists of a long list of words and parents are asked to mark which of those words their child produces, if any. The questionnaire includes a total of 817 words, divided in 24 categories: Sounds (17), Animals (56), Toys (24), Food and Drink (84), Vehicles (18), Home Objects (63), Furniture and Rooms (40), Clothes (34), Outside Things (34), People (39), Body Parts (30), Games and Routines (45), Verbs (96), Descriptive Words (50), Places to Visit (24), Quantitatives and Articles (21), Pronouns (27), Propositions and Words for Place (30), Colours and Shapes (14), Numbers (21), Modal and Auxiliary Verbs (18), Connectives (9), Words for Time (12) and Question Words (12). Although words are presented in isolation, some context is provided to parents as words are divided in different semantic categories. 'Grammatical' categories also exist, such as modal and auxiliary verbs or question words.

The CG-CDI is the adaptation of the CDI in CG containing both SMG and CG forms. As far as the lexicons of the two varieties are concerned, a large proportion of the lexicon is shared, but differences between CG and SMG might be found both lexically and phonologically. So there are three ways a concept might behave across the two varieties. First, a concept might be lexically the same, for example, the words for *hand* or *mouth*, where the word could further be phonologically different (SMG ['çeri] and CG ['ʃeri] for *hand*) or identical (['stomɐ] in both varieties for *mouth*). A second possibility is that a single concept might be lexically different in CG and SMG, for example, the word for *head* ([ce'fɐli] in SMG and [cʰ:el:e] in CG). Finally, a concept could exist in only one of the two varieties, for example, [tʰ:oros] in CG is equivalent to *bath towel*, which does not exist as a single word in SMG, where instead the word [pe't͡setɐ] for *towel* is generally used.

In the CG-CDI, we list as separate entries only items which differ lexically. For this, we include both concepts with different words in the two varieties and concepts which can be found in only one variety. Words which differed phonologically in the two varieties were entered in the CG-CDI as a single entry, for example, the above ['çeri] and ['ʃeri] for *hand*, and where possible the two different pronunciations were provided. Parents were asked to mark which pronunciation their child uses.

The CG-CDI contains a total of 817 words (110 words found only in CG, and 717 words found in SMG but also common to CG) for 729 concepts. Fewer concepts exist than words because a single concept can correspond to both a CG and an SMG word, as described above. There are thus 91 such TE pairs, with words from both varieties that correspond to a single meaning. The number of words included in this adaptation is remarkably higher than other monolingual versions, such as the American English CDI. The number is also fairly much lower than bilingual CDIs, which include two different lists of words, one from each language. The CG adaptation includes words from both varieties in one long list. The reason is that CG (as well as SMG) is a variety of Greek, and CG and SMG share a big portion of their lexicon. This results in very few CG-only words in the CG-CDI, and a large number of shared words.

The second section of Part I includes five questions on the child's frequency of word use, and parents need to answer them on a 3-point scale ('never' – 'sometimes' – 'often') depending on how often their child uses the word in the particular way. These questions relate to the use of words in the absence of the actual object or event: if the child uses the word to refer to the past or the future, if the child talks about absent objects, if the child will bring an object when someone asks for it, and if the child will talk about someone's object in the absence of the person to which the object belongs.

Part II: Sentences & Grammar and Word combinations

This part consists of several sections designed to study the use of morphosyntax by young children. Section 1, *Use of grammar*, includes seven questions which could be answered on a 3-point scale (never – sometimes – often) about the use of different grammatical markers by the child. These include the use of plural, genitive possessive, subjunctive, past tense prefix ε-/*e*-, gender agreement between nouns and adjectives, person agreement between subject and verb, diminutive, and case agreement in different sentence slots.

Sections 2–5 investigate grammar in more detail, with questions targeting several aspects of Greek morphology. Greek morphology, both CG and SMG, is rich in the sense that different semantic relations are expressed in the form of bound morphemes, often endings, which are attached onto verbs and nouns. In the following, we provide the original written form in Greek which, where necessary, we transliterate (in italics) and translate (in single quotes). For transliteration conventions, we employ the Latin alphabet where there is correspondence to English (e.g. the Greek 'θ' corresponds to the voiceless 'th' in English or the diphthong 'ου' to romanized 'u') and the original Greek where they do not (e.g. Greek 'δ' or 'γ').

Verb stems and endings encode information about person, number, tense, voice and duration of the action. For example, the form *αγαπ-ώ* (*aγapo* 'I love') is the first person, singular, present tense and active voice of the verb 'to love', while *αγαπ-ούμε* (*aγapume* 'we love') is the first person, plural, present tense and active voice of the same verb. On the other hand, *αγαπ-ιέμαι* (*aγapieme* 'I am loved') is the first person, singular, present tense, passive voice of the verb. The first person, singular, active voice, past tense, completed form of the verb is *αγάπ-**ησ-α*** (*aγapisa* 'I loved'), where -*ησ*- is the past tense suffix and -*α* the first person singular ending, while the first person, singular, active voice, past tense but continuous form is *αγαπ-**ούσ-α*** (*aγapusa* 'I was loved'), where -*ούσ*- is the past tense continuous suffix and -*α* the first person singular ending. Nouns also encode different kinds of information in their endings, such as gender, number and case. The word *αγάπ-η* (*aγapi* 'love') is singular, feminine, nominative/accusative case, while *αγάπ-ες* is the equivalent in plural. All nouns are accompanied by articles (definite or indefinite), which also encode the same kind of information: gender, number and case. Adjectives also need to agree with nouns in the same dimensions, encoded in their endings. For example, in the phrase *τον τεράστιο ελέφαντα* (*ton terastio elefada*), the definite article *τον* 'the', as well as the adjective *τεράστιο* 'huge' both agree in number (singular), gender (masculine) and case (accusative) with the noun *ελέφαντα* 'elephant'. Although CG and SMG morphology coincide in many forms, there are differences in the formation of certain types of verbs and nouns, with different suffixes in the two varieties. When this occurred in the CG-CDI, the different options were provided for participants to choose from.

Table 6.1 shows sections 2–5, the type of questions used and the grammatical points targeted in detail. The first question of each section is always a yes–no question and involves whether the child had already began using the grammatical point, while a different question asks parents whether the child makes any mistakes in creating the right grammatical form and, if so, to give some examples. Section 2, *Plural*, focuses on the way children form the plural of nouns, by asking parents to judge which ending the child would use for specific words belonging to three different genders (masculine, feminine and neutral) and different inclinations. In this grammatical aspect, there were no differences between CG and SMG forms. Section 3 focuses on verbs and is divided into four sub-sections: *Present*, *Past*, *Future* and *Duration*. For the *present* form of the verbs, parents are asked if the child changes the endings of verbs to denote person, as is typical in Greek morphology, and also to choose between different ways to form the present, including CG and SMG forms, for active and passive voice. For *past*, several ways for past tense formation are provided and parents are asked to choose how their child would form the past tense for different types of verbs. A separate question also asks parents whether the child opts to consistently add the past tense prefix *ε-* in past tense forms, which is always added in verbs for forming the past tense in CG but not in SMG forms. For the *future tense*, parents are only asked to choose which future tense particle the child would use for forming the future, having to choose between particles in CG (*εννά/enna*) and SMG (*θα/tha*). For *duration*, a multiple choice question provides various verb forms in the past/present progressive or completed, and parents are asked to choose which ones the child would produce for different types of verbs. No differences between the two varieties are targeted in this section. Section 4 is about *negation*, and this also involves several particles for expressing negation, from which parents need to choose the one(s) their child produces, including CG (*μεν/men*, *εν/en*, *έντζιαι/entʃe*) and SMG (*μην/min*, *δεν/ðen*) forms. In Section 5 several grammatical categories which typically accompany *Nouns* are targeted: *Articles*, *Adjectives* and *Comparatives*. Regarding *articles*, a multiple choice question asks parents which article their child would use with

Table 6.1 Detailed description of each section of Part II with the types of questions and grammatical points investigated

Section	*Grammatical feature*	*Type of question*	
(2) Plural	Noun plural	Yes/no question for use Multiple choice Errors – examples	masculine in *-ος, -ης, -ας, -ους* feminine in *-α, -η, -ου* neutral in *-ο, -ι, -α, -ως*
(3) Verbs	Present tense	Yes/no question for use Multiple choice	active – passive voice
	Past tense	Yes/no question for use Multiple choice Errors – examples	verbs in *-ω, -ώ, -ίζω, -άζω, -νω, -αίνω, -ζω* + irregular (*βλέπω/ vlepo* 'to see') use of past tense prefix *-ε*
	Future tense	Yes/no question for use Multiple choice	future particle *θα/εννά* (*tha/ enna*), subjunctive particle *να* (na)
	Duration	Yes/no question for use Multiple choice Errors – examples	progressive or completed verbs in *-ω, -ώ, -ίζω, -άζω, -βω, -λω, -νω, -χω* + irregular (*τρώω/troö* 'to eat')
(4) Negation	Verbal negation	Yes/no question for use Multiple choice Errors – examples	negation particle *όχι* (*ochi*), *δεν/εν* (*δen/en*), *μην/μεν* (*min/men*), *έντζιαι* (*entντ*)
(5) Nouns	Articles (definite and indefinite)	Yes/no question for use Multiple choice Errors – examples	article used with nouns: masculine ending in *-ος, -ας, -ης, -ους*; feminine nouns ending in *-η, -α, -ου*; neutral nouns ending in *-ο, -ι*
	Adjectives	Yes/no question for use Errors – examples	
	Comparatives	Yes/no question for use Multiple choice Errors – examples	*καλύτερο* (*kalitero* 'better'), *πιο καλό* (*pjo kalo* 'even better'), *πιο καλύτερο* (*pjo kalitero* 'best')
(6) Sentence complexity	Three longer sentences produced by the child		

different kinds of nouns. For *adjectives* the question only involves whether the child produces combinations with noun-adjective agreement (gender, number, case). Finally, for *comparatives*, parents are provided with a number of choices as to how to form the comparative form of nouns and are asked which one their child uses. In this section there are no differences between the two varieties.

Demographic questions

Several demographic factors have been shown to affect the size of children's expressive vocabulary in the past, such as birth order and parents' education levels (see, for example, Fenson *et al.*, 2007). Also, demographic information was collected in order to select participants on the basis of their health history and their family's language situation as well as history of language impairments. For the purposes of the current study a shorter version of the *Developmental and Language Background Questionnaire* was created, which is based on the ALEQ and ALDeQ questionnaires originally developed by Paradis *et al.* (2010, 2011) and subsequently modified in COST Action IS0804 (Tuller, 2015). The questionnaire had been translated into Greek for a previous CG-CDI study, in order to control for the different factors which could affect children's lexical development (Taxitari *et al.*, 2015).

The LexiKyp project version included general information about the child (name, birth date, gender, order of birth in family), followed by the child's health history (frequent ear infections or other illnesses), his or her exposure to other languages (if and how much the child is exposed to another language, whether there is a housemaid from another country in the household, or if one of the parents comes from another country), the educational level of mother and father, and any history of language difficulties or impairments in the family.

Procedure

The contact details of all volunteers in the study were registered in the LexiKyp database, which stored contact details and birth dates of children at different ages. Parents (exclusively mothers) were contacted when their child reached the right age for the study in one of five age groups: 18, 21, 24, 27 and 30 months. They were reminded about the project and the procedure, and asked if they would still like to take part. Parents who agreed to participate received an email which contained instructions as to how to access the online version of the CG-CDI on the SurveyMonkey website, along with a password for entering the study and a unique participant code for each parent. The first page of the online questionnaire gave the parent all the necessary information about the CG-CDI and asked for the parent's consent to proceed. Each parent participated in only one age group; if, however, parents did not complete the questionnaire after the first contact, they were contacted again at a later age unless they explicitly asked otherwise. Prior to the study, full ethical approval was obtained from the Cyprus National Bioethics Committee.

Parents were asked to complete the CG-CDI at their own time and place, but preferably when they would be uninterrupted. If they needed to stop and continue later, they could save their responses, sign out, and continue the completion at a later time. They were asked not to talk to other people or to the child herself while completing the questionnaire, and solely rely on their own knowledge about their child's language and communicative skills.

In Part I, the vocabulary checklist of the CG-CDI, parents were instructed to mark the field if their child produces a word, or leave it unmarked otherwise. They were also informed that they would find some words in CG in the word list and that they would sometimes find a word for an object in both CG and SMG. They were instructed to mark the version their child uses or mark both if the child uses both. They were also instructed to accept different pronunciations of the word from the child, as long as the word is systematically used by the child to refer to the concept in question.

In Part II, for each morphosyntactic feature, parents were asked if their child has started producing that specific element; if the parent answered yes, they would then proceed to more detailed questions. If they answered no, they would skip the remaining questions related to the particular element, and proceed to the next.

Reliability

Although this was not the main focus of the study, a small percentage (10%) of mothers was re-tested with the tool on average 46.8 days from their first completion of the form in order to test for intra-rater reliability. In addition, a small percentage of fathers (13.5%) was tested as well along with the mothers in order to test for inter-rater reliability in the age group of 21 months.

Scoring

For every item in the CG-CDI vocabulary checklist that the parent reported their child produced, a single point was given; fields left unmarked received no points. Extra words that the parent added were not considered, since this constituted a subjective listing of words from the parents' behalf and was optional when filling in the questionnaire. Words in the two varieties which correspond to the same concept were marked as TEs – for example, SMG [pɐsxɐˈli͡tsɐ] and CG [pɐpɐˈrunɐ] for *ladybird*. There are 91 such pairs in the CG-CDI; each word received one point to yield a total vocabulary score for each child. In order to calculate a conceptual vocabulary score, all TEs received one point, irrespective of whether the child produced only the CG word, only the SMG word, or both. Following de Houwer *et al.*'s (2006) terminology, CG and SMG words which make up a TE pair are called *members* of that pair. So, when a child produces only the CG or only the SMG member, she is said to produce a *singlet*; when, on the other hand, the child produces both members of the pairs, she is said to produce a *doublet*.

For every item in Part II (Sentences and Grammar) that the parent reported their child produced, a single point was given for up to 10 points.

Measures

In order to test children's expressive vocabulary in the bilectal CG-CDI, two measures were calculated, *total vocabulary score* (the total number of words the child can say, coming from both SMG and CG) and *total conceptual vocabulary* (by subtracting the number of doublets a child says from her total vocabulary score). Also, the number of TE pairs produced was measured as well as the number of singlets and doublets produced in these pairs. Additionally, a *total CG score* and a *total SMG score* were calculated from the TE pairs. Total scores were also calculated for the following grammatical categories: Nouns (animals, food & drink, vehicles, toys, house objects, outside objects, body parts, places to visit, clothes, furniture & rooms, people, numbers, colours & shapes), Verbs (verbs, modal & auxiliary verbs), Function words (pronouns, quantitatives & articles, questions, prepositions & words for place, connectives & particles), Adjectives (descriptive words), Adverbs (words for time), and Other (sounds, games & routines).

For Part II of the CG-CDI a *total morphosyntactic score* was calculated as a measure of grammatical complexity, on the basis of the number of morphosyntactic features the parent reported their child producing.

On the basis of the demographic information parents provided, children in each age group were divided into two categories depending on their birth order in the family (first-borns versus later-borns). A score from 1 to 7 was also calculated for each of the parents' level of education based on the European Social Survey (REF) using a 7-point Likert scale with Primary School Graduate as (1) and PhD holder as (7) on the scale. Table 6.2 shows the mean and standard deviation for each age group's maternal and paternal education scores.

Analysis

The main statistical analysis employed was an Analysis of Variance (ANOVA) comparing *production* (total, doublets, singlets, SMG, CG, grammatical categories, birth order and grammatical complexity) across age groups and gender. Pearson *r* correlations were also run between the different grammatical category scores and the total production scores in the CDI, as well as

Table 6.2 Maternal and paternal education for each age group separately

Age group	*Maternal education Mean (SD)*	*Paternal education Mean (SD)*
18	5.44 (0.89)	5.00 (1.49)
21	5.67 (0.72)	5.31 (1.17)
24	5.22 (0.91)	4.97 (1.10)
27	5.38 (0.94)	4.90 (1.32)
30	5.46 (0.92)	4.88 (1.30)

between the *total vocabulary score* and the *total morphosyntactic score*. The latter analysis was also performed for each age group separately, investigating the relationship between total production scores and maternal/paternal education levels, and also for testing inter- and intra-rater reliability.

Results

Development of the lexicon

Vocabulary production

A univariate ANOVA with total vocabulary score as a dependent variable, and age group and gender (male versus female) as fixed factors, revealed significant main effects of age group, $F_{(4,173)} = 44.65$, $p < 0.001$, $\eta^2 = 1$, and an interaction between age group and gender, $F_{(4,173)} = 2.72$, $p < 0.05$, $\eta^2 = 0.74$, and only a marginal main effect of gender, $F_{(1,173)} = 3.33$, $p = 0.70$, $\eta^2 = 0.44$. Figure 6.1 shows the increase in vocabulary production across ages and

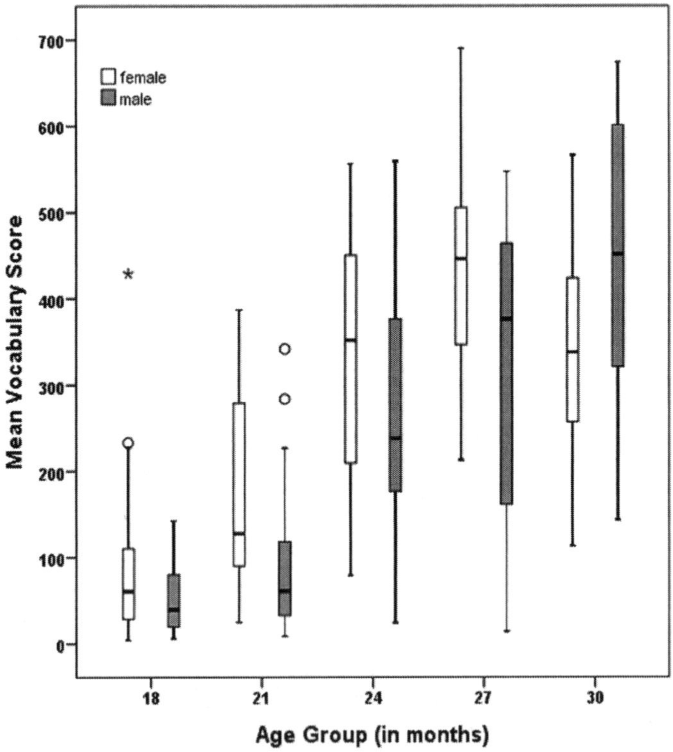

Figure 6.1 Increase in total vocabulary production score across ages, by gender (significant increase in total vocabulary by age, $F_{(4,173)} = 44.65$, $p < 0.001$, $\eta^2 = 0.52$)

Table 6.3 Participants' information for the five age groups (mean age, gender distribution and mean vocabulary score)

Age group	*Mean age in months (SD)*	*Number (female/male)*	*Mean vocabulary score (SD)*	*Mean conceptual vocabulary score (SD)*
18	17.85 (0.35)	44 (24/20)	72.97 (78.69)	71.23 (75.97)
21	20.78 (0.36)	36 (18/18)	142.47 (112.26)	139.31 (109.49)
24	23.91 (0.36)	32 (12/20)	289.16 (147.82)	283.25 (142.97)
27	26.92 (0.33)	28 (16/12)	385.07 (158.52)	373.82 (155.37)
30	29.76 (0.40)	33 (11/22)	411.82 (188.58)	400.61 (182.27)

separately for each gender; Table 6.3 shows the mean vocabulary score for each age group separately, collapsed for gender.

In order to further investigate the main effect of age group, planned post hoc comparisons showed significant differences in vocabulary production between all ages (ps < 0.05), except for age groups 18 and 21 months, as well as age groups 27 and 30 months.

In order to further investigate the interaction between gender and age group, independent-samples t-tests were run for each age group independently comparing word production in boys and girls. Only at age 21 months was there a significant difference between boys and girls, with the latter producing more words than boys, $t_{(34)} = 2.21$, $p < 0.05$. No significant differences were found between the other four groups (ps > 0.05). In order to test for intra- and inter-rater reliability, a percentage of mothers was re-tested with the tool as well as a percentage of fathers, and the data were correlated with the first time mothers completed the CG-CDI. Spearman Rho correlations showed that both the mothers who were re-tested and the fathers who were tested along with the mother showed positive significant correlations between their reports: intra-rater, $r_s = 0.37$, $p < 0.01$/inter-rater, $r_s = 0.28$, $p < 0.01$.

Production of different concepts

As with the total vocabulary score, a univariate ANOVA with total conceptual vocabulary score as a dependent variable, and age group and gender (male versus female) as fixed factors, was run. As for the previous analysis, it revealed a significant main effect of age group, $F_{(4,173)} = 45.68$, $p < 0.001$, $\eta^2 = 0.53$, and an interaction between age group and gender, $F_{(4,173)} = 2.76$, $p < 0.05$, $\eta^2 = 0.63$, and only a marginal main effect of gender, $F_{(1,173)} = 3.39$, $p = 0.07$. Table 6.3 shows the increase in conceptual vocabulary across ages.

Grammatical class

Univariate ANOVAs were run separately for each of the five grammatical classes, with percentage of the total vocabulary as a dependent variable and age as a fixed factor. A significant increase in the percentage of the children's total vocabulary was shown for: Nouns, $F_{(4,173)} = 7.24$, $p < 0.001$, $\eta^2 = 0.15$; Verbs, $F_{(4,173)} = 13.40$, $p < 0.001$, $\eta^2 = 0.24$; Adjectives, $F_{(4,173)} = 18.67$, $p < 0.001$, $\eta^2 = 0.31$; and Adverbs, $F_{(4,173)} = 12.79$, $p < 0.001$, $\eta^2 = 0.23$. A significant decrease was found for: Other Words, $F_{(4,173)} = 33.47$, $p < 0.001$, $\eta^2 = 0.44$; and no change in the percentage as a fraction of the total for Function Words, $F_{(4,173)} = 0.29$, $p = 0.89$. Figure 6.2 presents the grammatical classes as a fraction of the total vocabulary across ages in a pie chart plot.

However, because of the high variability in children's profiles and total vocabulary scores at these early stages of lexical development, a second analysis was run without the division in age groups but taking into account only the children's vocabulary scores. These were correlated with the percentage of each grammatical class as a fraction of the total vocabulary in Pearson r correlations. As with the ANOVA, total vocabulary score correlated positively with: Nouns, $r_{(173)} = 0.25$, $p < 0.01$; Verbs, $r_{(173)} = 0.71$, $p < 0.01$; Adjectives, $r_{(173)} = 0.76$, $p < 0.01$; and Adverbs, $r_{(173)} = 0.55$, $p < 0.01$; and negatively with Other Words, $r_{(173)} = -0.71$, $p < 0.01$. However, unlike the ANOVAs, there was a marginal correlation with Function Words, $r_{(173)} = 0.14$, $p = 0.07$.

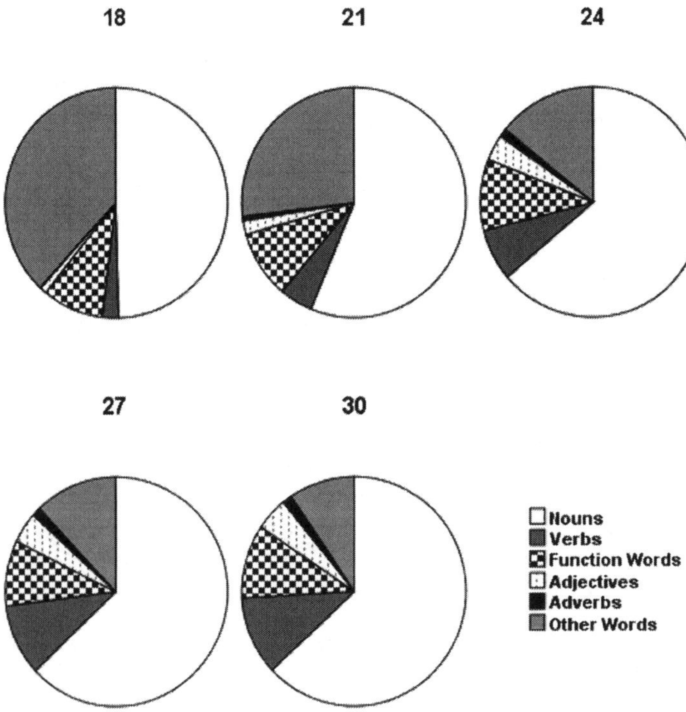

Figure 6.2 Percentage of each grammatical class as a fraction of children's total vocabulary

Morphosyntactic production

A univariate ANOVA with grammatical complexity as a dependent variable, and age group and gender (female versus male) as fixed factors, showed significant main effects of age, $F_{(4,173)} = 34.91$, $p < 0.001$, $\eta^2 = 0.46$, and gender, $F_{(1,173)} = 7.78$, $p < 0.001$, $\eta^2 = 0.05$, with an advantage of girls over boys in grammatical complexity. No interaction between age group and gender was found, $F_{(4,173)} = 2.13$, $p = 0.08$, $\eta^2 = 0.05$. Figure 6.3 shows the number of morphosyntactic features produced separately for each age group and gender.

In order to further investigate the main effect of age, Bonferroni post hoc comparisons showed that at 18 and 21 months children differed from all the rest of the groups ($ps < 0.01$), but not between ($p = 1$). The same was found for the 27- and 30-month-olds, who performed higher than the rest of the groups ($ps < 0.05$), but not differently from each other ($p = 1$). In order to then assess the main effect of gender, and on the basis of the pronounced difference in grammatical complexity between girls and boys at ages 27 and 30 months shown in Figure 6.4, one-way ANOVAs with grammatical complexity as a

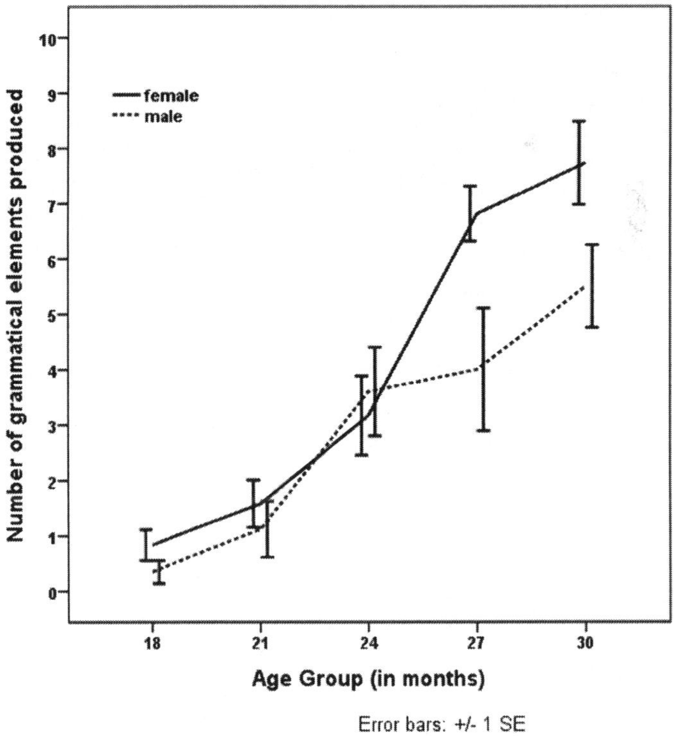

Figure 6.3 Number of morphosyntactic features produced shown separately for each age group and gender

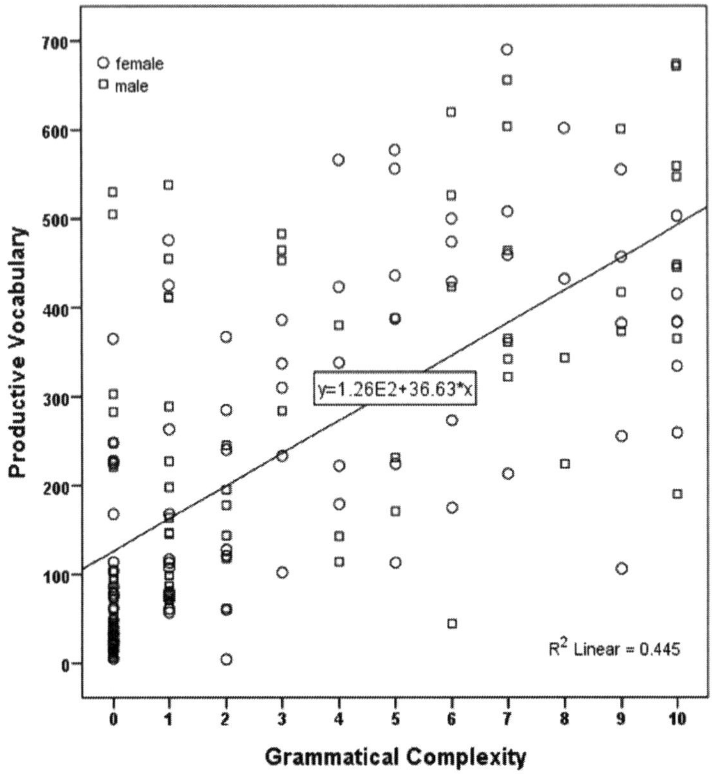

Figure 6.4 Positive correlation between the size of the children's lexicons as reported by parents, and their morphosyntactic ability, $r_{(173)} = 0.67$, $p < 0.01$

dependent variable and gender as grouping factor were run for each age group separately. Only at 27 months was there a significant difference in grammatical complexity with an advantage of girls over boys, $F_{(1,26)} = 6.40$, $p < 0.05$, while a marginal difference was noted at 30 months, $F_{(1,32)} = 3.53$, $p = 0.07$.

Relationship between vocabulary and morphosyntax

To test the relationship between the size of children's lexicons and their morphosyntactic ability, a Pearson *r* correlation was run comparing total vocabulary score and grammatical complexity. This was shown to correlate positively, $r_{(173)} = 0.67$, $p < 0.01$, as can be seen shown in Figure 6.4.

Interplay between Cypriot Greek and Standard Modern Greek

In order to investigate the early interplay between CG and SMG in children's early lexicons, an analysis of TE pairs was run comparing the production of singlets and doublets, as well as the production of CG and SMG words.

A univariate ANOVA with TE pair production as a dependent variable, and age group and member type (single versus doublet) as fixed factors, showed significant main effects of age, $F_{(4,346)} = 55.32$, $p < 0.001$, $\eta^2 = 0.38$, and member type, $F_{(1,346)} = 280.15$, $p < 0.001$, $\eta^2 = 0.46$, as well as an interaction between age group and member type, $F_{(4,346)} = 15.36$, $p < 0.001$, $\eta^2 = 0.16$. Figure 6.5 shows the number of singlets and doublets produced across ages. Further one-way ANOVAs for doublets and singlets separately showed a significant increase in production for both across ages (singlets, $F_{(4,172)} = 43.00$, $p < 0.001$; doublets, $F_{(4,172)} = 13.12$, $p < 0.001$). In order to further investigate the interaction between age and member type, Bonferroni post hoc comparisons showed that singlet production at 18 and 21 months differed from all other age groups (ps < 0.05), as well as singlet production at 24 and 30 months ($p < 0.05$). The production of doublets at ages of 18, 21 and 24 months differed from doublet production at 27 and 30 months.

A second analysis of the TE pairs focused on which variety the members in those pairs came from. A univariate ANOVA with number of TE pairs

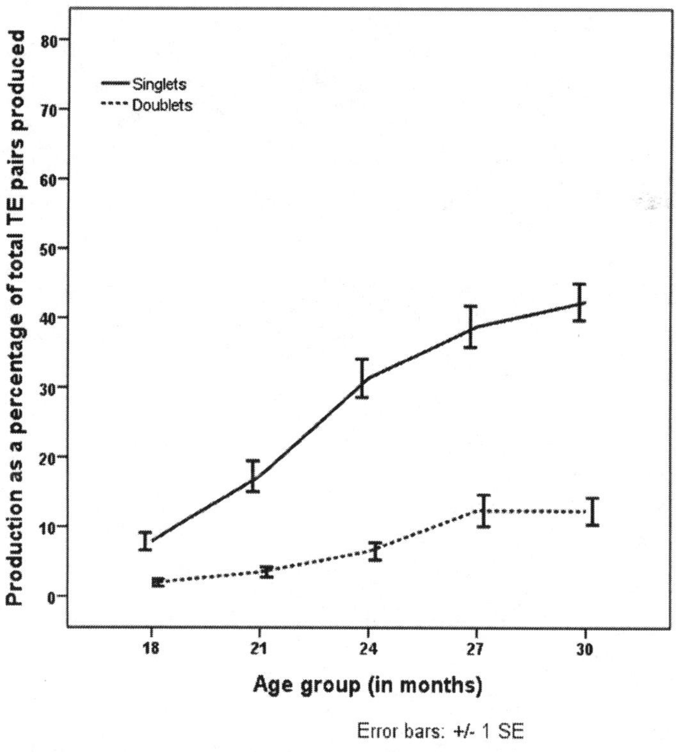

Figure 6.5 TE pairs produced across ages, shown as singlets and doublets separately

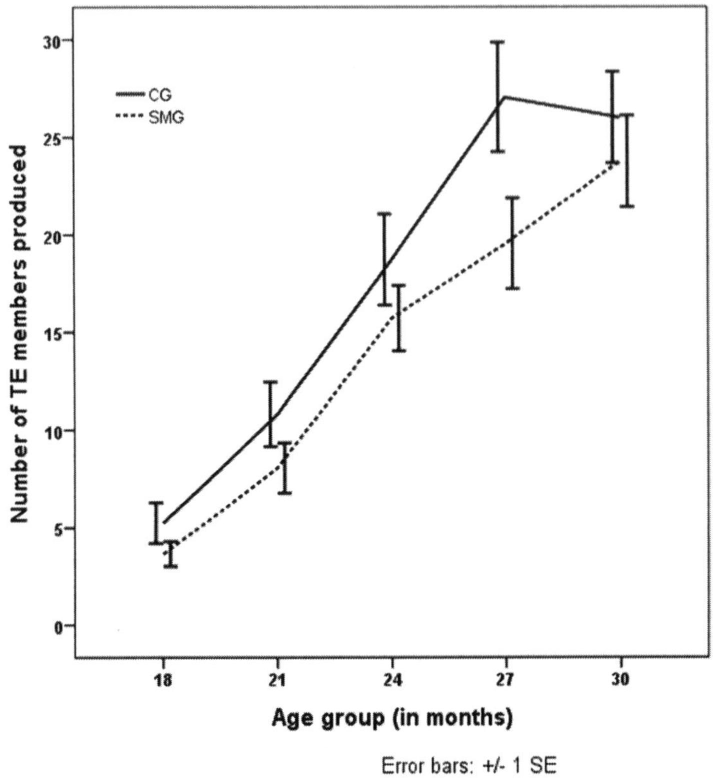

Figure 6.6 TE members produced from each variety across ages

produced as a dependent variable, and age group and variety (CG and SMG) as fixed factors, revealed a main effect of age, $F_{(4,336)} = 49.67$, $p < 0.001$, $\eta^2 = 0.37$, as well as a main effect of variety, $F_{(1, 336)} = 8.68$, $p < 0.01$, $\eta^2 = 0.03$, but no interaction between the two, $F_{(4,336)} = 0.74$, $p = 0.57$. Figure 6.6 shows the production of CG and SMG words as part of TE pairs across ages.

Demographic factors

Birth order in the family as well as maternal and paternal education levels were tested as factors affecting both the children's expressive vocabulary and their morphosyntactic skills on the basis of previous findings in other languages (Fenson *et al.*, 2007). In order to test how birth order affected the size of the expressive vocabulary/grammatical complexity, a Univariate ANOVA with total vocabulary/morphosyntactic score as a dependent variable, and age group and birth order as fixed factors, revealed, as expected, a significant main effect of age group for both vocabulary, $F_{(4,173)} = 46.50$, $p < 0.001$, $\eta^2 = 0.53$, and grammar, $F_{(5,173)} = 25.02$, $p < 0.001$, $\eta^2 = 0.44$. It also revealed a marginal main effect of birth order for vocabulary, $F_{(1,173)} = 3.86$, $p = 0.05$, $\eta^2 = 0.02$, with first-borns ($M = 273.16$, $SE = 12.81$) producing more words than later-borns ($M = 232.84$, $SE = 15.95$) on average, but no such main effect for grammar, $F_{(1,173)} = 1.08$, $p = 0.30$, $\eta^2 = 0.01$. It also showed no interaction between the two for vocabulary, $F_{(4,173)} = 1.12$, $p = 0.35$, $\eta^2 = 0.03$, or grammar, $F_{(4,173)} = 0.02$, $p = 1.00$, $\eta^2 = 0.00$.

In order to investigate how parents' education affected vocabulary and grammar development, Pearson *r* correlations were run for each age group separately with total vocabulary/morphosyntactic score and maternal/paternal education levels. The correlations did not show any meaningful relationship between maternal or paternal education levels and total vocabulary/morphosyntactic score in any of the age groups ($ps > 0.05$).

Discussion

The first aim of this study was the investigation of language development in children who grow up as bilectal speakers in the diglossic community of Greek-speaking Cyprus. The children studied fell into five age groups spanning from 18 to 30 months of age with three-month intervals. In terms of lexical development, the collected data showed a clear increase in word production across these ages, similar to other CDI adaptations and to what can be expected from the word learning literature (see the Wordbank website for data from several languages). This suggests that the CDI, which has been adapted for many languages (and cultures), is proving a suitable and powerful tool for the study of early language development in Cyprus as well.

Children growing up in the bilectal community of Greek-speaking Cyprus are shown at 18 months to have on average a productive vocabulary of around 70 words; this doubles at 21 months and doubles again at 24 months of age, until it reaches over 400 words at 30 months. This trajectory in word production is similar to the trajectory exhibited by toddlers exposed to other languages in Europe, such as German (Szagun *et al.*, 2006), Italian (Caselli *et al.*, 1999) or Turkish, or outside Europe, such as American English or Quebec French (see Wordbank website for data from different languages). It appears then that we can use the CDI to extract crosslinguistic regularities in the development of the lexicon in toddlers and that the size of the lexicon might not be affected to a high degree by language-specific characteristics, as other aspects of language are, such as morphosyntactic development. The size of the lexicon seems to be in line with children growing up as bilinguals as well. The literature provides conflicting information about whether bilinguals have lexicons of similar sizes to monolinguals, with some studies supporting that they are similar if the total vocabulary from both languages is taken into account and other studies supporting that bilinguals lag behind monolinguals (see, for example, De Houwer *et al.*, 2014; Pearson &

Fernández, 1994). Recent data from bilingual CDIs, however, support that monolinguals and bilinguals have similar productive vocabularies if the total expressive vocabulary score from both languages is taken into account (Hoff *et al.*, 2012; Neofytou *et al.*, 2015), further supporting an overall crosslinguistic similarity in the development of the lexicon.

A well-known fact in the study of lexical development (and language development in general) is the high variance of children within and across ages (e.g. Fenson *et al.*, 1994, 2000). Our five age groups also exhibited high variance, which became higher as children grew from 18 to 30 months of age. For this reason, an additional correlational analysis was run which did not include any pre-division of children into age groups, but instead compared the size of their lexicons (total vocabulary score) and the percentages of the different grammatical categories. This showed a pattern very similar to the analysis of the five age groups, apart from the category of *function words*, which has shown a trend for a positive correlation with total vocabulary score not evident in the ANOVA. This suggests that, besides the high variance, age groupings are legitimate in the analysis of lexical development, but they could be obscuring certain patterns which are not immediately visible when children are grouped with children of the same age instead of the same language ability. Our groupings included children with a three-month age difference and this could have allowed for the comparable results between the two analyses; groupings with smaller intervals (of the scale of one month) might not be equally informative, and instead a correlation analysis which takes into account the size of the lexicon might be more appropriate. All in all, variability in the acquisition of language is now considered the norm – children may pass through the same stages during their development but they seem to do so at different ages and paces. The CDI then can give us an indication of the degree to which variability can be normal (Szagun *et al.*, 2014), and this can be used in clinical practice to identify children at risk early on.

Several factors might affect this variability in early language development. Previous studies using the CDI have shown an effect of maternal education on vocabulary as well as morphosyntactic production (Fenson *et al.*, 2007; Huttenlocher *et al.*, 2010; Jackson-Macdonado *et al.*, 2013). Previous studies have also shown an effect of birth order in the family, with first-borns having an advantage over later borns (Fenson, 2007), although this effect was shown not to be as strong a predictor as education level (Huttenlocher *et al.*, 2010). The size of the lexicon, as well as grammatical complexity, were not shown in the current study to be affected by maternal or paternal education levels but, as expected, did show a marginally significant effect of birth order. However, it needs to be acknowledged that parents in the current study came from the higher end of the socio-economic scale on the basis of their education levels, as shown in Table 6.2. This absence, therefore, of a significant relationship between parents' education level and vocabulary/morphosyntactic production could be an artefact of the low number of parents with low education levels and the vast majority of parents at the high end of the scale. In order to further investigate this in the future, a study with a balanced number of parents from different socio-economic and educational levels needs to be designed which will evaluate the actual effect of socio-economic status on toddlers' language development. Such a study will also allow for a better clinical use of the questionnaire, which is not available with the current data as the socio-economic status of the parents was not controlled for.

A division of children's expressive vocabulary into grammatical categories also showed a progression from low variability within children's early lexicons to high variability as children become more advanced word learners. The categories of words from which their lexicons are composed are in agreement with Caselli *et al.*'s (1999) four-stage model of lexical development. In Stage 1, lexicons are composed of *routines and word games*, which correspond to our Other Words category. Stage 2 involves *reference*, and occurs between 50 and 200 words when lexicons are mainly composed of nominals – just as the lexicons of 18- and 21-month-olds in the CG-CDI study are mainly composed of Nouns (as well as Other Words). Stage 3 involves *predication*, and begins to develop after children have accumulated vocabularies of 100–200 words, similar to the significance increase in Verb and Adjective production as the lexicon grew larger, as found in this study. Finally, Stage 4 involves *grammatical function words*, and occurs after children have accumulated vocabularies of more than 400 words. Although we cannot directly observe this stage in our data because our 30-month-olds are on average just reaching the 400-word stage, we did note a trend for an increase in *function words* between 18 and 30 months of age in the correlational analysis. This is possibly due to the fact that these young children's lexicons have not grown large enough yet to exhibit a statistically significant increase in function words; however, function words are present from very early on, and are thought to be memorized routines rather than actual grammatical markers (Caselli *et al.*, 1999). According to Caselli and colleagues (1999), Stage 4 holds strongly in English, where function words rise suddenly after the 400-word threshold, but the increase in function words was found to be linear in Italian from 0 to 600 words. This was thought to be due to the fact that Italian is a morphologically rich language, and children exhibit an advantage in morphosyntactic production earlier than children learning English. With the CG data and the marginal correlation between vocabulary size and function words, we are not certain which of the two is true for the bilectal children growing up in Cyprus. It is possible, however, that the correlation will become stronger if more ages are added to the dataset so that we can follow development without the three-month intervals between ages present in the current dataset.

In terms of morphosyntactic development, grammatical complexity was also shown to exhibit an increase from 18 to 30 months of age. Interestingly, there is a pronounced increase in grammatical complexity between the ages of 21 and 24 months and a second one between 24 and 27 months, which beg for an explanation. The first transition could indicate children's entrance into to 200-word stage, where *predication* develops and verbs and adjectives increase. In a language with rich inflectional morphology such as Greek, this might indicate the simultaneous production of different clitic morphemes in both verbs and nominals. The second transition is possibly related to Stage 4, where more function words are added and the morphosyntactic abilities of children seem to further improve. This explanation is supported by the results of the correlational analysis between vocabulary size and grammatical complexity. Grammatical development in Greek Cypriot children was shown to correlate significantly with the size of their lexicons; this is a relationship widely reported in the literature and present for different languages, such as English, Spanish, Italian, Hebrew and Japanese (see Devescovi *et al.*, 2003), Swedish (Berglund & Eriksson, 2000) and German (Szagun *et al.*, 2006). Devescovi *et al.* (2003) used data from the English and Italian CDIs to argue that vocabulary size is actually a better predictor of grammatical development than both age and gender. This relationship between grammar and vocabulary has been used to support non-modular accounts of language development, where there is a strong interdependence of the different linguistic systems and variability is the key universal characteristic in this process (Marchman *et al.*, 2004; Szagun *et al.*, 2006; Thordardottir *et al.*, 2002).

Devescovi *et al.* (2003) also reported an early advantage in grammatical complexity for Italian over English due to the rich inflectional morphology of the Italian language. Early grammatical development was also noted by Szagun *et al.* (2006) for German, and it can also be seen in the CG data with some morphosyntactic elements produced from 18 months of age. However, more analyses of the grammatical abilities of children and comparisons with children exposed to languages with less rich morphology will need to be carried out before we can argue the same for children exposed to CG.

Both the vocabulary analysis and the grammatical analysis showed gender differences with an advantage for girls (interaction between age group and gender in vocabulary analysis and main effect of gender in morphosyntax analysis). In the CG-CDI, when the vocabulary production of boys and girls was compared individually in each age group, gender differences were only evident at 21 months. Similarly, for grammatical development, robust differences were only traced at 27 months. This is also a well-known effect reported in the literature; gender differences are reported in some languages, such as German (Szagun *et al.*, 2006) and English (Fenson *et al.*, 2000), although they are not found in other languages, such as Swedish (Berglund & Eriksson, 2000) or Hebrew (Maital *et al.*, 2000). In a recent study with 10 non-English languages, the advantage for girls was evident for communicative gestures, productive vocabulary and word combinations, and increased with age. This led the researchers to suggest that the advantage for girls is caused by robust factors that are not specific to each linguistic community, possibly biological in nature, although social factors cannot be ruled out due to an absence of data for gender stereotypes in the linguistic communities under study (Eriksson *et al.*, 2012). Studies with the American English CDI report differences between boys and girls which place girls on average about one month ahead of boys, but these differences account for less than 2% of the variation found within and across ages, and they are mainly limited to production (Fenson *et al.*, 2000). The fact that no differences are found for comprehension in the American English CDI, or in the CDIs of other languages, might suggest that gender differences are actually an artefact of the cultural environment in which the child is raised. Studies by Huttenlocher and her colleagues support that language input from parents and caregivers is a stronger predictor of language skills, both lexical and syntactic, than both gender and SES, suggesting that environmental factors in the form of parental behaviour play a strong role in shaping young children's language abilities, over and above biological gender differences (see Huttenlocher *et al.*, 2010). In other words, exposure to how parents and caregivers speak, and the kind of language they use, determines how children will develop their own language abilities and predicts children's language profiles a few years later. The effects of social variables could then be evident in the linguistic behaviour of children, not only in terms of how much they speak, but also as motivation for using more complex language, both in terms of different lexical items and in terms of complex syntactic structures.

A final analysis involved children's conceptual vocabulary and TE pairs. When *doublets* were taken away from the children's total vocabulary, their conceptual vocabulary showed the same pattern as their total word production. An increase in concept production was noted with increased age, and girls overall produced more concepts than boys. The TE pairs analysis showed the simultaneous production of both *singlets* and *doublets* in every age group, and both of them increased with age. Children in Greek-speaking Cyprus from as young as 18 months of age can produce one or two words for a single concept coming from either variety of the language, with an advantage for CG words which is possibly due to the fact that children acquire CG in daily interactions. But they also produce a high number of SMG words, increasing with age, which cannot be solely attributed to more formal routes of communication, such as the media, cartoons or education. A possible explanation for this could be that parents opt for more standard forms of the language when communicating with their infants and toddlers, thus bringing child-directed speech closer to SMG irrespective of what they themselves use for other types of daily interactions. Additionally, as these bilectal children grow older, they learn more singlets (i.e. more concepts), but they also learn more doublets (i.e. two words for the same concept). This is in agreement with previous findings for bilectal children who acquire CG (Taxitari *et al.*, 2015), but also with bilingual children who comprehend and produce words from two languages for a single concept (de Houwer *et al.*, 2006). Although we cannot be certain that the two words produced refer to the same concept at this young age, they are still used in the early lexicons of children, and in the case of bilinguals at least, they coincide with the absence or a weak form of mutual exclusivity.

This flexibility then of both bilingual and bilectal children to use more than one label for a single concept is taken as evidence against mutual exclusivity, the bias which has been shown to guide monolingual children's language development. Bilectal children are shown here to exhibit similar behaviour to bilingual children, found both in experimental studies and in other CDI studies, which might suggest that bilingual and bilectal children could be closer on the monolingualism–bilingualism continuum than previously thought. Our analysis of TE pairs shows that words for singlets and doublets come from both varieties and there are both dialectal words and standard Greek words in the lexicons of infants even at the early age of 18 months, and they both increase as children grow. This poses a number of theoretical questions about the development of bilectal children's language systems: Do they have a single lexicon, or language system in general, for both varieties of the language, as monolinguals do, or do they form two completely different lexicons, or even systems, as bilinguals do for the two languages? And if they have two, when in development and how do they develop?

Further research is needed to answer these questions, which will combine the current CDI data with other methods of investigation, such as behavioural or physiological data, allowing for more robust conclusions to be drawn, and for studying other aspects of children's linguistic and cognitive development, such as, for example, executive functions. It is also important, especially for the clinical uses of the CDI, that the questionnaire is tested for inter- and intra-rater reliability, and that it is cross-validated with other experimental methods of investigation, so we are confident that the parents in Cyprus provide us with reliable information and that the questionnaire measures what it is designed to measure. Having said that, the fact that we have obtained in the current study results comparable to monolingual and bilingual CDIs in other languages should allow for the current set of data to be used with confidence by researchers, and possibly also by clinicians on the island.

Conclusion

The LexiKyp project is the first large-scale investigation of language development in the bilectal community of Cyprus. Here we present data from five age groups, from 18 to 30 months of age. It is a first effort to study language development on the island, through parental reports on their child's lexical and grammatical development. We aim to create a semantic as well as a grammatical profile, and to study the relationship between vocabulary and grammar in a morphologically rich language, such as Greek. The findings are comparable to data obtained in other languages, documenting the high variability in early language development and the close interdependence between the lexicon and morphology. The CG-CDI is expected to become a valuable tool for researchers and clinicians on the island and the Greek-speaking world in general. Additionally, the study contributes to the understanding of bilectal development in general. We aim to provide answers to the question of where these children are on an assumed monolingualism–bilingualism continuum, applying the idea of comparative bilingualism (Grohmann, 2014) to much younger children; some initial evidence from the use of TE pairs suggests that there could be many similarities between bilectal and bilingual children, which could extend beyond the vocabulary to other aspects of language acquisition and cognitive development.

References

Au, T.K. and Glusman, M. (1990) The principle of mutual exclusivity in word learning: To honor or not to honor? *Child Development* 61 (5), 1474–1490.

Berglund, E. and Eriksson, M. (2000) Communicative development in Swedish children 16–28 months old: The Swedish early communicative development inventory – words and sentences. *Scandinavian Journal of Psychology* 41, 133–144.

Caselli, C., Casadio, P. and Bates, E. (1999) A comparison of the transition from first words to grammar in English and Italian. *Journal of Child Language* 26 (1), 69–111.

Clark, E.V. (2004) How language acquisition builds on cognitive development. *Trends in Cognitive Sciences* 8 (10), 472–478.

De Houwer, A., Bornstein, M.H. and De Coster, S. (2006) Early understanding of two words for the same thing: A CDI study of lexical comprehension in infant bilinguals. *International Journal of Bilingualism* 10 (3), 331–347.

De Houwer, A., Bornstein, M.H. and Putnik, D.L. (2014) A bilingual–monolingual comparison of young children's vocabulary size: Evidence from comprehension and production. *Applied Psycholinguistics* 35 (6), 1189–1211.

Devescovi, A., Caselli, M.C., Marchione, D., Reilly, J. and Bates, E. (2003) A cross-linguistic study of the relationship between grammar and lexical development. *Journal of Child Language* 32 (4), 759–786.

Durrant, S., Delle Luche, C., Cattani, A. and Floccia, C. (2015) Monodialectal and multidialectal infants' representation of familiar words. *Journal of Child Language* 21 (1), 447–465.

Erikkson, M., Marschik, P.B., Tulviste, T. *et al.* (2012) Differences between girls and boys in emerging language skills: Evidence from 10 language communities. *British Journal of Developmental Psychology* 30, 326–343.

Fenson, L., Dale, P.S., Reznick, J.S., Bates, E., Thal, D. and Pethick, S. (1994) Variability in early communicative development. *Monographs of the Society for Research in Child Development* 59 (5), 1–185.

Fenson, L., Bates, E., Dale, P.S., Goodman, J., Reznick, J.S. and Thal, D. (2000) Measuring variability in early child language: Don't shoot the messenger. *Child Development* 71 (2), 323–328.

Fenson, L., Marchman, V.A., Thal, D.J., Dale, P.S., Reznick, J.S. and Bates, E. (2007) *MacArthur-Bates Communicative Development Inventories: User's Guide and Technical Manual* (2nd edn). Baltimore, MD: Paul H. Brookes.

Golinkoff, R.M., Hirsh-Pasek, K. and Hollich, G. (1999) Emerging cues for word learning. In B. MacWhinney (ed.) *The Emergence of Language* (pp. 305–330). Hillsdale, NJ: Lawrence Erlbaum.

Grohmann, K.K. (2011) Some directions for the systematic investigation of the acquisition of Cypriot Greek: A new perspective on production abilities from object clitic placement. In E. Rinke and T. Kupisch (eds) *The Development of Grammar* (pp. 179–203). Amsterdam: John Benjamins.

Grohmann, K.K. (2014) Towards comparative bilingualism. *Linguistic Approaches to Bilingualism* 4, 336–341.

Grohmann, K.K. and Kambanaros, M. (2016) The gradience of multilingualism in language development: Positioning bilectalism within comparative bilingualism. *Frontiers in Psychology: Language Sciences* 7 (37), doi:10.3389/fpsyg.2016.00037.

Grohmann, K.K. and Leivada, E. (2012) Interface ingredients of dialect design: Bi-*x*, sociosyntax of development, and the grammar of Cypriot Greek. In A.M. Di Sciullo (ed.) *Towards a Biolinguistic Understanding of Grammar: Essays on Interfaces* (pp. 239–262). Amsterdam: John Benjamins.

Hoff, E., Core, C., Place, S., Rumiche, R., Señor, M. and Parra, M. (2012) Dual language exposure and early bilingual development. *Journal of Child Language* 39 (1), 1–27.

Huttenlocher, J., Waterfall, H., Vasilyeva, M., Vevea, J. and Hedges, L.V. (2010) Sources of variability in children's language growth. *Cognitive Psychology* 61 (4), 343–365.

Jackson-Maldonado, D., Marchman, V. and Fernald, L. (2013) Short-form versions of the Spanish MacArthur-Bates Communicative Development Inventories. *Applied Psycholinguistics* 34, 837–868.

Jørgensen, R.N., Dale, P.S., Bleses, D. and Fenson, L. (2010) CLEX: A cross-linguistic lexical norms database. *Journal of Child Language* 37 (2), 419–428.

Kambanaros, M., Grohmann, K.K., Michaelides, M. and Theodorou, E. (2012) Comparing multilingual children with SLI to their bilectal peers: Evidence from object and action picture naming. *International Journal of Multilingualism* 10, 1–22.

Kambanaros, M., Grohmann, K.K., Michaelides, M. and Theodorou, E. (2014) On the nature of verb–noun dissociations in bilectal SLI: A psycholinguistic perspective from Greek. *Bilingualism: Language and Cognition* 17 (1), 169–188.

Maital, S.L., Dromi, E., Saqi, A. and Bornstein, M.H. (2000) The Hebrew Communicative Development Inventory: Language-specific properties and cross-linguistic generalizations. *Journal of Child Language* 27 (1), 43–67.

Marchman, V.A., Martínez-Sussmann, C. and Dale, P. (2004) The language-specific nature of grammatical development: Evidence from bilingual language learners. *Developmental Science* 7 (2), 212–224.

Markman, E.M. and Hutchinson, J.E. (1984) Children's sensitivity to constraints on word meaning: Taxonomic versus thematic relations. *Cognitive Psychology* 16 (1), 1–27.

Markman, E.M., Wasow, J.L. and Hansen, M.B. (2003) Use of the mutual exclusivity assumption by young word learners. *Cognitive Psychology* 47 (3), 241–275.

Neofytou, E., Roch, N., Bailey, L.M., Kiryakova, R. and Mills, D. (2015) Comparison of monolingual and bilingual versions of Welsh and English CDI: Preliminary toddler norms. Poster presented at the *Biennial Meeting of the Society for Research in Child Development*, Philadelphia, PA.

Paradis, J., Emmerzael, K. and Duncan, T.S. (2010) Assessment of English language learners: Using parent report on first language development. *Journal of Communication Disorders* 43 (6), 474–497.

Paradis, J., Genesee, F. and Crago, M. (2011) *Dual Language Development and Disorders: A Handbook on Bilingualism and Second Language Learning* (2nd edn). Baltimore, MD: Paul H. Brookes.

Pearson, B.Z. and Fernández, S.C. (1994) Patterns of interaction in the lexical growth in two languages of bilingual infants and toddlers. *Language Learning* 44, 617–653.

Rowe, C. and Grohmann, K.K. (2013) Discrete bilectalism: Towards co-overt prestige and diglossic shift in Cyprus. *International Journal of the Sociology of Language* 142, 119–142.

Szagun, G., Steinbrink, C., Franik, M. and Stumper, B. (2006) Development of vocabulary and grammar in young German-speaking children assessed with a German language development inventory. *First Language* 26 (3), 259–280.

Szagun, G., Stumper, B. and Schramm, S.A. (2014) *German Communicative Development Inventory: An Adaptation of the MacArthur-Bates for Toddlers*. Frankfurt am Main: Peter Lang.

Taxitari, L., Kambanaros, M. and Grohmann, K.K. (2015) A Cypriot Greek adaptation of the CDI: Early production of translation equivalents in a bi-(dia)lectal context. *Journal of Greek Linguistics* 15, 122–145.

Thordardottir, E.T, Weismer, S.E. and Evans, J.L. (2002) Continuity in lexical and morphological development in Icelandic and English-speaking 2-year-olds. *First Language* 22 (1), 3–28.

Tsiplakou, S. (2014) How mixed is a 'mixed' system? The case of the Cypriot Greek *koiné*. *Linguistic Variation* 14, 161–178.

Tuller, L. (2015) Clinical use of parental questionnaires in multilingual contexts. In S. Armon-Lotem, J. de Jong and N. Meir (eds) *Assessing Multilingual Children: Disentangling Bilingualism from Language Impairment* (pp. 301–330). Bristol: Multilingual Matters.

Werker, J.F. and Byers-Heinlein, K. (2008) Bilingualism in infancy: First steps in perception and comprehension. *Trends in Cognitive Sciences* 12 (4), 144–151.

Part 3

Language Acquisition in the Presence of a Disorder

7 Obstructive Sleep Apnoea Syndrome: Does It Really Affect Language Acquisition during Early Childhood?

Georgia Andreou and Matina Tasioudi

Introduction

History and definition

Obstructive sleep apnoea syndrome (OSAS) in children was first reported almost 40 years ago (Guilleminault *et al.*, 1976) as a rare condition, and this first research focused mainly on the syndrome's severe form and its comorbidities, e.g. cor pulmonale. In 2002 the American Academy of Pediatrics (AAP) published a technical report on the diagnosis and management of childhood OSAS using the following definition of the syndrome:

> OSAS in children is a disorder of breathing during sleep characterized by prolonged partial upper airway obstruction and/or intermittent complete obstruction (obstructive apnea) that disrupts normal ventilation during sleep and normal sleep patterns. It is associated with symptoms including habitual (nightly) snoring, sleep difficulties, and/or daytime neurobehavioral problems. Complications may include growth abnormalities, neurologic disorders, and cor pulmonale, especially in severe cases. (AAP, 2002)

This definition is still considered valid today. According to the American Academy of Sleep Medicine Manual (AASM, 2012), when assessing sleep and associated events an obstructive apnoea in children is scored when there is an absence (or >90% reduction) of airflow that lasts for two or more missed breaths and is associated with maintained inspiratory effort. An obstructive hypopnoea is described as having a >30% reduction in airflow associated with a ≥4% decrease in oxygen desaturation and/or arousal and also lasts for two or more missed breaths with preservation of respiratory effort. OSAS is considered the most important manifestation of the spectrum of sleep-disordered breathing (SDB), which includes several disorders such as primary snoring and upper airway resistance syndrome, among others (Nespoli *et al.*, 2013). The syndrome's prevalence during childhood varies in different epidemiological studies between 1% and 6% and it peaks between two and eight years of age (Balbani *et al.*, 2005; Lumeng & Chervin, 2008; Marcus *et al.*, 2012).

Pathophysiology

When it comes to the pathophysiology of OSAS, the main cause is considered to be nasopharyngeal obstruction due to excess of lymphoid tissues (adenoids and tonsils), since it alters the head's posture in order to facilitate breathing and therefore influences the craniofacial structure and the dentofacial development accordingly (Ellingsen *et al.*, 1995; Katz & Marcus, 2012). More specifically, OSAS during early childhood or infancy causes, among other things, changes in facial bone growth (e.g. anterior and inferior position of the hyoid bone) (Vieira *et al.*, 2011). Furthermore, there is an important percentage of children with OSAS who do not improve significantly after adenotonsillectomy, suggesting that there must also be other contributing factors (Apostolidou *et al.*, 2008; Tauman *et al.*, 2006). Childhood obesity was not considered an important predisposing factor for childhood OSAS, since most of the patients in the early studies had normal BMI indices. However, as the incidence of obesity increases in children, literature has shifted in acknowledging childhood obesity as an important risk factor for the occurrence of OSAS (Dayyat *et al.*, 2007, 2009; Narang & Mathew, 2012). There are also studies that relate childhood OSAS to neuromotor abnormalities, such as abnormal central nervous system processing of upper airway signals (Huang *et al.*, 2008; Tapia *et al.*, 2010).

The pattern of breathing during sleep is different in children with OSAS compared to adults. Children do not wake up as frequently in response to apnoeas and they preserve a more normal sleep architecture (Goh *et al.*, 2000), resulting in less incidents of daytime sleepiness than adults do (Gozal *et al.*, 2001). In children, only 50% of non-REM and 35% of REM obstructions end in arousal, and the percentages are even smaller for infants (McNamara *et al.*, 1996). On the other hand, children with OSAS present 'obstructive hypoventilation' (American Thoracic Society, 1996), which is described as persistent partial airway obstruction leading to gas exchange abnormalities (hypercapnia and/or hypoxemia).

Diagnosis

Loud snoring, presented almost every night, is the first indicator for paediatric SDB, but does not always imply OSAS (Preutthipan *et al.*, 2000).

Therefore, standardized screening questionnaires have been created for diagnosing OSAS (Brouillette *et al.*, 1984; Croft *et al.*, 1990; Suen *et al.*, 1995; van Someren *et al.*, 1990, 2000), but the application of such questionnaires alone has not been successful in distinguishing children with OSAS from normal children (Aljadeff *et al.*, 1996; Gold *et al.*, 1986; Tal *et al.*, 1988). The results of such questionnaires have also been doubted by polysomnography (PSG) findings (van Someren *et al.*, 1990, 2000). There are also some questionnaires (e.g. OSA-18) that have been adapted for the Greek paediatric population, and despite their consistency and reliability they poorly predicted OSAS severity (Mousailidis *et al.*, 2014). However, the results of other questionnaires adapted to Greek, such as OSD-6, were significantly correlated to the PSG results and can be used to add more aspects to the PSG findings (Lachanas *et al.*, 2014).

Since clinical history alone has been found insufficient for the accurate diagnosis of OSAS for most patients, PSG sleep recordings are characterized as the gold standard (Marcus *et al.*, 2012). The measurement of apnoeas and hypopnoeas during PSG allows us to quantify the severity of OSAS in children using the combined number of apnoeas and hypopnoeas per hour, known as the Apnoea/Hypopnoea Index (AHI), along with other measurements such as the severity of gas exchange abnormalities and the amount of sleep disruption. An AHI >1 is considered abnormal according to the American Academy of Sleep Medicine, while immediate treatment is recommended for any child with an AHI >5. Severe childhood OSAS is defined as having an AHI >10. Nevertheless, we should not ignore that the fact that detailed questionnaires on day and night symptoms and complete physical examination are also necessary for a proper diagnosis, classification of the severity and treatment of the syndrome (Urquhart, 2013).

Treatment and consequences

Adenotonsillectomy (AT) is the most common and effective way to treat paediatric OSAS and helps at least two-thirds of OSAS children (Helfaer *et al.*, 1996; Mitchell, 2007; Nixon *et al.*, 2005; Tami *et al.*, 1987). However, in many cases, while there is significant improvement, residual OSAS remains (Apostolidou *et al.*, 2008; Tauman *et al.*, 2006). Therefore, orthodontic treatment and orofacial muscle reinforcing physiotherapy should also be considered in certain cases, along with treatment of obesity, if present (Marcus *et al.*, 2012). For patients who do not improve significantly with AT, a continuous positive airway pressure (CPAP) via a face mask or nasal mask during sleep has also been proven to have good results and is mostly recommended for children with OSAS and obesity (Marcus *et al.*, 2012).

If childhood OSAS is left untreated there are several morbidities associated with its presence in children described in the literature. Excessive daytime sleepiness, even though quite common in adult patients, is not as frequent for children and ranges between 7% and 49% in different studies (Carroll *et al.*, 1995; Chervin *et al.*, 2006; Gozal *et al.*, 2001). However, it affects some of these children, who appear to be relatively sleepier than typically developing children (Melendres *et al.*, 2004). Increased plasma tumour necrosis factor-alpha (TNF-α) levels have been associated with increased frequency of excessive daytime sleepiness in adults, but this is not the case for children since high TNF-α levels cannot be used as a predictor for the presence of daytime sleepiness based on paediatric findings (Alexopoulos *et al.*, 2013).

However, the local and systemic inflammation, the intermittent hypoxemia and sleep defragmentation events that are present in paediatric OSAS are associated with elevated serum levels of TNF-α (Entzian *et al.*, 1996; Kataoka *et al.*, 2004), C-reactive protein (CRP; Gozal *et al.*, 2012), and interleukin-6 and -8 (IL-6/IL-8; Entzian *et al.*, 1996; Maeder *et al.*, 2015; see also McNicholas, 2009, for a review). Genetic variation in the IL-6/CRP pathway was also found to be associated with increased risk for OSAS in European and American children and may account for the higher CRP levels found in paediatric OSAS (Kaditis *et al.*, 2014). Impaired insulin-like growth factor-1 (IGF-1) is also found in OSAS children (Nieminen *et al.*, 2002) and is strongly linked to delayed growth and development (Capdevila & Gozal, 2008). In addition, among the most important consequences are also some cardiovascular complications linked to childhood OSAS, such as abnormal heart rate variability (Shouldice *et al.*, 2004), hypertension (Marcus *et al.*, 1998), ventricular dysfunction (Amin *et al.*, 2005; Itzhaki *et al.*, 2005; Kaditis *et al.*, 2010), and pulmonary hypertension (Aljadeff *et al.*, 1996; Marcus *et al.*, 1995; Nieminen *et al.*, 2000). Besides that, in a cohort of Greek children with OSAS, HDL cholesterol levels were found to be inversely related to severity of OSAS in non-obese participants (Alexopoulos *et al.*, 2011). Nevertheless, thanks to early diagnosis and proper treatment the severe cardiovascular morbidities in OSAS children have presented with lower frequency during recent years (Nespoli *et al.*, 2013).

Besides the pathological comorbidities of childhood OSAS, neurocognitive deficits are also a major consequence of the syndrome and present as neurobehavioural problems (aggressive/depressive behaviour, emotional lability), learning difficulties, poor school performance, ADHD (Chervin *et al.*, 2005), and even lower IQ compared to the healthy population (see also Bass *et al.*, 2004; Gottlieb *et al.*, 2004; Kohler *et al.*, 2009; Kurnatowski *et al.*, 2006; Rosen, 2004). Childhood OSAS patients are also found to have reduced auditory processing in dichotic digits tests (Ziliotto *et al.*, 2006), slower information processing, insufficient encoding and verbal memory problems (Spruyt *et al.*, 2009). What is quite promising, on the other hand, is that preliminary data suggest that some of these cognitive deficits may be reversible following treatment of mild sleep apnoea in children; however, factors such as age at treatment time, duration of SDB, pre-morbid intellectual level, socio-economic status or the effectiveness of treatment may adversely affect the long-term outcome (Landau *et al.*, 2012; Montgomery-Downs *et al.*, 2005).

Most of the research so far has focused only on cognitive functions such as attention and memory, and there are only a few studies that have focused on language abilities (Andreou & Agapitou, 2007; Honaker *et al.*, 2009; Landau *et al.*, 2012; Liukkonen *et al.*, 2012; Yorbik *et al.*, 2014; see also de Castro Correa *et al.*, 2016, for a review). However, the prevalence for childhood OSAS peaks between two and eight years of age which is a critical period for the acquisition and development of language (Nelson *et al.*, 2006). All the studies mentioned above examined oral language ability among other measurements, and found mainly reduced verbal fluency levels. For the Greek language, the study of Andreou and Agapitou (2007) found significant semantic and phonemic language deficits, along with poor school performance in Greek language lessons, in adolescents with SDB. Following this study our team tested the morphosyntactic ability of children with OSAS (Andreou & Tasioudi, 2015), since there were no data for this language level for the Greek language. According to our results, children with OSAS had significantly lower performance in morphosyntactic production but we found no statistically significant difference in morphosyntactic comprehension compared to a typically developing group of participants.

The cause of cognitive decline in OSAS seems to be complicated and the data in the literature largely address the adult population. Significant correlation has been found between cognitive impairment and daytime sleepiness (Verstraeten, 2007), and there are also studies mainly blaming the nocturnal hypoxia for the same effects (Aloia *et al.*, 2003; Greneche *et al.*, 2011). Memory consolidation is postulated to occur during REM sleep (Diekelmann & Born, 2010); therefore sleep fragmentation could be one of the reasons affecting cognitive functions in children with OSAS. Other researchers also claim that OSAS results in damage to certain brain structures if left untreated (O'Brien & Gozal, 2002). More specifically, it causes a decrease in grey matter in the hippocampus, in the anterior cingulate, in the cerebellum and in the frontal, parietal and temporal lobes (Gale & Hopkins, 2004; Macey *et al.*, 2002; Morrell *et al.*, 2003) and in the hippocampal volume (Fung *et al.*, 2007). In addition, the frontal and parietal cortices become abnormal and it is also considered the cause for decreased mean neuronal metabolite ratio of *N*-acetyl aspartate to choline in the left hippocampus and right frontal cortex (Halbower *et al.*, 2006). Paediatric research has also found that there is a shared pathogenetic mechanism between endothelial dysfunction caused by OSAS and neurocognitive impairment (Gozal *et al.*, 2010). Another model proposed is the microvascular theory suggesting that a vascular compromise might exist in the small vessels of the brain (Aloia *et al.*, 2004). Another theory suggests that sleep defragmentation and hypoxia effects are synergistic and they interact with vulnerable brain regions such as hippocampus, prefrontal cortex, and subcortical grey and white matter (Beebe, 2006;

Beebe & Gozal, 2002; for a more detailed review see Andreou *et al.*, 2014; Lal *et al.*, 2012). However, existing data are limited and more research is required.

Based on the above facts, we see that several studies have found that general cognitive ability and language are affected by the occurrence of OSAS, but until now research has mostly examined the general language ability without focusing on specific language areas. Therefore, our goal is to investigate the main language areas that are quite challenging for Greek children with developmental language disorders, namely morphosyntax, phonology and semantics (Stavrakaki, 2005) in order to examine which of these areas are also challenging for children with OSAS. We also decided to examine the non-verbal ability of children with OSAS since, as mentioned above, children with SDB and OSAS were found to have lower non-verbal ability than typically developing children (O'Brien *et al.*, 2004, among others). Moreover, we wanted to make sure that all our participants did not suffer from serious decline of non-verbal ability that could possibly affect their results on the language tests.

Method

Participants and examination procedure

In the present study, the participants were 25 children with OSAS (Apnoea/Hypopnoea Index/hour (AHI) = 5.25, *SD* = 3.26) referred to the Sleep Laboratory of the Pulmonary Clinic of the University Hospital of Larissa, Greece, for breathing problems during the night. The OSAS diagnosis was based on PSG findings. The age of the OSAS group of participants was 4.1–6.11 years (mean chronological age [MCA] = 5.6, *SD* = 1.02). To test our hypothesis, we formed a control group of 25 typically developing children (TDC) of the same chronological age (MCA = 5.7, *SD* = 1.16/AHI = 0) who did not have breathing disorders during sleep. All children in our study lived in cities or rural areas of Central Greece (Larisa, Volos, Karditsa, Trikala, Lamia) during the experimental procedure. The conditions of the experimental procedure were the same for both groups.

After the diagnosis, we informed the parents about the study and with their written consent we moved to the individual examination at children's homes which lasted one to two hours, on one or two consecutive days. During the examination, language and non-verbal ability tests were administered to our participants. The same tests were administered to the control group of children. The examination for each participant took place in a quiet and comfortable environment, mostly at their homes, in order to cause the least possible anxiety and distractions. The researcher was sitting next to or opposite the child in order to observe and write down the answers on the Individual Test Sheet.

Assessments

Raven's Coloured Progressive Matrices

In order to assess the non-verbal ability of our participants, each child completed the Raven's Coloured Progressive Matrices Test (RCPM; Raven, 2008/2015) standardized for the Greek population. We chose to use a non-verbal ability test along with the language assessment so as to ensure that the performance of each group on the language test is not a result of a decline in general cognitive ability. Therefore, children with low results on RCPM (below 70) were excluded from our sample.

RCPM is one of the most widely used and extensively researched non-verbal tests employed in educational and clinical practice worldwide (Jensen, 1980; Raven, 2000, among others) and assesses the two main components of general cognitive ability (*g*) identified by Spearman (1927): (i) the *eductive* ability (the ability to make meaning out of confusion and to handle complexity; and (ii) the *reproductive* ability (the ability to absorb, recall and reproduce explicit information). This test is also considered appropriate for research since it demonstrated good inter-item consistency and split-half reliability across all age levels tested in normative studies (Cotton *et al.*, 2005). It is also considered easy to administer and to interpret (Raven, 2000; Pueyo *et al.*, 2008) and a fast way for identifying academic potential even in students with limited language ability. It is also suitable for the evaluation of individuals from different cultural and linguistic backgrounds as it is not affected significantly by the sociocultural background of students. Nevertheless, it appears to hold more promise as a general screening instrument which should be used in conjunction with other tests in order to acquire the full academic potential of a child (Everatt *et al.*, 2004; Georgas, 1971; Mills & Tissot, 1995).

RCPM is standardized for children aged 4–12 years and consists of 36 items, divided into three groups (A, AB, B), each of which includes 12 items. Each group is formed by a series of designs with a missing part and beneath these designs there are six smaller designs for completing the major one. Those taking the test are expected to select the correct small design to complete the bigger design. Each test group requires the extraction of a different rule or sequence for the proper completion of the design. The difficulty level increases gradually. Each participant required 15–30 minutes for completing the test. All correct answers were scored out of a maximum score of 36 (one point for each correct answer) and then turned into percentiles based on the age-related norms of the manual.

L-a-T-o I: Psychometric test for language ability

To assess the language ability of children with OSAS we administered to all participants a standardized language ability test for the Greek language which examines all levels of language and speech forms (L-a-T-o I: Psychometric test for language ability; Tzouriadou *et al.*, 2008). L-a-T-o I was designed based on the developmental approach on language acquisition (Bloom, 1975; Bloom & Lahey, 1978) and is a combination of the developmental psychological approach and the cognitive approach (Markman, 1981; Markman & Gorin, 1981; Rabinowitz & Glaser, 1985). It is suitable for children 4, 0–7, 11 years old. It examines all aspects of speech involved in the learning process and has some unique characteristics for the Greek language:

- it assesses the adequacy, the strengths and weaknesses of the participants in all main linguistic levels (phonology, morphosyntax, semantics);
- it assesses comprehension, organization and expression of both oral and written language;
- it is standardized for the Greek population, and is thus reliable and valid for testing Modern Greek;
- it provides norms based on a representative sample of the Greek population;
- it is relatively fast and well paced, in order to make the examination process easy for both the researcher and the participant.

L-a-T-o I consists of 10 sub-tests as follows:

(a) *Picture Vocabulary*. It assesses the child's ability to understand everyday words. It consists of 23 items. The researcher presents the child a page with four pictures and asks him to point two of them.
e.g. *Show me tree. / Show me baby.*

(b) *Semantic Association Vocabulary*. It assesses the child's ability to understand and semantically associate words – pictures which share a common semantic element. It consists of 15 items. The stimuli are presented on a page with pictures. At the top of the page there is a box with three pictures-words with semantic association (e.g. *they are all 'food'*). Below the box there are four pictures. The researcher says *Show me the pictures that best match those found at the top of the page* and the child is required to select two of them to match those inside the box (e.g. *two more 'foods'*). Children are not required to name the items.

(c) *Receptive Vocabulary*. It assesses the child's ability to find common words based on their description. It consists of 12 items. The child is presented with a page of four pictures and is asked to point the one that the researcher refers to or describes.
e.g. *Show me something that we wear in summer.* / The child should say: *Bathing suit*.

(d) *Expressive Vocabulary*. It consists of two parts. In the first part, which consists of 14 items, the child is asked to find words based on their oral description and on their first syllable.

e.g. *Tell me a word that begins with du- and is a bird that does quack-quack.* /The child should say: *duck.*

In the second part, which consists of 15 items, the researcher asks the child to give simple definitions of common words.

e.g. *What is a dog?*

(e) *Articulation.* It consists of two parts and evaluates the child's ability to articulate properly the most challenging Modern Greek consonants and consonant clusters. In the first part, which consists of 13 items, the researcher says a sentence and stops at the word that the child should pronounce using the picture as a visual aid.

e.g. *Tom is a boy. Mary is a ...* / The child should say: *girl.*

In the second part, which consists of 16 items, the procedure is the same but this time there are only semantic stimuli, not pictures. The researcher utters a sentence with a missing word and the child is asked to complete it orally.

e.g. *Mary is a woman. Tom is a ...* / The child should say: *man.*

(f) *Phoneme Blending/Completion.* It consists of 30 items and evaluates the child's ability to complete words or pseudowords using individual phonemes. The presentation rate was about two phonemes per second, using natural tone, rhythm and pauses.

e.g. *The researcher says: /c-a-t/.* The child should say: *cat.*

(g) *Phoneme Analysis/Segmentation.* It consists of 29 items and assesses the child's ability to analyze words or pseudowords in individual phonemes. This process is directly related to reading ability.

e.g. *The researcher says: dog* / The child should say: */d-o-g/.*

(h) *Phoneme Distinction.* It consists of two parts and evaluates the ability to distinguish phonemes along with interpreting semantic clues (combination of semantic and phonemic awareness). In the first part, which consists of 14 items, the researcher utters two words that differ in a single phoneme, along with a small sentence describing one of them. The child is asked to choose one of them based on the semantic content of the sentence said by the researcher.

e.g. *The researcher says: money – honey: we use it to pay* / The child should say: *money.*

The second part consists of 21 items and evaluates prosody, focusing on the speed perception of similar phonemes combinations. The researcher says to the child the initial, the final or the middle phonemes of a word and then presents the child with two options to choose the correct one.

e.g. *The researcher says: he-: did I say 'here' or 'tear'?* / The child should say: *here.*

(i) *Morphosyntactic Comprehension.* It consists of 13 items and evaluates receptive morphosyntactic ability. The child is presented with three similar pictures and should choose which one best fits the sentence uttered by the researcher.

e.g. *Show me the picture that fits best the sentence: Many dogs are sitting down.*

(j) *Morphosyntactic Completion/Production.* It consists of 13 items and examines expressive morphosyntactic ability. The researcher utters a sentence while presenting two pictures and pauses at the point where the child has to continue with the appropriate word that matches the picture pointed to by the researcher.

e.g. The researcher says: *This truck carries many boxes. This one carries only …* / The child should say: *One box.*

In order to answer correctly in both Morphosyntactic Comprehension and Production, the child should be able to understand or form singular and plural number of regular nouns in different cases, singular and plural number of regular and common irregular verbs in present, past and future tenses, to produce nouns out of verbs, to use the passive participle, to use the comparative forms of common adjectives, and to use ordinal numbers.

Each linguistic area consists of the following sub-tests:

- *Phonology*: Articulation, Phoneme Blending/Completion, Phoneme Analysis/Segmentation, Phoneme Distinction.
- *Semantics*: Picture Vocabulary, Semantic Association Vocabulary, Receptive Vocabulary, Expressive Vocabulary.
- *Morphosyntax*: Morphosyntactic Comprehension, Morphosyntactic Completion/Production, Articulation.

Articulation is part of the morphosyntax area since it requires more than just the proper articulation of the experimental words. In order to find the experimental word, especially in the second part, the child has to understand the sentences uttered by the researcher.

L-a-T-o I has more sub-tests evaluating the phonological and the semantic level of the language since during the ages 4–7, 11 oral abilities develop rapidly. Moreover, phonological and phonemic awareness are expected to be fully developed by the age of eight years (Guasti, 2007). The performance in this part of the test can be considered as a reliable indicator for reading readiness.

The duration of the examination for L-a-T-o I was between 50 and 70 minutes and was administered throughout a single meeting. In case of fatigue of the participant the administration of the test was paused and we continued during the next meeting, according to the instructions of the manual, along with the RCPM administration. Children were given about 10–15 seconds to answer each question. In all sub-tests, the administration started from the first question and continued until the last, or until the child reached the upper limit of three consecutive wrong answers.

The 10 sub-tests of L-a-T-o I were scored separately. Each correct answer was scored with 1 grade. The scores were added for each language area and then were transformed into percentiles based on the age-related norms of the manual. In this way we acquired the separate evaluation of the phonological, morphosyntactic and semantic areas of language (mean performance = 10, *SD* = 3). The sum of the correct answers in form of percentiles also led to the general language ability ratio (mean performance = 100, *SD* = 15).

Statistical analysis

In the first place, an exploratory data analysis was conducted to determine whether the score distribution of various tests was normally distributed. Results based on the Kolmogorov–Smirnov test for normality indicated that the score distribution for all the tests we performed did not deviate significantly from a normal distribution. More specifically, the results for normal distribution were above the statistical significance ($\alpha < 0.05$), as shown below: Raven's Non-Verbal Ability Test ($\alpha = 0.20$), semantics ($\alpha = 0.035$), phonology ($\alpha = 0.20$), morphosyntax ($\alpha = 0.059$), general language ability ratio ($\alpha = 0.20$). Based on these findings, we decided to perform parametric tests to compare the mean performance of the two groups of participants. More specifically, we performed a One-way ANOVA to compare the effect of the experimental group on all five variables tested. Subsequently, we conducted independent sample *t*-tests to verify our results using a between-group analysis. The significance threshold was set at 0.01, to eliminate the possibility of false findings due to the small number of participants. The effects of rural versus urban area of residence have not been factored in since most of the participants came from urban areas (43 urban versus seven rural). According to the answers of the parents to a short questionnaire on their studies and working status, which had been completed prior to the beginning of the study, all of them had attended at least high school or had higher studies and characterized themselves as either employees, business owners or home-staying mothers. The statistical analysis was performed using SPSS Statistics 21.

Results

Our results are presented in Table 7.1 where we can see the mean performance, along with the standard deviation, of each group in general language ability, semantics, phonology, morphosyntax and non-verbal ability.

As we can see by comparing the mean performance of the two groups of participants, the OSAS group performed worse than the TDC group in all language levels tested and had lower overall non-verbal ability. Especially in morphosyntax, the mean performance of the OSAS group was lower than 1 *SD* below the mean score for this age, as described in L-a-T-o I (Mean = 10, *SD* = 3). The scoring in phonology was also quite low, while the OSAS group performed better in semantics, but still worse than the TDC group.

Table 7.1 Mean performance and *t*-test results of the groups in the language and the non-verbal ability test

	Typically Developing Children (TDC) Mean (SD)	*Obstructive sleep apnoea syndrome (OSAS) Mean (SD)*	*t-value*	*p-value*
Semantics	10.9 (1.76)	8.4 (2.44)	3.05	0.004*
Phonology	10.7 (1.95)	7 (1.91)	5.34	0.000*
Morphosyntax	10.4 (2.11)	6.7 (1.70)	5.79	0.000*
General language ability ratio	107 (13.48)	86 (11.18)	4.94	0.000*
Raven's Non-Verbal Ability	107.3 (9.34)	94.8 (15.22)	2.51	0.017

Notes: *Statistically significant result, $p < 0.01$. SD = standard deviation.

The general language ability ratio was also lower for OSAS children, but also still within the normal range of results (Mean = 100, $SD = 15$). The OSAS group had lower performance than the TDC group on Raven's Coloured Progressive Matrices for non-verbal ability.

Specifically, the results from the one-way ANOVA analysis showed a significant effect of the group of participants on all language areas tested on the language test: on semantics (F (1, 48) = 9.33, $p = 0.004$), on phonology (F (1, 48) = 28.51, $p = 0.000$) and on morphosyntax (F (1, 48) = 33.51, $p = 0.000$). A significant effect of the group of participants was also found for the general language ability ratio with the OSAS group performing significantly lower than the TDC group (F (1, 48) = 24.40, $p = 0.000$). Nevertheless, the effect of the group of participants on non-verbal ability (F (1, 48) = 6.31, $p = 0.017$) just failed to be significant. The one-way ANOVA findings were also confirmed using independent sample *t*-tests and indicated that the OSAS children scored significantly below the TDC controls in each language domain tested and in general language ability but not in non-verbal ability, as seen in Table 7.1.

Discussion

Childhood OSAS research has focused so far mainly on the syndrome's behavioural and cognitive effects while the effects on language development are scarcely examined (Kohler *et al.*, 2009; Kurnatowski *et al.*, 2006, among others). However, our research findings provide evidence that children with OSAS lag behind their peers without OSAS in all language domains. As can be seen in our results, participants with OSAS had significantly lower general language ability scores on the L-a-T-o I test in comparison to TDC and our findings are in accordance with previous literature findings that revealed deficits in language and general cognitive problems (Gozal, 2008; Halbower & Mahone, 2006; Kohler *et al.*, 2009; Kurnatowski *et al.*, 2006). We also suggest that the reduced language ability that we found even in early childhood is one of the main factors leading to poor academic performance in older children with OSAS or SDB (Andreou & Agapitou, 2007; Gozal & Pope, 2001) since it can lead to difficulties in processing complex verbal instructions and in poor expressive language at both oral and written level.

However, when it comes to the results of the non-verbal ability test that we performed the difference between them was not statistically significant despite the fact that the OSAS group performed worse than the TDC group. The findings of the literature show diversity of results on non-verbal ability. There are studies like ours that did not find any significant difference between OSAS and TDC groups in non-verbal ability or IQ (Pietropaoli *et al.*, 2015), while in others the OSAS group performed significantly worse (O'Brien *et al.*, 2004; Ziliotto *et al.*, 2006, among others). These diverse findings are also supported by our results, since the standard deviation of the OSAS performance in RCPM was quite large (almost 15), indicating inconsistency in the non-verbal ability. We purport that our findings are consistent with the literature findings that show decline in cognition (verbal and non-verbal, see also Bass *et al.*, 2004; Gottlieb *et al.*, 2004; Kohler *et al.*, 2009; Kurnatowski *et al.*, 2006; Rosen, 2004) and the reason for the lack of statistical significance on non-verbal ability could be possibly attributed to the different assessment tool that we used.

Besides general language ability in childhood OSAS, we also examined the performance of our participants in the three main linguistic areas of phonology, morphosyntax and semantics. These areas are, so far, the most examined areas in language disorders and in typical development (Guasti, 2007; Stavrakaki, 2005). As we mentioned earlier, there is only sporadic evidence on the effects of OSAS in these areas specifically and our purpose was to approach the language effects of the syndrome in a more systematic way and to the full extent. We found statistically significant results that reveal the effect of OSAS on all language areas examined as shown in Table 7.1. More specifically, the phonology tasks revealed effects of OSAS on phonological development, since the OSAS group performed significantly worse than the TDC group, in the borderline of normal performance. Our results in this part of the test are also consistent with the literature which has revealed problems in phonemic fluency (Andreou & Agapitou, 2007) and reduced verbal abilities in children with OSAS (Honaker *et al.*, 2009). These findings could be a result of the reduced auditory processing (Ziliotto *et al.*, 2006), suggesting possible auditory processing disorder. In the same study, participants with OSAS were also found to have low performance in a memory test for non-verbal sounds. These findings suggest problems in the phoneme-decoding process which could explain the low performance in the phonology sub-tests found in our research for the OSAS group. Moreover, the problems that we found in phonemic production could also be attributed to the early changes in facial bone growth (e.g. anterior and inferior position of the hyoid bone, increased total and inferior anterior heights of the face; Vieira *et al.*, 2011) and the higher incidence of open lip and lower tongue position, and of hypotonia of the upper and lower lips, tongue and buccinator muscles which are found in children with OSAS and enlarged adenoids and tonsils (Valera *et al.*, 2003). These changes cause problems in mastication and deglutition in OSAS children and we suggest that they could also contribute to poor articulation of demanding phomemes. However, there are no studies so far addressing this issue.

Through the examination of the semantic development in childhood OSAS we also found a significant difference of performance between the two groups of participants. Semantics is, so far, the most studied linguistic area for adults with OSAS, and seems to be affected by its presence (see Andreou & Makanikas, 2014, for a review). Nevertheless, there are a few studies in children and adolescents with OSAS that have shown impairments in semantic development in the form of dysfunction in semantic fluency or receptive and expressive vocabulary (Andreou & Agapitou, 2007; see also Halbower & Mahone, 2006, for a review). Therefore, our results seem to be consistent with the literature findings indicating lower performance in this semantic area, and we also suggest that a possible reason for having this kind of finding is the slower information processing and insufficient encoding, along with the verbal memory problems found in children with OSAS (Spruyt *et al.*, 2009).

The last linguistic area we examined was morphosyntax, in which we also found statistically significant lower performance of the OSAS group of participants. This is also the only area in which the OSAS participants performed slightly lower than the normal range of results as described in our standardized test, and seems to be the most affected in our study. However, there are no studies in childhood OSAS addressing the effects on this area apart from the one performed by our team (Andreou & Tasioudi, 2015), which found lower morphosyntactic ability in expression but not in comprehension. There are also some studies that have found insufficient encoding and difficulties in processing verbal instructions of increasing linguistic complexity that could be considered the aetiology for our results (Honaker *et al.*, 2009; Spruyt *et al.*, 2009). Nevertheless, morphosyntax is the most studied area in children with language disorders in Greek and seems to be the most challenging for them (Stavrakaki, 2005), and according to our results it is also challenging for children with OSAS.

Based on our findings, we see that OSAS affects language acquisition in early childhood and we could also suggest, based on the findings of the literature, that there is a complex mechanism affecting several brain areas behind the aetiology of these results. Our findings could be attributed to sleep defragmentation and hypoxaemia, since these pathologic situations affect the function of the hippocampus, prefrontal cortex, frontal lobes and subcortical white matter, and these brain regions are highly associated in the literature with language functions and memory (Nagy *et al.*, 2004; Vigneau *et al.*, 2006, among others). Based on these findings and on the fact that childhood OSAS is also associated with general cognitive decline and neurobehavioural problems (see also Bass *et al.*, 2004; Gottlieb *et al.*, 2004; Kohler *et al.*, 2009; Kurnatowski *et al.*, 2006; Rosen, 2004), we suggest that the language effect of OSAS could result from impairments in language speed processing, memory or perception (Kail, 1994; Leonard *et al.*, 2007; Tallal *et al.*, 1993, among others). Nevertheless, to confirm that kind of hypothesis, more research should be conducted combining language testing, using online tests preferably, and simultaneous brain activity monitoring. Moreover, it would be quite interesting to examine whether the language effects of OSAS can also be explained based on linguistic theories for language impairment, but that would require more targeted language testing and crosslinguistic research to highlight possible differences between the performance in different languages. Besides that, we emphasize that there should also be more research based on a multidisciplinary approach to examine different aspects of the syndrome's effects. Moreover, medical treatment should be combined with early language intervention in order to avoid the risk of poor language development and consequent school failure.

Conclusion

We studied the effects of OSAS in early childhood since the existing research data on language abilities in OSAS patients do not clearly indicate which are the language domains mostly affected and to what extent. Our findings reveal a significant effect of OSAS in all the administered language tasks (general language ability, phonology, semantics and morphosyntax). Therefore, we suggest that more research is needed in the field considering factors other than the severity of symptoms, such as the age of the participants, because it has been suggested that OSAS occurrence during the critical ages of brain growth and development such as childhood and adolescence may cause notable language decline. Multidisciplinary approaches and brain monitoring techniques could also give new perspectives in finding the aetiology, in diagnosing and in treating OSAS during childhood.

References

AAP (American Academy of Pediatrics) (2002) Clinical practice guideline: Diagnosis and management of childhood obstructive sleep apnea syndrome. *Pediatrics* 109 (4), 704–712.

AASM (American Academy of Sleep Medicine) (2012) *AASM Manual for the Scoring of Sleep and Associated Events Rules: Terminology and Technical Specifications*, Version 2.0. Darien, IL: AASM.

Alexopoulos, E.I., Gletsou, E., Kostadima, E., Kaditis, D., Zakynthinos, E., Gourgoulianis, K. and Kaditis A. (2011) Effects of obstructive sleep apnea severity on serum lipid levels in Greek children with snoring. *Sleep and Breathing* 15 (4), 625–631.

Alexopoulos, E.I., Theologi, V., Malakasioti, G., *et al.* (2013) Obstructive sleep apnea, excessive daytime sleepiness, and morning plasma TNF-α levels in Greek children. *Sleep* 36 (11), 1633–1638.

Aljadeff, G., Gozal, D., Bailey-Wahl, S.L., Burrell, B., Keens, T.G. and Ward, S.L. (1996) Effects of overnight supplemental oxygen in obstructive sleep apnea in children. *American Journal of Respiratory and Critical Care Medicine* 153 (1), 51–55.

Aloia, M.S., Ilniczky, N., Di Dio, P., Perlis, M.L., Greenblatt, D.W. and Giles, D.E. (2003) Neuropsychological changes and treatment compliance in older adults with sleep apnea. *Journal of Psychosomatic Research* 54 (1), 71–76.

Aloia, M.S., Arnedt, T.J., Davis, J.D., Riggs, R.L. and Byrd, D. (2004) Neuropsychological sequelae of obstructive sleep apnea-hypopnea syndrome: A critical review. *Journal of the International Neuropsychological Society* 10, 772–785.

American Thoracic Society (1996) Standards and indications for cardiopulmonary sleep studies children. *American Journal of Respiratory and Critical Care Medicine* 153, 866–878.

Amin, R.S., Kimball, T.R., Kalra, M., *et al.* (2005) Left ventricular function in children with sleep-disordered breathing. *American Journal of Cardiology* 95 (6), 801–804.

Andreou, G. and Agapitou, P. (2007) Reduced language abilities in adolescents who snore. *Archives of Clinical Neuropsychology* 22 (2), 225–229.

Andreou, G. and Makanikas, K. (2014) Obstructive sleep apnea syndrome and its impact on verbal abilities from childhood to adulthood. In G. Andreou (ed.) *Language and Special Education: A Psycholinguistic Approach* (pp. 185–213). Thessaloniki: Giachoudis.

Andreou, G. and Tasioudi, M. (2015) Obstructive sleep apnea syndrome and morphosyntactic development in children. *Proceedings of the 6th ISEL Conference ExLing 2015* (pp. 5–8). Athens: ISEL Editions.

Andreou, G., Vlachos, F. and Makanikas, K. (2014) Effects of chronic obstructive pulmonary disease and obstructive sleep apnea on cognitive functions: Evidence for a common nature. *Sleep Disorders* 2014, 1–18.

Apostolidou, M.T., Alexopoulos, E.I., Chaidas, K., Ntamagka, G., Karathanasi, A., Apostolidis, T.I., Gourgoulianis, K. and Kaditis, A.G. (2008) Obesity and persisting sleep apnea after adenotonsillectomy in Greek children. *Chest* 134 (6), 1149–1155.

Balbani, A.P., Weber, S.A., Silke, A.T. and Montovani J.C. (2005) Update in obstructive sleep apnea syndrome in children. *Revista Brasileira de Otorrinolaringologia* 71 (1), 74–80.

Bass, J.L., Corwin, M., Gozal, D., *et al.* (2004) The effect of chronic or intermittent hypoxia on cognition in childhood: A review of the evidence. *Pediatrics* 114 (3), 805–816.

Beebe, D.W. (2006) Neural and neurobehavioral dysfunction in children with obstructive sleep apnea. *PLoS Medicine* 3 (8), e323.

Beebe, D.W. and Gozal, D. (2002) Obstructive sleep apnea and the prefrontal cortex: Towards a comprehensive model linking nocturnal upper airway obstruction to daytime cognitive and behavioral deficits. *Journal of Sleep Research* 11, 1–16.

Bloom, L. (1975) *Language Development*. Chicago, IL: University of Chicago Press.

Bloom, L. and Lahey, M. (1978) *Language Development and Language Disorders*. Hoboken, NJ: John Wiley.

Brouillette, R., Hanson, D., David, R., Klemka, L., Szatkowski, A., Fernbach, S. and Hunt, C. (1984) A diagnostic approach to suspected obstructive sleep apnea in children. *Journal of Pediatrics* 105 (1), 10–14.

Capdevila, O.S. and Gozal, D. (2008) Neurobiological consequences of sleep apnea syndrome in children. *Revista de Neurologia* 47 (12), 659–664.

Carroll, J.L., McColley, S.A., Marcus, C.L., Curtis, S. and Loughlin, G.M. (1995) Inability of clinical history to distinguish primary snoring from obstructive sleep apnea syndrome in children. *Chest* 108 (3), 610–618.

Chervin, R.D., Ruzicka, D.L., Archbold, K.H. and Dillon, J.E. (2005) Snoring predicts hyperactivity four years later. *Sleep* 28 (7), 885–890.

Chervin, R.D., Weatherly, R.A., Ruzicka, D.L., *et al.* (2006) Subjective sleepiness and polysomnographic correlates in children scheduled for adenotonsillectomy vs. other surgical care. *Sleep* 29 (4), 495–503.

Cotton, S.M., Kiely, P.M., Crewther, D.P., Thomson, B., Laycock, R. and Crewther, S.G. (2005) A normative and reliability study for the Raven's Coloured Progressive Matrices for primary school aged children from Victoria, Australia. *Personality and Individual Differences* 39 (3), 647–659.

Croft, C.B., Brockbank, M.J., Wright, A. and Swanston, A.R. (1990) Obstructive sleep apnea in children undergoing routine tonsillectomy and adenoidectomy. *Clinical Otolaryngology and Allied Sciences* 15, 307–314.

Dayyat, E., Maarafeya, M.M.A., Capdevila, O.S., Kheirandish-Gozal, L., Montgomery-Downs, H.E. and Gozal, D. (2007) Nocturnal body position in sleeping children with and without obstructive sleep apnea. *Pediatric Pulmonology* 42, 374–379.

Dayyat, E., Kheirandish-Gozal, L., Sans Capdevila, O., Maarafeya, M.M.A. and Gozal, D. (2009) Obstructive sleep apnea in children: Relative contributions of body mass index and adenotonsillar hypertrophy. *Chest* 136 (1), 137–144.

de Castro Corrêa, C., Cavalheiro, M.G., Maximino, L.P., Silke, A. and Weber, T. (2016) Obstructive sleep apnea and oral language disorders. *Brazilian Journal of Otorhinolaryngology* 82 (1), 98–104.

Diekelmann, S. and Born, J. (2010) The memory function of sleep. *Nature Reviews Neuroscience* 11, 114–126.

Ellingsen, R., Vandevanter, C., Shapiro, P. and Shapiro, G. (1995) Temporal variation in nasal and oral breathing in children. *American Journal of Orthodontics & Dentofacial Orthopedics* 107, 411–417.

Entzian, P., Linnemann, K., Schlaak, M. and Zabel, P. (1996) Obstructive sleep apnea syndrome and circadian rhythms of hormones and cytokines. *American Journal of Respiratory and Critical Care Medicine* 153 (3), 1080–1086.

Everatt, J., Smythe, I., Ocampo, D. and Gyarmathy, E. (2004) Issues in the assessment of literacy-related difficulties across language backgrounds: A cross-linguistic comparison. *Journal of Research in Reading* 27, 141–151.

Fung, S.J., Xi, M.C., Zhang, J.H., Sampogna, S., Yamuy, J., Morales, F.R. and Chase, M.H. (2007) Apnea promotes glutamate-induced excitotoxicity in hippocampal neurons. *Brain Research* 1179, 42–50.

Gale, S.D. and Hopkins, R.O. (2004) Effects of hypoxia on the brain: Neuroimaging and neuropsychological findings following carbon monoxide poisoning and obstructive sleep apnea. *Journal of the International Neuropsychological Society* 10 (1), 60–71.

Georgas, J. (1971) *Georgas I.Q. Test for Children*. Athens: Kedros.

Goh, D.Y., Galster, P. and Marcus, C.L. (2000) Sleep architecture and respiratory disturbances in children with obstructive sleep apnea. *American Journal of Respiratory and Critical Care Medicine* 162 (2, Part 1), 682–686.

Gold, A.R., Schwartz, A.R., Bleecker, E.R. and Smith P.L. (1986) The effect of chronic nocturnal oxygen administration upon sleep apnea. *American Review of Respiratory Disease* 134 (5), 925–929.

Gottlieb, D.J., Chase, C., Vezina, R.M., Heeren, T.C., Corwin, M.J., Auerbach, S.H., Weese-Mayer, D.E. and Lesko, S.M. (2004) Sleep-disordered breathing symptoms are associated with poorer cognitive function in 5-year-old children. *Journal of Pediatrics* 145 (4), 458–464.

Gozal, D. (2008) Obstructive sleep apnea in children: Implications for the developing of central nervous system. *Seminars in Pediatric Neurology* 15 (2), 100–106.

Gozal, D. and Pope, D. (2001) Snoring during early childhood and academic performance at ages thirteen to fourteen years. Pediatrics 107 (6), 1394–1399.

Gozal, D., Wang, M. and Pope, D.W. (2001) Objective sleepiness measures in pediatric obstructive sleep apnea. *Pediatrics* 108 (3), 693–697.

Gozal, D., Kheirandish-Gozal, L., Bhattacharjee, R. and Spruyt, K. (2010) Neurocognitive and endothelial dysfunction in children with obstructive sleep apnea. *Pediatrics* 126 (5), e1161–e1167.

Gozal, D., Kheirandish-Gozal, L., Bhattacharjee, R. and Kim, J. (2012) C-reactive protein and obstructive sleep apnea syndrome in children. *Frontiers in Bioscience* (Elite edn) 4, 2410–2422.

Greneche, J., Krieger, J., Bertrand, F., Erhardt, C., Maumy, M. and Tassi, P. (2011) Short-term memory performances during sustained wakefulness in patients with obstructive sleep apnea-hypopnea syndrome. *Brain and Cognition* 75 (1), 39–50.

Guasti, M. (2007) *L'acquisizione del Linguaggio: Un'Introduzione*. Milano: Cortina.

Guilleminault, C., Eldridge, F., Simmons, F.B. and Dement, W.C. (1976) Sleep apnea in eight children. *Pediatrics* 58, 23–30.

Halbower, A. and Mahone, M. (2006) Neuropsychological morbidity linked to childhood sleep-disordered breathing. *Sleep Medicine Reviews* 10 (2), 97–107.

Halbower, A.C., Degaonkar, M., Barker, P.B., Earley, C.J., Marcus, C.L., Smith, P.L., Prahme, M.C. and Mohone M.E. (2006) Childhood obstructive sleep apnea associates with neuropsychological deficits and neuronal brain injury *PLoS Medicine* 3 (8), e301.

Helfaer, M.A., McColley, S.A., Pyzik, P.L., *et al.* (1996) Polysomnography after adenotonsillectomy in mild pediatric obstructive sleep apnea. *Critical Care Medicine* 24 (8), 1323–1327.

Honaker, S.M., Gozal, D., Bennett, J., Capdevila, O.S. and Spruyt, K. (2009) Sleep-disordered breathing and verbal skills in school-aged community children. *Developmental Neuropsychology* 34 (5), 588–600.

Huang, J., Colrain, I.M., Melendres, M.C., *et al.* (2008) Cortical processing of respiratory afferent stimuli during sleep in children with the obstructive sleep apnea syndrome. *Sleep* 31 (3), 403–410.

Itzhaki, S., Lavie, L., Pillar, G., Tal, G. and Lavie, P. (2005) Endothelial dysfunction in obstructive sleep apnea measured by peripheral arterial tone response in the finger to reactive hyperemia. *Sleep* 28 (5), 594–600.

Jensen, A.R. (1980) *Bias in Mental Testing*. London: Methuen.

Kaditis, A.G., Alexopoulos, E.I., Dalapascha, M., Papageorgiou, K., Kostadima, E., Kaditis, D.G., Gourgoulianis, K. and Zakynthinos, E. (2010) Cardiac systolic function in Greek children with obstructive sleep-disordered breathing. *Sleep Medicine* 11 (4), 406–412.

Kaditis, A.G., Gozal, D., Khalyfa, A., *et al.* (2014) Variants in C-reactive protein and IL-6 genes and susceptibility to obstructive sleep apnea in children: A candidate-gene association study in European American and Southeast European populations. *Sleep Medicine* 15 (2), 228–235.

Kail, R. (1994) A method for studying the generalized slowing hypothesis in children with specific language impairment. *Journal of Speech and Hearing Research* 37, 418–421.

Kataoka, T., Enomoto, F., Kim, R., *et al.* (2004) The effect of surgical treatment of obstructive sleep apnea syndrome on the plasma TNF-alpha levels. *Tohoku Journal of Experimental Medicine* 204 (4), 267–272.

Katz, E. and Marcus, C. (2012) Obstructive sleep apnea: Children versus adults. In A. Pack (ed.) *Sleep Apnea: Pathogenesis, Diagnosis and Treatment* (pp. 370–398). London: Informa Healthcare.

Kohler, M.J., Lushington, K., van den Heuvel, C.J., Martin, J., Pamula, Y. and Kennedy, D. (2009) Adenotonsillectomy and neurocognitive deficits in children with sleep disordered breathing. *PLoS One* 4 (10), e7343.

Kurnatowski, P., Putynski, L., Lapienis, M. and Kowalska, B. (2006) Neurocognitive abilities in children with adenotonsillar hyperthrophy. *International Journal of Pediatric Otorhinolaryngology* 70, 419–424.

Lachanas, V.A., Mousailidis, G.K., Skoulakis, C.E., Papandreou, N., Exarchos, S., Alexopoulos, E.I. and Bizakis, J.G. (2014) Validation of the Greek OSD-6 quality of life questionnaire in children undergoing polysomnography. *International Journal of Pediatric Otorhinolaryngology* 78 (8), 1342–1347.

Lal, C., Strange, C. and Bachman, D. (2012) Neurocognitive impairment in obstructive sleep apnea. *Chest* 141 (6), 1601–1610.

Landau, Y.E., Bar-Yishay, O., Greenberg-Dotan, S., Goldbart, A.D., Tarasiuk, A. and Tal, A. (2012) Impaired behavioral and neurocognitive function in preschool children with obstructive sleep apnea. *Pediatric Pulmonology* 47, 180–188.

Leonard, L.B., Weismer, S.E., Miller, C.A., Francis, D.J., Tomblin, J.B. and Kail, R.V. (2007) Speed of processing, working memory, and language impairment in children. *Journal of Speech, Language, and Hearing Research* 50 (2), 408–428.

Liukkonen, K., Virkkula, P., Haavisto, A., Suomalainen, A., Aronen, E.T., Pitkäranta, A. and Kirjavainen, T. (2012) Symptoms at presentation in children with sleep-related disorders. *International Journal of Pediatric Otorhinolaryngology* 76, 327–333.

Lumeng, J.C. and Chervin, R.D. (2008) Epidemiology of pediatric obstructive sleep apnea. *Proceedings of the American Thoracic Society* 5, 242–252.

Macey, P.M., Henderson, L.A., Macey, K.E., *et al.* (2002) Brain morphology associated with obstructive sleep apnea. *American Journal of Respiratory and Critical Care Medicine* 166 (10), 1382–1387.

Maeder, M.T., Strobel, W., Christ, M., *et al.* (2015) Comprehensive biomarker profiling in patients with obstructive sleep apnea. *Clinical Biochemistry* 48 (4–5), 340–346.

Marcus, C.L., Carroll, J.L., Bamford, O., Pyzik, P. and Loughlin, G.M. (1995) Supplemental oxygen during sleep in children with sleep-disordered breathing. *American Journal of Respiratory and Critical Care Medicine* 152 (4, Part 1), 1297–1301.

Marcus, C.L., Greene, M.G. and Carroll, J.L. (1998) Blood pressure in children with obstructive sleep apnea. *American Journal of Respiratory and Critical Care Medicine* 157 (4, Part 1), 1098–1103.

Marcus, C.L., Brooks, L.J., Ward, S.D., *et al.* (2012) Diagnosis and management of childhood obstructive sleep apnea syndrome. *Pediatrics* 130, e714–e755.

Markman, E. (1981) Comprehension monitoring. In W.P. Dickson (ed.) *Children's Oral Communication Skills* (pp. 61–84). New York: Academic Press.

Markman, E. and Gorin, L. (1981) Children's ability to adjust their standards for evaluating comprehension. *Journal of Educational Psychology* 73, 320–325.

McNamara, F., Issa, F.G. and Sullivan C.E. (1996) Arousal pattern following central and obstructive breathing abnormalities in infants and children. *Journal of Applied Physiology* 81 (6), 2651–2657.

McNicholas, W.T. (2009) Obstructive sleep apnea and inflammation. *Progress in Cardiovascular Diseases* 51 (5), 392–399.

Melendres, M.C., Lutz, J.M., Rubin, E.D. and Marcus, C.L. (2004) Daytime sleepiness and hyperactivity in children with suspected sleep-disordered breathing. *Pediatrics* 114, 768–775.

Mills, J.C. and Tissot, S.L. (1995) Identifying academic potential in students from under-represented populations: Is using the Ravens Progressive Matrices a good idea? *Gifted Child Quarterly* 39, 209–217.

Mitchell, R.B. (2007) Adenotonsillectomy for obstructive sleep apnea in children: Outcome evaluated by pre- and postoperative polysomnography. *Laryngoscope* 117 (10), 1844–1854.

Montgomery-Downs, H., Crabtree, V.M. and Gozal, D. (2005) Cognition, sleep and respiration in at-risk children treated for obstructive sleep apnea. *European Respiratory Journal* 25 (2), 336–342.

Morrell, M.J., McRobbie, D.W., Quest, R.A., Cummin, A.R., Ghiassi, R. and Corfield, D.R. (2003) Changes in brain morphology associated with obstructive sleep apnea. *Sleep Medicine* 4 (5), 451–454.

Mousailidis, G.K., Lachanas, V.A., Skoulakis, C.E., Sakellariou, A., Exarchos, S.T., Kaditis, A.G. and Bizakis, J.G. (2014) Cross-cultural adaptation and validation of the Greek OSA-18 questionnaire in children undergoing polysomnography. *International Journal of Pediatric Otorhinolaryngology* 78 (12), 2097–2102.

Nagy, Z., Westerberg, H. and Klingberg, T. (2004) Maturation of white matter is associated with the development of cognitive functions during childhood. *Journal of Cognitive Neuroscience* 16 (7), 1227–1233.

Narang, I. and Mathew, J. (2012) Childhood obesity and obstructive sleep apnea. *Journal of Nutrition and Metabolism* 2012, 134202; doi:10.1155/2012/134202.

Nelson, H.D., Nygren, P., Walker, M. and Panoscha, R. (2006) Screening for speech and language delay in preschool children: Systematic evidence review for the US preventive services task force. *Pediatrics* 117, 298–310.

Nespoli, L., Caprioglio, A., Brunetti, L. and Nosetti, L. (2013) Obstructive sleep apnea syndrome in childhood. *Early Human Development* 89 (Suppl. 3), S33–S37.

Nieminen, P., Tolonen, U. and Löppönen, H. (2000) Snoring and obstructive sleep apnea in children: A 6-month follow-up study. *Archives of Otolaryngology – Head & Neck Surgery* 126 (4), 481–486.

Nieminen, P., Löppönen, T., Tolonen, U., Lanning, P., Knip, M. and Löppönen, H. (2002) Growth and biochemical markers of growth in children with snoring and obstructive sleep apnea. *Pediatrics* 109 (4), e55.

Nixon, G.M., Kermack, A.S., McGregor, C.D., Davis, G.M., Manoukian, J.J., Brown, K.A. and Brouillette, R.T. (2005) Sleep and breathing on the first night after adenotonsillectomy for obstructive sleep apnea. *Pediatric Pulmonology* 39, 332–338.

O'Brien, L.M. and Gozal, D. (2002) Behavioural and neurocognitive implications of snoring and obstructive sleep apnoea in children: Facts and theory. *Paediatric Respiratory Reviews* 3 (1), 3–9.

O'Brien, L.M., Mervis, C.B., Holbrook, C.R., Bruner, J.L., Smith, N.H., McNally, N., Catherine McClimment, M. and Gozal, D. (2004) Neurobehavioral correlates of sleep-disordered breathing in children. *Journal of Sleep Research* 13, 165–172.

Pietropaoli, N., Supino, M.C., Vitelli, O., Rabasco, J., Evangelisti, M., Forlani, M., Parisi, P. and Villa, M.P. (2015) Cognitive function in preschool children with sleep-disordered breathing. *Sleep and Breathing* 19 (4), 1431–1437.

Preutthipan, A., Chantarojanasiri, T., Suwanjutha, S. and Udomsubpayakul, U. (2000) Can parents predict the severity of childhood obstructive sleep apnoea? *Acta Paediatrica* 89, 708–712.

Pueyo, R., Junqué, C., Vendrell, P., Narberhaus, A. and Segarra, D. (2008) Raven's coloured progressive matrices as a measure of cognitive functioning in cerebral palsy. *Journal of Intellectual Disability Research* 52, 437–445.

Rabinowitz, M. and Glaser, R. (1985) Cognitive structure and process in highly competent performance. In F.D. Horowitz and M. O'Brien (eds) *The Gifted and Talented:*

Developmental Perspectives (pp. 75–98). Washington, DC: American Psychological Association.

Raven, J. (2000) The Raven's progressive matrices: Change and stability over culture and time. *Cognitive Psychology* 41, 1–48.

Raven, J.C. (2008/2015) *Raven's Educational Coloured Progressive Matrices* (Greek version). Athens: Motivo Axiologisi.

Rosen, C.L. (2004) Obstructive sleep apnea syndrome in children: Controversies in diagnosis and treatment. *Pediatric Clinics of North America* 51 (1), 153–167.

Shouldice, R.B., O'Brien, L.M., O'Brien, C., de Chazal, P., Gozal, D. and Heneghan, C. (2004) Detection of obstructive sleep apnea in pediatric subjects using surface lead electrocardiogram features. *Sleep* 27 (4), 784–792.

Spearman, C. (1927) *The Nature of 'Intelligence' and the Principles of Cognition* (2nd edn). London: Macmillan.

Spruyt, K., Capdevila, O.S., Kheirandish-Gozal, L. and Gozal, D. (2009) Inefficient or insufficient encoding as potential primary deficit in neurodevelopmental performance among children with OSA. *Developmental Neuropsychology* 34 (5), 601–614.

Stavrakaki, S. (2005) Greek neurolinguistics: The state-of-the-art. *Journal of Greek Linguistics* 5, 181–228.

Suen, J.S., Arnold, J.E. and Brooks, L.J. (1995) Adenotonsillectomy for treatment of obstructive sleep apnea in children. *Archives of Otolaryngology – Head & Neck Surgery* 121 (5), 525–530.

Tal, A., Leiberman, A., Margulis, G. and Sofer, S. (1988) Ventricular dysfunction in children with obstructive sleep apnea: Radionuclide assessment. *Pediatric Pulmonology* 4 (3), 139–43.

Tallal, P., Miller, S. and Fitch, R. (1993) Neurobiological basis of speech: A case for the preeminence of temporal processing. *Annals of the New York Academy of Sciences* 682, 27–47.

Tami, T.A., Parker, G.S. and Taylor, R.E. (1987) Post-tonsillectomy bleeding: An evaluation of risk factors. *Laryngoscope* 97, 1307–1311.

Tapia, I.E., Bandla, P., Traylor, J., Karamessinis, L., Huang, J. and Marcus, C.L. (2010) Upper airway sensory function in children with obstructive sleep apnea syndrome. *Sleep* 33 (7), 968–972.

Tauman, R., Gulliver, T.E., Krishna, J., Montgomery-Downs, H.E., O'Brien, L.M., Ivanenko, A. and Gozal, D. (2006) Persistence of obstructive sleep apnea syndrome in children after adenotonsillectomy. *Journal of Pediatrics* 149 (6), 803–808.

Tzouriadou, M., Singolitou, E., Anagnostopoulou, E. and Vakola, I. (2008) *Psychometric Criterion of Language Adequacy (L-a-T-o-1)*. Thessaloniki: Aristotle University of Thessaloniki and Ministry of Education.

Urquhart, D. (2013) Investigation and management of childhood sleep apnoea. *Hippokratia* 17 (3), 196–202.

Valera, F., Travitzki, L., Mattar, S., Matsumoto, M., Elias, A.M. and Anselmo-Lima, W. (2003) Muscular, functional and orthodontic changes in pre-school children with enlarged adenoids and tonsils. *International Journal of Pediatric Otorhinolaryngology* 67 (7), 761–770.

van Someren, V.H., Hibbert, J., Stothers, J.K., Kyme, M.C. and Morrison, G.A.J. (1990) Identification of hypoxaemia in children having tonsillectomy and adenoidectomy. *Clinical Otolaryngology and Allied Sciences* 15, 263–271.

van Someren, V.H., Burmesterc, M., Alusib, G. and Laned, G. (2000) Methodology: Are sleep studies worth doing? *Archives of Disease in Childhood* 83, 76–78.

Verstraeten, E. (2007) Neurocognitive effects of obstructive sleep apnea syndrome. *Current Neurology and Neuroscience Reports* 7 (2), 161–166.

Vieira, B.B., Itikawa, C.E., de Almeida, L.A., Fernandes, R.M., Anselmo-Lima, W.T. and Valera, F.C. (2011) Cephalometric evaluation of facial pattern and hyoid bone position in children with obstructive sleep apnoea syndrome. *International Journal of Pediatric Otorhinolaryngology* 75, 383–386.

Vigneau, M., Beaucousin, V., Hervé, P.Y., Duffau, H., Crivello, F., Houdé, O., Mazoyer, B. and Tzourio-Mazoyer, N. (2006) Meta-analyzing left hemisphere language areas: Phonology, semantics, and sentence processing. *NeuroImage* 30 (4), 1414–1432.

Yorbik, O., Mutlu, C., Koc, D. and Mutluer, T. (2014) Possible negative effects of snoring and increased sleep fragmentation on developmental status of preschool children. *Sleep and Biological Rhythms* 12, 30–36.

Ziliotto, K.N., dos Santos, M.F., Monteiro, V.G., *et al.* (2006) Auditory processing assessment in children with obstructive sleep apnea syndrome. *Brazilian Journal of Otorhinolaryngology* 72 (3), 321–327.

8 Language Impairment in 22q11.2 Deletion Syndrome: A Case Study from Cyprus

Maria Kambanaros, Loukia Taxitari, Eleni Theodorou, Marina Varnava and Kleanthes K. Grohmann

Introduction

Crosslinguistic research describing the language and cognitive abilities of children with rare syndromes is sparse. The aim of the present case study is to report on the language abilities of a school-aged boy genetically confirmed with 22q11.2 deletion syndrome (22q11.2DS). This syndrome follows an autosomal dominant inheritance pattern; a child only needs to get the abnormal gene from one parent in order to inherit the disease. However, only around 10% of all cases of 22q11.2DS are inherited, while the majority of occurrences are due to a random mutation (Shprintzen, 2008). Our participant falls into the latter category.

22q11.2DS results from a submicroscopic hemizygous deletion: one of the two copies of chromosome 22 is missing at position 11 (Woodin *et al.*, 2001). Historically, it has also been known by many other names, including DiGeorge syndrome, Shprintzen syndrome and velocardiofacial syndrome. Now that researchers have found the unifying genetic cause of these conditions, the term 22q11.2 deletion syndrome is preferred (http://www.22q.org/awareness-events/awareness/same-name-campaign). It is an increasingly common genetic disorder affecting at least 1 in 2000–7000 live births (Shprintzen, 2008). The phenotypic description is quite varied, with close to 200 clinical features identified so far as relating to abnormalities of the heart, palate, velopharyngeal mechanism, immune system, central nervous system and brain morphology (see Woodin *et al.*, 2001 and references within). However, each child is affected differently and the symptoms can vary widely, ranging from less severe to severely affected. Children with 22q11.2DS tend to have similar facial features, including a long, narrow face, wide-set almond-shaped eyes, a broad nasal bridge and bulbous nose tip, a small mouth, small, low-set ears that are folded over at the top, and an irregular skull shape (see an older description from www.nhs.uk/conditions/digeorge-syndrome). Furthermore, there is evidence that 22q11.2DS remains undiagnosed in many children as an isolated speech and language disorder or a developmental delay in the presence of few or no physical abnormalities (Niklasson *et al.*, 2001).

There is a large body of research literature on the behavioural and psychiatric profiles of individuals with 22q11DS (see Scandurra *et al.*, 2013 and references within); however, within the paediatric population information is limited. The large variation of the phenotype can make diagnosis more difficult. According to some researchers, the median age of diagnosis is 6.5 years (Solot *et al.*, 2000).

The majority of individuals with 22q11.2DS show relatively mild cognitive deficits, sometimes including intellectual impairment (IQ 51–70), with verbal IQ often significantly higher than performance IQ and/or non-verbal IQ. However, there are reports of individuals with low normal intelligence (IQ 71–85) and some with an IQ in excess of 85 (Niklasson *et al.*, 2001). Individuals with 22q11.2DS show relative strengths in verbal ability, rote processing, verbal memory, reading and spelling. In addition, there are reported weaknesses in language abilities, attention, working memory, executive functions, visuospatial memory and psychosocial functioning (see Woodin *et al.*, 2001 and references within for both points).

In particular, research on the manifestations of speech and language disorders in children with 22q11.2DS is not prominent, despite communication impairment hailed as an outstanding deficit, with an estimated 90% of children having some type of speech-language deficit. Pre-school children with 22q11.2DS often show smaller vocabularies, word-finding deficits, reduced length of sentences, delayed use of grammatical structures and difficulties with discourse (Persson *et al.*, 2006). Moreover, expressive language delays are often more severe than receptive language delays. Furthermore, specific language impairment (SLI) was also reported for individual children in a large 22q11.2DS cohort from the US (Solot *et al.*, 2000, 2001) and in smaller case studies involving Dutch children (Goorhuis-Brouwer *et al.*, 2003). SLI is a term applied to children whose speech and language is substantially below age level for no apparent reason, in the absence of neurological damage, impaired sensorimotor abilities, and so on (i.e. with normal intelligence levels, hearing, vision, etc.). The reader is referred to Bishop (2014) for a more recent definition of SLI.

Of direct relevance to our research is Persson *et al.*'s (2006) study involving Swedish pre-schoolers and school-aged children with 22q11.2DS. The study assessed receptive vocabulary knowledge using the Swedish version of the Peabody Picture Vocabulary Test (PPVT; Dunn & Dunn, 1981), narrative retell performance using the Bus Story Test (BST; Renfrew, 1997) modified for Swedish, and articulation abilities based on Swedish norms in 19 children (10 girls and nine boys) between the ages of five and eight years genetically diagnosed with 22q11.2DS. The mean full-scale IQ of the group was 78 and in addition six children had autism spectrum disorder, attention deficit/hyperactivity disorder, or a combination of the two. For the PPVT, results revealed that the majority of children who participated on this task ($n = 14$) scored moderately low on receptive vocabulary, revealing more difficulties with understanding single words beyond that expected based on performance/non-verbal IQ. With regard to the BST, the majority of the 22q11.2DS children scored below the mean on the information score of the task. Of clinical interest was the finding of a negative correlation between age and the information score. In other words, the older the children were, the more difficulties they had recalling information on the BST. Furthermore, all but one participant had a shorter average sentence length than expected according to chronological age norms. In contrast, five participants produced subordinate clauses within normal limits, while 14 had a lower number of subordinate clauses according to chronological age norms revealing low grammatical abilities. The type of qualitative errors analyzed from the group with 22q11.2DS on the BST included grammatical errors (e.g. errors of prepositions, gender, definite articles) and incomplete utterances. Finally, articulation abilities were within the normal range for the majority of children with 22q11.2DS, with the remaining children showing mild deficits. Based on their findings, the researchers concluded that the vast majority of participants had language impairments, and difficulties were found in all language areas investigated for the group with 22q11.2DS. Persson and colleagues did not opt for the term SLI to describe the language performance of their group of participants with 22q11.2DS given that the non-linguistic characteristics of the group were quite diverse (e.g. behavioural difficulties including autism spectrum disorders and attention deficit/hyperactivity disorder or palatal/velopharyngeal anomalies) and that the notion of 'specific' language impairment is in the context of otherwise normal development (see Bishop, 2014).

However, three studies were found in the literature reporting SLI in children with 22q11.2DS. A brief description of the studies is reported in Table 8.1. According to Solot *et al.* (2000), nearly all children with 22q11DS in the US cohort were speaking by school age. Nevertheless, persistent difficulties were noted in syntax, vocabulary, knowledge of concepts, word finding and organization of discourse. However, the exact number of individuals with these difficulties and their age were not detailed. Similarly, Solot *et al.* (2001) report on persistent language impairment, particularly in expressive skills, among five- to 16-year-olds with 22q11.2DS. Furthermore, four of 11 (36%) had SLI, defined as language impairment, beyond what could be expected from their general level of ability.

Table 8.1 Summary of published research describing specific language impairment (SLI) in children with 22q11.2DS

Study	*Solot et al. (2000)*	*Solot et al. (2001)*	*Goorhuis-Brouwer et al. (2003)*
No. of participants	305	79	4
Language of investigation	English	English	Dutch
Age range	≤ 5 ≥	0;7–16;7	5;0–6;8
IQ range	Not provided	For pre-school children: Bayley Scales of Infant Development (BSID; *mental scale score*) 68.6 ± 13.3; WIPSI: 84.5 ± 10.4 For school-aged children: WISC-III, VIQ: 77.8 ± 13.6; PIQ: 71.7 ± 12.8; FSIQ: 73.0 ± 12.6	Non-verbal IQ (normal range: 90–112)
Language testing	(a) Pre-school Language Scales-3 (PLS-3) (b) Clinical Evaluation of Language Fundamentals-Revised (CELF-R) (c) Goldman-Fristoe Test of Articulation (d) Peabody Picture Vocabulary Test-Revised (e) Expressive One Word Vocabulary Test-Revised	(a) PLS-3 (b) CELF-R	(a) Language Comprehension (Dutch version of the Reynell Test of Language Development) (b) Language production (test for sentence development) (c) Spontaneous speech sample (d) Articulation and diadochokinetic (DDK) rates
Linguistic deficit	(1) severe delays in expressive language in 53% of the children (2) receptive language delays in 25% of the children (3) difficulties in a variety of linguistic domains (syntax, vocabulary, concepts, word-finding, discourse organization)	(1) expressive language skills significantly worse than receptive language (2) SLI pattern in 36% of the school-aged children (3) speech abnormalities of varying kinds in 75.9% of the school-aged children	(1) long sentences produced *or* (2) two- and three-word utterances produced only *or* (3) primarily non-verbal communication
Conclusion	Delays cannot be explained by cognitive factors, but as the **presence of specific speech and language impairment.** Presence/absence of cardiac or palatal abnormalities: no effect on development outcome.	An **SLI pattern of disorder**: (a) delayed emergence of language and (b) persistent speech and language disorders.	**Children were characterized as SLI**: phonological programming deficit syndrome (2/4) or verbal dyspraxia (2/4).

Goorhuis-Brouwer *et al.* (2003) report on four children out of 18 that failed to develop adequate speech and language production after more than two years of speech and language therapy despite non-verbal IQ in the normal range (90–106). Each child showed some medical condition in line with the 22q11.2DS phenotype (e.g. conductive hearing loss, velopharyngeal insufficiency, submucous cleft palate, heart problems). The children were re-assessed post-therapy between five years and 6;8 on the comprehension subtest of the Reynell Language Developmental Scales adapted for Dutch (yields a language comprehension quotient), a spontaneous language measure (MLU), a language production task at the sentence level, and on articulation abilities. The oldest participant (P1), a girl aged 6;8, on assessment showed normal language comprehension skills, produced long sentences (six words or more), but speech was overall unintelligible despite successful pharyngoplasty and speech and language therapy. The second child (P2), a boy aged six, had normal language comprehension but production consisted of two- to three-word utterances and speech remained unintelligible. A second boy (P3), also aged six, at follow-up assessment, remained unintelligible with speech characterized by severe hypernasality and undifferentiated articulation. The fourth child (P4), a girl aged five at the time of re-assessment, showed unintelligible speech because of severe hypernasality and a severe articulation disorder.

Based on language performance after testing, the researchers claim that the four children with 22q11.2DS fulfilled the criteria of a linguistic subtype of SLI (as termed by Bishop & Leonard, 2000): for P1 and P3 a phonological programming deficit, and for P2 and P4 a verbal dyspraxia. In verbal dyspraxia, language comprehension is adequate but speech is extremely limited, with impaired production of speech sounds and short utterances. With regard to phonological programming deficit, children are argued to have intact language comprehension and form long utterances but speech is hard to understand. In both cases, the difficulty with producing speech cannot be accounted for in terms of dysarthria (i.e. muscle weakness because of brain damage).

To our knowledge, our report is the first to describe the linguistic manifestations of a language deficit associated with this particular genetic syndrome for Greek, and in the context of bilectalism (Rowe & Grohmann, 2013). Bilectalism is used here to characterize the situation in Cyprus in which children of Greek Cypriot parents, with Cypriot Greek-speaking family and friends, grow up, yet get exposed to Standard Modern Greek from an early age – first through media such as TV cartoons, later through public schooling starting in nursery and kindergarten, becoming gradually more systematic in primary school. In the absence of a separate Cypriot Greek orthographic system, Greek can only be taught through the medium of the standard variety in order to teach children how to read and write. We take this to be the standard path of language development by Greek Cypriot children, as relevant for our study.

A core area of investigation will be the performance of our participant with 22q11.2DS on structural language, that is, his morphosyntactic abilities and performance on more complex language tasks. Our testing battery contains several measures for probing structural language, ranging from comprehension of complex structures (e.g. Wh-questions), morphosyntactic properties (agreement relations) and other phenomena (object clitic production and placement) to the production of structurally complex clauses (including subordinates and relatives) on a narrative retell task. But the entire testing battery goes well beyond structural language. As the first research on language abilities in 22q11.2DS for (Cypriot) Greek, we take a broader angle and also investigate global language abilities, non-verbal IQ, as well as receptive and expressive vocabulary skills. Furthermore, to decipher the issue of comorbidity with SLI, the performance of our participant with 22q11.2DS on all measures will be compared to two groups of typically developing children of the same chronological age and a group of children with a clinical diagnosis of SLI. Taking the lead from Rice (2016), we will present the outcome of our detailed testing in a comparative conceptual framework of a 2 × 2 design comparing the linguistic performance of children with SLI and those with typical language development (TLD) to our participant with 22q11.2DS.

Aims

The purpose of the present study is to profile the language abilities of one male child with 22q11.2DS (P.I.) and compare his performance to that reported for children of the same chronological age with TLD and ones with a diagnosis of SLI across a battery of linguistic tests. The aims of the study are five-fold:

(1) to investigate P.I.'s receptive and expressive language abilities, with an emphasis on structural language performance;
(2) to compare P.I.'s language performance across all measures with that of children with TLD of the same chronological age;
(3) to compare P.I.'s language performance across all measures with that of children of the same chronological age diagnosed with SLI;
(4) to determine whether error patterns on structural language tasks differentiate P.I. from TLD and/or SLI peers;
(5) to shed light on the 22q11.2DS ± SLI debate based on the findings.

Method

Participant

Our participant, P.I., was a pre-school boy aged 5;11 when the study began and enrolled in the pre-school education programme of a public school in Nicosia, Cyprus. He was not receiving special education services. All tests were conducted at this age except comprehension of and exhaustivity in simple and multiple Wh-questions, which were conducted at 6;5.

P.I. was diagnosed with 22q11.2DS by the head geneticist of the Makarios Hospital Genetics Clinic in Nicosia using the fluorescence *in situ* hybridization test (FISH). The FISH test is specially designed to look for small groups of genes that are deleted and in the case of 22q11.2DS shows whether the region of chromosome 22 is present. If only one copy of chromosome 22 *lights up* with fluorescent DNA dye, rather than both copies, the FISH test is positive for 22q11 deletion. Hearing was tested by the Makarios Hospital Audiology Clinic and reported to be within normal limits. Also, the hospital reported no positive assessment of autism spectrum disorder symptoms or any other psychiatric condition.

P.I. was born from healthy, unrelated parents who are both highly educated with university degrees, the mother in an allied health profession and the father in information technology. P.I. also has a healthy brother who is older by three years. An oral-peripheral motor examination administered by a certified speech and language therapist (first author) revealed no structural abnormalities of the speech mechanism including the palate. At the time of the study, he was receiving private speech therapy for voice quality (e.g. hypernasality) and mild misarticulations. P.I. presented with hoarseness and reduced vocal volume but generally intelligible speech during the time of the study. Testing across all measures was conducted over a six-month period.

Comparative groups

For our comparison with P.I., a total of 27 bilectal children participated in this study. For selection purposes, we considered 'bilectal' those children whose parents are both Greek Cypriots, who were born and raised in Cyprus, and who did not spend any large amount of time outside the island, including Greece. We did not control any more specifically for balanced input or age of exposure to Cypriot Greek and Standard Modern Greek but assumed the standard path of language development laid out above (see Grohmann & Kambanaros, 2016). The children were divided into three groups, one group including children with SLI of the same chronological age as P.I. and two control groups with TLD (five- to six-year-olds and six- to seven-year-olds). Table 8.2 reports the background information of all the participants from the comparative groups.

All children came from the Limassol district and the majority attended public pre-primary or primary schools. Parental consent forms and an information letter that explained the purpose of the study were distributed, and only children whose parents gave written consent participated in the study. The consent form provided additional information such as demographics, the education level of each of the parents, and the parents' occupations (see

Table 8.2 Participant details for the comparative groups

Group	*Mean age (SD)*	*Gender*	*Non-verbal IQ (SD)*	*SES*
TLD 5- to 6-year-olds	5;8 (0;6)	6M, 4F	90 (12.5)	4.4 (1.08)
TLD 6- to 7-year-olds	6;4 (0;3)	3M, 5F	N/A	4.5 (0.76)
SLI	5;6 (0;3)	7M, 2F	100.5 (12.8)	3.67 (0.50)

Notes: TLD = typical language development; SLI = specific language impairment; SD = standard deviation; SES = socio-economic status based on mother's level of education: 0 = did not complete primary education, 1 = primary education, 2 = high school, 3 = lyceum, 4 = diploma, 5 = university degree, 6 = masters, 7 = doctorate; M = male; F = female; N/A = not available.

Theodorou *et al.*, 2016 for participant details). The exclusion criteria which restricted individual participation were: (i) a known history of neurological, emotional, developmental or behavioural problems; (ii) hearing and vision not adequate for test purposes after school screening at the beginning of the school year; (iii) non-verbal performance not in the broad range of normal; (iv) gross motor difficulties; and (v) low socio-economic status. All information was obtained from the speech-language therapists and teachers or from the children's parents.

Language-impaired children (five- to six-year-old SLI group)

Nine children with SLI (seven boys and two girls), aged between 4;11 and 5;11 with a mean age of 5;6 (*SD* 0;3), served as the language-impaired comparative group. Children were diagnosed with SLI by certified speech and language therapists based on case history information, informal testing of comprehension and production abilities, analysis of spontaneous language samples and clinical observation. SLI diagnosis was confirmed by further testing on tools used for diagnostic purposes in Cyprus (Theodorou, 2013; Theodorou *et al.*, 2016). Children with SLI included in the study were receiving speech and language therapy services by practitioners in private settings.

Typically language developing children (five- to seven-year-old TLD groups)

Ten children (six boys and four girls) with TLD, aged between 4;5 and 6;6 with a mean age of 5;8 (*SD* 0;6), served as the chronological age-matched group for all tests, except Wh-question Comprehension and Wh-question Exhaustivity. For the latter, a second group of eight children (three boys and five girls) with a mean age of 6;4 (*SD* 0;3) served as the chronological age-matched group (P.I.'s age was 6;5 at the time). According to the classroom teacher and parent reports, each participant in the control groups was typically developing in all respects. No control child was previously referred to or had received treatment by a speech and language therapist.

Socio-economic status

All children came from families with a medium to high socio-economic status, as measured by mothers' education level using the European Social Survey (2010) database. We compared P.I.'s mother's education level (undergraduate degree from university) to the education levels of the mothers of the other three groups. Her education level did not differ from that of the TLD five- to six-year-olds group mothers ($t_{(9)} = -0.52$, $p = 0.62$) or the TLD six- to seven-year-olds group mothers ($t_{(7)} = 0.62$, $p = 0.28$), but it did from the SLI group ($t_{(8)} = 2.47$, $p < 0.05$), whose mothers' education levels had a lower mean than P.I.'s mother's.

Non-verbal IQ

Prior to the study proper, children from the TLD five- to six-year-olds group and the SLI group were tested on the Raven's Coloured Progressive Matrices (RCPM; Raven *et al.*, 2000), following the Greek norms of Sideridis *et al.* (2015). Raw scores were converted into standard scores, which provided each child's non-verbal IQ. This requirement was satisfied for each child separately and only applied to the children to be compared on chronological age.

Materials and procedures

All language measures were administered to P.I. and the two groups of children, those with a clinical diagnosis of SLI and those that had TLD. Of the TLD children, the five- to six-year-olds were tested on measures (A–E) as were the group of children with SLI, while the TLD six- to seven-year-olds were tested on measures (F–G) to correspond with P.I.'s chronological age at the time of testing. Each of the measures (A–G) is described in detail below.

(A) Diagnostic Verbal IQ Test

Children's global language abilities were measured using the Diagnostic Verbal IQ Test (DVIQ; Stavrakaki & Tsimpli, 2000), modified for Cypriot Greek (Theodorou, 2013). This test is used by language researchers and clinicians to assess language abilities for Greek-speaking children; while it is not yet standardized, it is in the process of undergoing standardization in Greece. The DVIQ has five subtests: expressive vocabulary, comprehension of morphosyntax, production of morphosyntax, comprehension of metalinguistic concepts and sentence repetition. The production of morphosyntax subtest includes diverse grammatical properties and markers such as nominal and verbal suffixes, object clitics, articles, agreement relations and relative clauses, among others.

Each child was tested individually on all subtests, which involved naming and showing pictures as well as completing and repeating sentences. Children's responses were recorded on the answer sheets, and later analyzed and scored. Each correct response received 1 point, with the exception of the sentence repetition subtest, which was scored according to the number of errors in each repetition (maximum score of 3 points correct for each sentence). The original DVIQ has been used in published studies for the identification of children with SLI in Greece (Mastropavlou *et al.*, 2011) and Cyprus (Mastropavlou *et al.*, 2011; Petinou & Okalidou, 2006); the Cypriot Greek-adapted version has also been tested widely in Cyprus by our research team (see, among others, Kambanaros *et al.*, 2013, 2014).

(B) Bus Story Test

A topic-centred narrative, the Bus Story Test (BST; Renfrew, 1997) is used widely by speech and language therapists to assess narrative abilities in children ranging from three to eight years of age. It is translated into Greek and also used in Greece as a non-standardized measure. For this study, the Greek translation of the BST was used (with minor changes in phonology and morphology adapted to Cypriot Greek; cf. Theodorou & Grohmann, 2010), since Greek Cypriot children are accustomed to hearing stories in Standard Modern Greek rather than in Cypriot Greek from their pre-school years.

The experimenter told each child the story individually while the child looked at the picture strips illustrating the story. Afterwards, the child was requested to retell the story as close to the original as possible. Test administration was around 10 minutes. The narrative samples were transcribed and divided into sentences (*t*-units). Children's narrative productions were each evaluated with respect to five descriptors, three from the BST manual and two additional ones developed for our research purposes:

(1) *Information* (Renfrew, 1997). The number of relevant information pieces were tallied following the BST manual, where 'essential' information gets two points and 'subsidiary' information gets 1 point; the Information score is the total number of points accumulated.
(2) *Subordinate Clauses* (Renfrew, 1997). All subordinate clauses were identified and counted for a total score, as per BST manual.
(3) *A5LS*. The mean length of the five longest sentences was computed.
(4) *MLU-word*. In the absence of normative data for mean length of utterance (MLU) in Cypriot Greek, it was calculated based on words for each narrative (MLU-word); all words were added up and the sum was divided by sentences produced (MLU-word was chosen, since there is no study to support the use of a morpheme-based MLU in any variety of Modern Greek).
(5) *T-units* (Renfrew, 1997). The total number of sentences produced was added up, as suggested in the BST manual.

(C) Expressive Vocabulary Test

In order to assess naming abilities, the Expressive Vocabulary Test (EVT; Vogindroukas *et al.*, 2009) was administered. The EVT contains 50 concrete black-and-white pictures for naming. It is standardized in Greece and has norms for Standard Modern Greek. Because of the differences between the standard language and the dialect, 11 items have alternative words in Cypriot Greek (10 lexical alternatives and one phonological alternative); they were considered acceptable responses. Children were asked to name the object in the picture. Responses were recorded on the answer sheet and then scored as correct or incorrect on a word-by-word basis.

(D) Peabody Picture Vocabulary Test

In order to assess receptive vocabulary skills, the Greek version of the Peabody Picture Vocabulary Test (PPVT; Dunn & Dunn, 1981, adapted to Standard Modern Greek by Simos *et al.*, 2011), developed for research purposes in Greece and Cyprus, was used. The PPVT measures receptive vocabulary at the single word level.

The Greek version of the test consists of 228 items, equally distributed across 19 item sets. Each set contains 12 items of increasing difficulty. The examiner presented a quadrant of four numbered pictures and asked the child to point to or say the number of the picture of the spoken word.

(E) Clitics-in-Islands Test

The COST Action A33 Clitics-in-Islands Test (CIT; Varlokosta *et al.*, 2015), a testing tool designed to elicit clitic production, was used. The CIT is a production task for third-person singular accusative object clitics in which the target-elicited clitic is embedded within a *because*-clause (a so-called syntactic island):

(1) i mama xtenizi ti koɾua tʃe i koɾua en omoɾfi. ʝati i koɾua en omoɾfi? i koɾua en omoɾfi ʝati i mama tis… [xtenizi tin-CL].[1]

'Mommy is combing the girl and the girl is beautiful. Why is the girl beautiful? The girl is beautiful because her mommy… [combs her-CL].'

The CIT involved a total of 19 items: 12 target structures (i.e. test items) after two warm-ups, plus five unrelated fillers. All target structures were indicative declarative clauses formed around a transitive verb. All participating children were shown a coloured sketch picture on a laptop screen, depicting the situation that was described by the experimenter.

Participants heard the description of each picture that the experimenter provided and then had to complete the *because*-clause in which the use of a clitic was expected. The ideal response was a verb-clitic sequence (such as *xtenizi tin* 'combs her' in the above example), but some participants started with *because* on their own and others filled in right after the experimenter's prompt of *because*. The experiments were not audio- or video-taped, but answers were recorded by the researcher on a score sheet during the session.

(F) Wh-questions task I: Comprehension of d-linked and non-d-linked Wh-arguments

The design of the Comprehension of Wh-questions experimental tool was adapted from COST Action A33. The tool was designed to test subject and object questions, and *who*- versus *which*-questions, using a question-picture matching task. (For a detailed description of the tool, see Varnava & Grohmann, 2014.)

A total of 24 target questions were asked in random order (plus two trial questions during the lead-in phase). Each target question was accompanied by the appropriate slide on a computer-based MS PowerPoint presentation and verbalized by the experimenter. The task involved a sentence-picture selection. The child had to choose the appropriate picture out of four pictures in total (one target, three distracters) after the target question was asked. The distracter pictures involved reversed roles (agent of the action depicted as patient/theme), a semantic error picture (action depicted on the picture different from that of the target question), and a number error picture in which the character(s) involved do not agree in number with the target question (e.g. while in the target question *who*-singular is used, the distracter picture would depict two or more characters involved in the action). The child had to listen to a question, then look carefully at four pictures on the computer screen, and decide, verbally or by pointing, which picture appropriately answered the target question. The pictures on the slide were numbered from 1 to 4. The experimenter wrote down the picture number provided by the child for each target question on a score sheet. All data recorded on the score sheet were entered in an MS Excel sheet for further analysis. P.I. responded to all questions.

(G) Wh-questions task 2: The acquisition of exhaustivity in simple and multiple Wh-questions

The Comprehension of Exhaustivity in Wh-questions experiment was adapted from COST Action 33 (cf. Varnava & Grohmann, 2014). The tool was designed to test the comprehension of exhaustivity in four types of Wh-questions; Protocol B tested for *pci* 'who all'-questions only (i.e. Type 2), while Protocol A tested for the other three types of Wh-questions: Type 1: simple Wh-questions; Type 3: paired Wh-questions; Type 4: triple Wh-questions.

A total of 30 target questions were asked in Protocol A and 12 target questions in Protocol B. Each target question was accompanied by the appropriate slide on a computer-based PowerPoint presentation; the task involved a question-after-picture test. Each child's responses were recorded on a score sheet which were later entered in an MS Excel sheet for further analysis. P.I. responded to all questions.

Structural language probes

We consider structural language probes to be those that tap into morphosyntactic abilities and language complexity. For our purposes, the *comprehension and production of morphosyntax subtests* of the DVIQ, the *sentence repetition subtest* of the DVIQ, the *number of subordinate clauses produced* on the BST, *performance on the CIT*, and *comprehension of D-linked and non-D-linked Wh-questions and comprehension of exhaustivity in Wh-questions* serve as measures of structural language complexity for our analyses in this research.

Scoring and analysis

For all tests (e.g. PPVT, EVT, CIT), an *accuracy score* was calculated by summing up the number of correct responses. For all subcategories of the DVIQ, except sentence repetition, a single point was given for every correct response, and no points for every incorrect one. For sentence repetition, 3 points were given for every correct response, 2 points for every response with one error, 1 point for every response with two errors, and no points for responses with three or more errors. For the Wh-question Comprehension measure, 1 point was given for each correct answer and no points for errors; three types of errors were possible: reversal, semantic and number. Reversal errors are cases in which the participant's answer involves the opposite syntactic element, i.e. instead of subject the participant points to the object. Semantic errors are cases in which the participant chooses a picture in which the action depicted is different from that of the target question. Number errors are cases in which the character(s) involved in the action do not agree in number with that of the target question (e.g. while in the target question *who*-singular is used, the distracter picture would depict two or more characters involved in the action).

Results

The main statistical analysis used was the Crawford–Howell *t*-test (Crawford & Howell, 1998), a method developed in neuropsychology for the comparison of single cases with control groups (with small sample numbers). Using this method, P.I.'s accuracy scores were compared to the TLD and SLI groups using a one-tailed *t*-test. The results are reported in Table 8.3.

Non-verbal IQ

P.I.'s non-verbal IQ based on the RCPM was 69. There were no statistically significant differences in non-verbal IQ between the SLI and TLD five- to six-year-old groups (Mann-Whitney $U = 25.5$, $n_1 = 10$, $n_2 = 9$, $p = 0.11$ two-tailed). When P.I.'s performance was compared to the mean performance of each group (see Table 8.2), there was no significant difference from the TLD five- to six-year-old group ($t_{(9)} = -1.61$, $p = 0.07$), but his non-verbal IQ was significantly lower than that of the SLI group ($t_{(8)} = -2.29$, $p < 0.05$).

Table 8.3 Raw scores (DVIQ, PPVT, EVT, CIT, Wh-Qs) for P.I. (22q11.2DS) in comparison to the specific language impairment and typical language development groups

Test	*Subtest*	*Mean score*			*Cut-off scores*
		P.I. MA: 5;11	*TLD (SD) MA: 5;8*	*SLI (SD) MA: 5;6*	
DVIQ	Vocabulary (max. 27)	19	22.9 (2.2)	16.8 (2.8)	21
	Production: morphosyntax (max. 24)	9	19.8 (2.1)	13.9 (2.7)	17
	Comprehension: metalinguistic concepts (max. 25)	17	19.9 (1.8)	18 (3.9)	19
	Comprehension: morphosyntax (max. 31)	16	25.4 (2.6)	24.6 (3.8)	24
	Sentence repetition (max. 48)	35	45.5 (2.5)	40.9 (2.5)	43
	Total DVIQ Score (max. 155)	96	133.5 (7.6)	114.1 (10.5)	128
PPVT	(max. 212)	34	63.8 (11.7)	54.8 (16.6)	61
EVT	(max. 50)	25	33.3 (5.1)	21.7 (2.7)	29
CIT	(max. 12)	9	11.6 (1.3)	11 (1)	
BST	Information	17	35.8 (11.5)	21.8 (8.9)	31
	A5SL	5.4	8.44 (2.1)	5.4 (0.8)	7
	Subordinate clauses	1	7.8 (4.1)	1.7 (1.5)	5
	T-units	8	20.6 (3.9)	15.6 (3.8)	17
	MLU-word	4.6	4.7 (1.2)	3.4 (0.7)	4.3
		P.I MA: 6;5	*TLD (SD) MA: 6;4*		
Wh-Q comprehension	Subject *who* (max. 6)	3	4.3 (1.2)	n/a	n/a
	Subject *which* (max. 6)	2	3.6 (1.1)	n/a	n/a
	Object *who* (max. 6)	3	3.6 (1.2)	n/a	n/a
	Object *which* (max. 6)	2	3.8 (1.2)	n/a	n/a
Wh-Q exhaustivity	Simple (max. 8)	4	6.6 (2.6)	n/a	n/a
	Simple all (max. 8)	7	8 (0.2)	n/a	n/a
	Paired (max. 8)	0	3.8 (3.8)	n/a	n/a
	Triple (max. 4)	0	1.8 (1.9)	n/a	n/a

Notes: max = maximum; DVIQ = Diagnostic Verbal IQ Test; PPVT = Peabody Picture Vocabulary Test; EVT = Expressive Vocabulary Test; CIT = Clitics-in-Islands Test; BST = Bus Story Test; Wh-Q = Wh-questions; TLD = typical language development; SLI = specific language impairment; SD = standard deviation; MA = mean age (years;months); max = maximum score correct; n/a = not applicable.

Diagnostic Verbal IQ Test

P.I.'s comparison to the TLD group revealed that he performed significantly lower on three subtests of the DVIQ: (i) in the *production of morphosyntax* ($t_{(9)} = -4.9, p < 0.001$); (ii) in the *comprehension of morphosyntax* ($t_{(9)} = -3.46, p < 0.01$), and (iii) in the *sentence repetition* subtest ($t_{(9)} = -3.99, p < 0.01$). P.I. showed no significant difference from TLD peers on the remaining two subtests of the DVIQ, namely comprehension of metalinguistic concepts ($t_{(9)} = -1.55, p = 0.08$) and expressive vocabulary ($t_{(9)} = -1.71, p = 0.06$). Overall, his total DVIQ score was significantly lower than that of his TLD peers ($t_{(9)} = -4.69, p < 0.01$).

When P.I.'s performance was compared to that of the SLI group, he showed a significantly lower performance on two DVIQ subtests: (i) *comprehension of morphosyntax* ($t_{(8)} = -2.12, p < 0.05$) and (ii) *sentence repetition* ($t_{(8)} = -2.26, p < 0.05$). There was no significant difference between P.I. and the SLI group on the remaining DVIQ subtests, expressive vocabulary ($t_{(8)} = 0.75, p = 0.24$), comprehension of metalinguistic concepts ($t_{(8)} = -0.25, p = 0.41$), and production of morphosyntax ($t_{(8)} = -1.71, p = 0.06$). Overall, his total DVIQ score was not significantly different from the SLI group

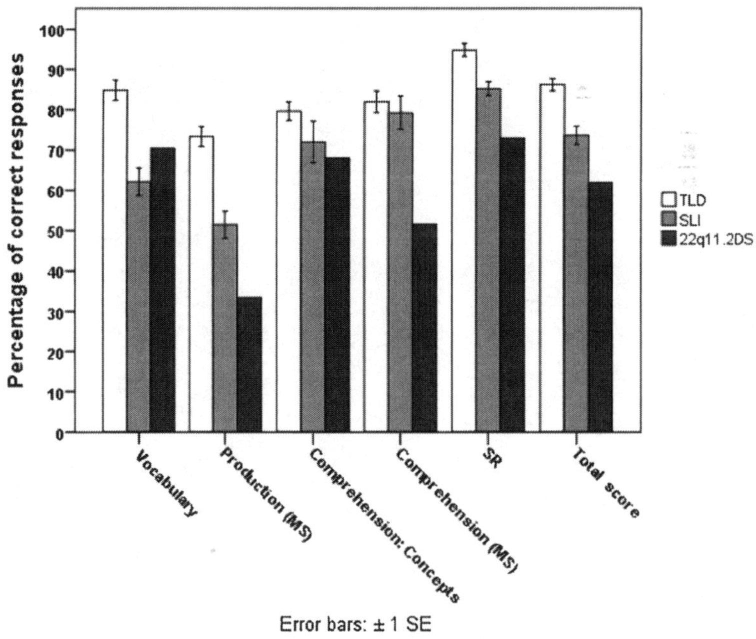

Key: MS = morphosyntax, SR = sentence repetition, TLD = typical language development, SLI = specific language impairment

Figure 8.1 Performance (% correct) of P.I. (22q11.2DS) in comparison to the TLD group and the SLI group on the five different subtests of the DVIQ

($t_{(8)} = -1.64$, $p = 0.07$). Figure 8.1 shows P.I.'s performance in comparison to the TLD and SLI groups on the subtests and total score on the DVIQ test.

Bus Story Test

When P.I.'s performance was compared to the TLD group on the BST, he showed a significantly lower performance only on the *number of sentences (t-units) produced* ($t_{(9)} = -3.09$, $p < 0.01$). There was no significant difference between P.I. and the TLD group for Information ($t_{(9)} = -1.55$, $p = 0.08$), A5LS ($t_{(9)} = -1.37$, $p = 0.1$), number of subordinate clauses produced ($t_{(9)} = -1.58$, $p = 0.07$), and MLU-word ($t_{(9)} = -0.06$, $p = 0.48$).

When compared to the SLI group, P.I. also only showed a significantly lower performance for *number of sentences (t-units) produced* ($t_{(8)} = -1.91$, $p < 0.05$). There were no significant differences between P.I. and the SLI group performance for Information ($t_{(8)} = -0.51$, $p = 0.31$), A5LS ($t_{(8)} = 0$, $p = 0.5$), number of subordinate clauses produced ($t_{(8)} = -0.42$, $p = 0.34$), and MLU-word ($t_{(8)} = 1.64$, $p = 0.07$).

Figure 8.2 shows P.I.'s performance compared to the TLD and SLI groups on the number of sentences (*t*-units) produced.

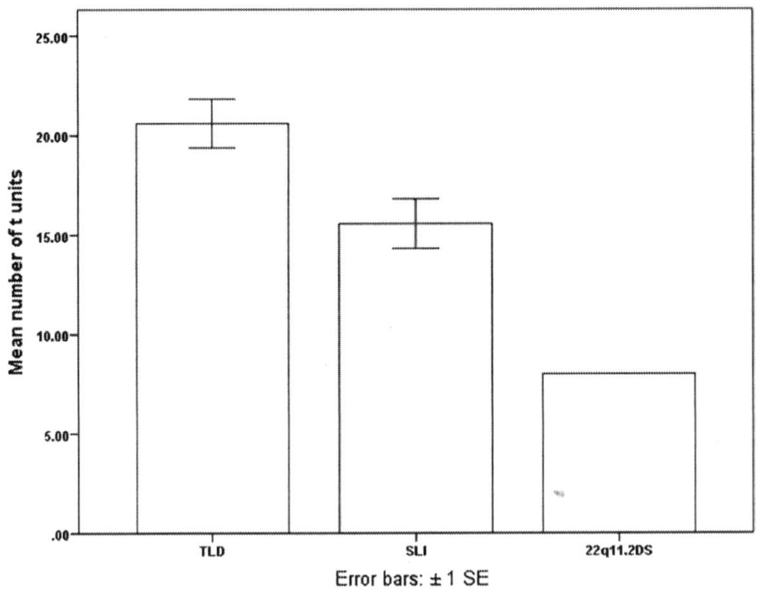

Key: TLD = typical language development, SLI = specific language impairment

Figure 8.2 Performance (% correct) of P.I. (22Q11.2DS) in comparison to the TLD group and the SLI group on the production of sentences (*t*-units) on the BST

Peabody Picture Vocabulary Test

For receptive vocabulary at the single word level, P.I. performed significantly lower compared to the TLD group ($t_{(9)} = -2.42, p < 0.05$), but not when compared to the SLI group ($t_{(8)} = -1.19, p = 0.13$).

Expressive Vocabulary Test

For expressive vocabulary, P.I. showed a similar performance on this task to both groups of children, those with TLD ($t_{(9)} = -1.54, p = 0.08$) and those with SLI ($t_{(8)} = 1.15, p = 0.14$).

Clitics-in-Islands Test

P.I. showed a significantly lower performance on this task than both groups of children, the children with TLD ($t_{(9)} = -1.95, p < 0.05$) and those with SLI ($t_{(8)} = -1.9, p < 0.05$).

Results from the PPVT, the EVT and the CIT across P.I. and the two comparative groups of children are graphically displayed in Figure 8.3.

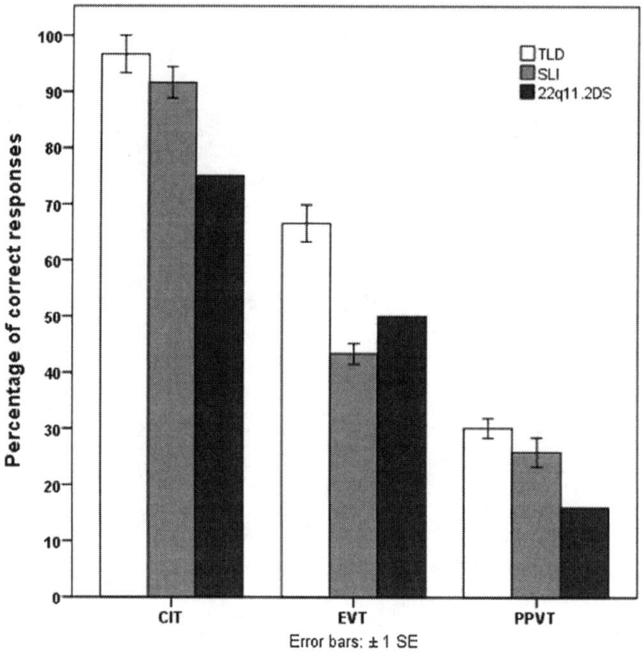

Key: TLD = typical language development, SLI = specific language impairment, CIT = Clitics-in-Islands Test, EVT = Expressive Vocabulary Test, PPVT = Peabody Picture Vocabulary Test

Figure 8.3 Performance (% correct) of P.I. (22Q11.2DS) in comparison to the TLD group and the SLI group on the CIT, the EVT and the PPVT

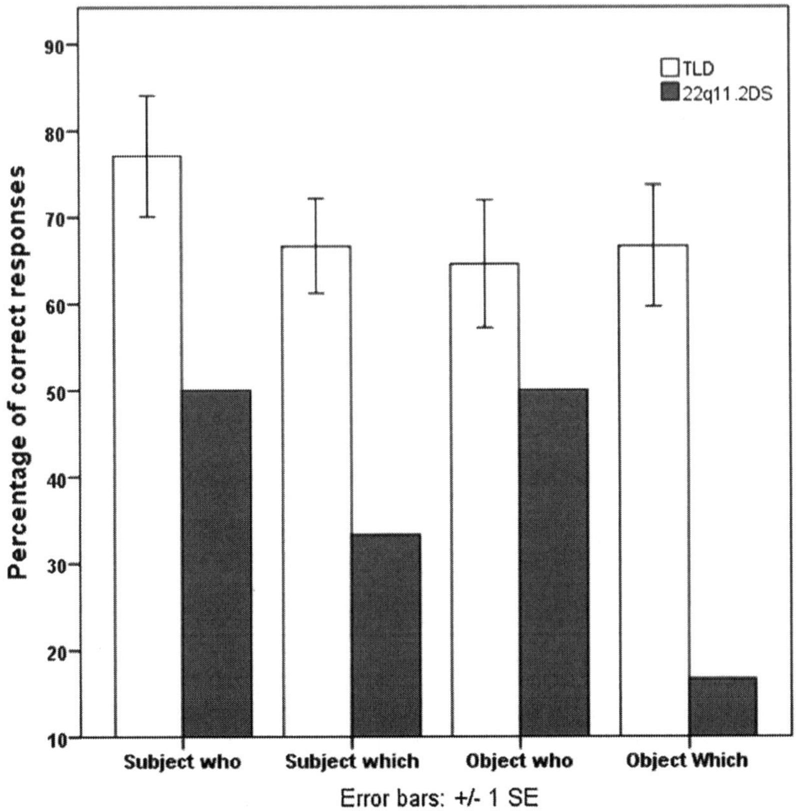

Figure 8.4 Performance (% correct) of P.I. (22q11.2DS) in comparison to the typical language development group on the Wh-questions comprehension test

Wh-question Comprehension

P.I.'s comparison to the TLD group (Figure 8.4) revealed that he performed significantly lower than the TLD group on the subject and the object *which*-questions (subject *which* $t_{(7)} = -2.03$, $p < 0.05$, object *which* $t_{(7)} = -2.36$, $p < 0.05$), but not the subject or object *who*-questions (subject *who* $t_{(7)} = -0.82$, $p = 0.22$, object *who* $t_{(7)} = -0.66$, $p = 0.26$).

Wh-question Exhaustivity

P.I.'s comparison to the TLD group revealed that he performed significantly lower only on one type of Wh-questions, namely simple *who all* ($t_{(7)} = -94.28$, $p < 0.001$). P.I. showed no significant difference from the TLD peers on the remaining three Wh-question types, namely simple ($t_{(7)} = -0.75$,

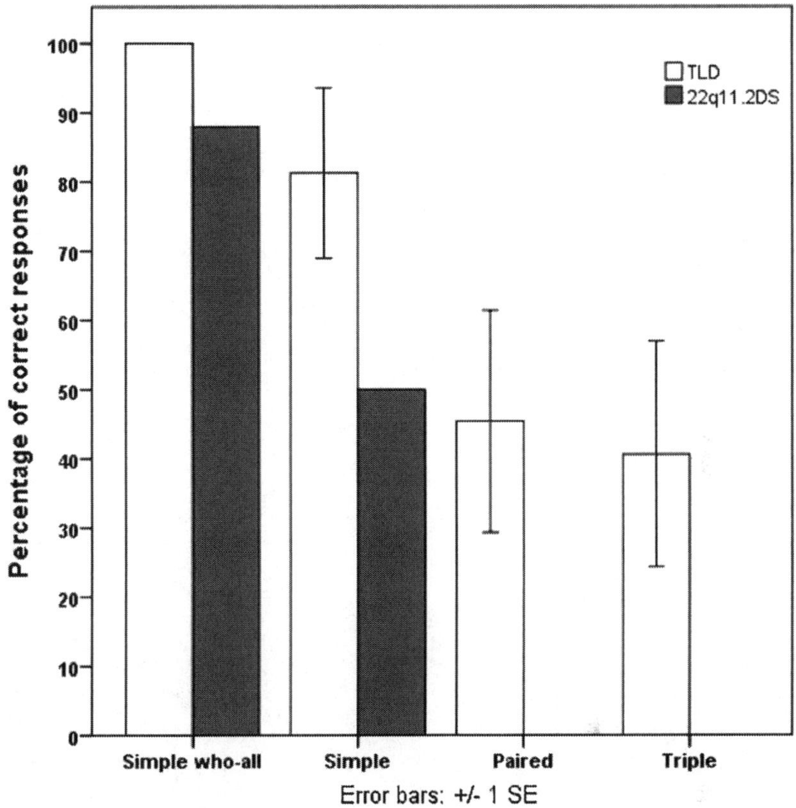

Figure 8.5 Performance (% correct) of P.I. (22q11.2DS) in comparison to the typical language development group on the Wh-questions exhaustivity test

$p = 0.24$), paired ($t_{(7)} = -0.95, p = 0.19$), and triple ($t_{(7)} = -0.83, p = 0.22$). Figure 8.5 shows the different types of Wh-questions for the TLD group and P.I.

Error Analyses

Comprehension and production of morphosyntax subtests of the Diagnostic Verbal IQ Test

In order to compare the errors of P.I. with the TLD and SLI groups, an items analysis was run by calculating the percentage of children who responded correctly to each item. Pearson *r* correlations revealed a significant positive relationship between the TLD and the SLI groups in terms of their performance on individual items for both morphosyntax production ($r_{(23)} = 0.66$, $p < 0.01$) and comprehension ($r_{(31)} = 0.78$, $p < 0.01$) as well as sentence repetition ($r_{(16)} = 0.84$, $p < 0.01$), although the SLI group show more variability in their errors. Figure 8.6 is a box plot of the performance of TLD and SLI children on the DVIQ subtests.

In order to identify the most problematic items, we looked at which items were given a correct response by less than 50% of children. That is, the majority of structures that were difficult for children with SLI (e.g. locative prepositions, subordinate and subjunctive clauses, future tense) were also problematic for P.I. with the exception of the past tense and the third-person plural, which were impaired only in the SLI group. We hasten to point out that the children with SLI do not form a homogeneous group, since they experience difficulties in different language levels. For comprehension of morphosyntax, P.I. and the children with SLI showed similar error patterns

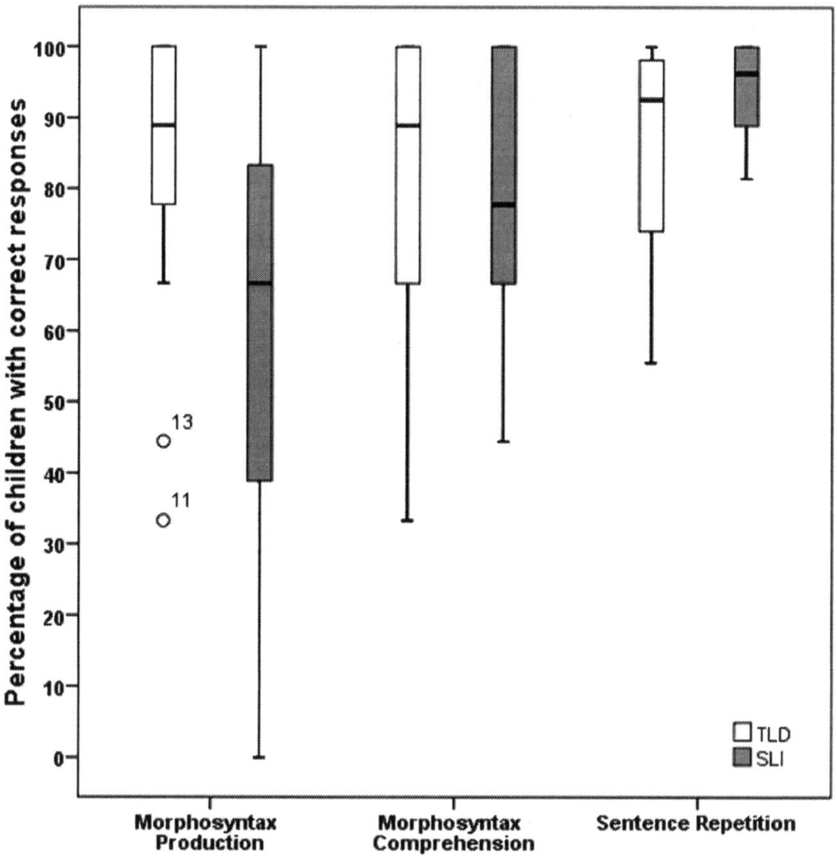

Figure 8.6 Percentage of children who responded correctly in the items analysis of DVIQ subtests Production of Morphosyntax, Comprehension of Morphosyntax, and Sentence Repetition

(e.g. #17: 'Show some of the cats.'; #18: 'Before you show the bear, show the cat.'; #21: 'I will show a big duck, and then you will show a small fox.').

Finally, for sentence repetition, all items ($n = 16$) were recalled correctly by more than 50% of children in both groups. However, the SLI group had two items which only 55% of children repeated correctly. P.I. repeated 10 sentences correctly, but for three sentences he received 0 points each, for one sentence he received 1 point, and for two sentences he received 2 points each.

Performance on the Clitics-in-Islands Test

Out of the 12 target structures, P.I. omitted the clitic two times, an error that is not found in the SLI group productions (see also Theodorou & Grohmann, 2015). He produced one more error that concerns the use of the corresponding full noun phrase instead of the expected clitic (Table 8.4).

Comprehension of Wh-questions

The different types of errors for the different question types are shown in Figures 8.7 and 8.8. We compared P.I.'s performance in subject and object *who*- and *which*-questions for the three error types separately using Crawford–Howell *t*-tests, in order to see if they made similar errors in the different question types.

There was a significantly higher number of number errors for P.I. than the control group in the subject *who*-questions ($t_{(7)} = 2.06$, $p < 0.05$), as well as a significantly higher number of reversal errors for P.I. than the control group in object *who*-questions ($t_{(7)} = 6.78$, $p < 0.01$) and in object *which*-questions ($t_{(7)} = 37.71$, $p < 0.01$).

Exhaustivity of Wh-questions

Error analysis of responses in Wh-questions Types 1 and 2 revealed that P.I.'s errors are of the singleton type only, whereas the children with TLD's errors are of singleton and plural types (see Table 8.5, where 64 is the total

Table 8.4 Correct and incorrect productions as well as error types for clitics

Response accuracy	*Response type*	*Score*		
		22q11.2DS	*Typical language development (SD)*	*Specific language impairment (SD)*
Correct (max. 12)	Proclisis	7	7 (5.04)	8.5 (4.59)
	Enclisis	2	5 (4.60)	2.5 (4.64)
Incorrect	Omission	2		
	Noun phrase	1		
	Other			1 (0.35)

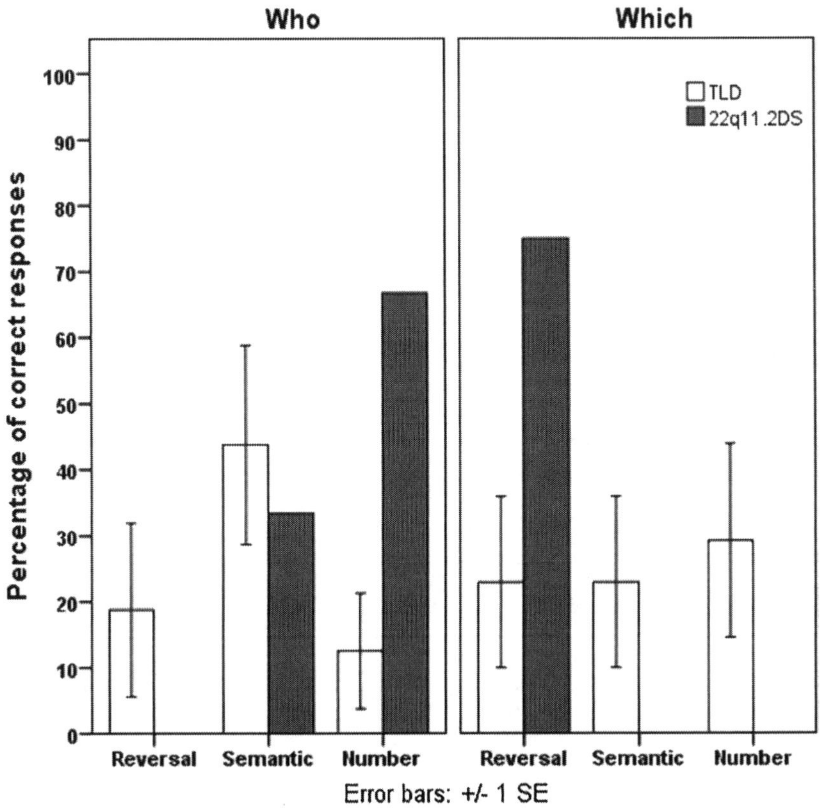

Figure 8.7 Error percentages of P.I. (22q11.2DS) in comparison to the typical language development group on the Wh-questions comprehension test for subject questions

number of items/responses in simple Wh-questions for the TLD group). P.I. did not achieve any correct target response in paired Wh-questions (Type 3) in contrast to children with TLD, who responded correctly on 29 occasions out of 64 items; P.I. did not respond correctly in triple Wh-questions (Type 4) either, in contrast to children with TLD who responded correctly on 13 occasions out of 32 items (see Table 8.6).

Discussion

The purpose of the present study was to profile, for the first time, the language abilities of a pre-school Greek-speaking child with 22q11.2DS and compare him to two groups of chronological age-matched children across a number of linguistic tools used for research purposes in Cyprus: two groups of children with TLD and another group of children with clinically

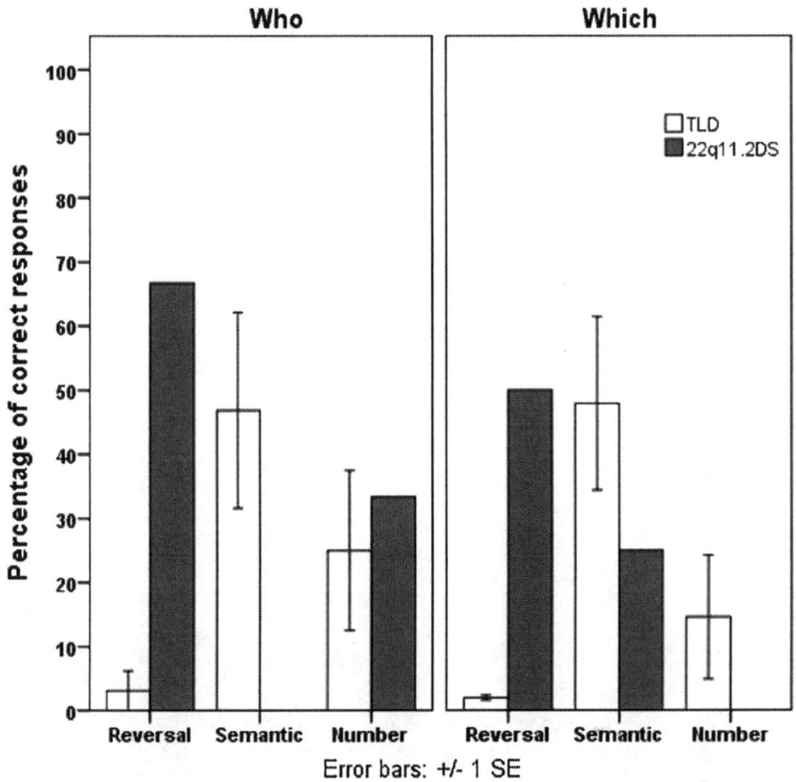

Figure 8.8 Error percentages of P.I. (22q11.2DS) in comparison to the typical language development group on the Wh-questions comprehension test for object questions

Table 8.5 Number of errors (out of the total number of errors committed) in simple Wh-questions (Types 1 and 2)

Question type	*Error type*	*22q11.2DS*	*Typical language development*
Simple Wh-Q (*pcos*) (max. 8)	Singleton	4/8	7/64
	Plural		5/64
'who all' Wh-Q (*pci*) (max. 8)	Singleton	1/8	
	Plural		

diagnosed SLI. Overall, the findings are relevant to clinical practice by demonstrating the value of language profiling in assisting in characterizing the pattern of language impairment in a given child with 22q11.2DS, with the ultimate aim of developing appropriate treatment plans. Also, by comparing our participant to a group of children with SLI, that is, with known profiles

Table 8.6 Number of errors (out of the total number of errors committed) in paired and triple Wh-questions (Types 3 and 4)

Question type	*Error type*	*22Q11.2DS*	*Typical language development*
Paired Wh-questions (max. 8)	Subject list		19/64
	1-subject	1/8	1/64
	1-object	6/8	15/64
	Other	1/8	
Triple Wh-questions (max. 4)	1-triple		1/32
	Plural triples		4/32
	Subject list		7/32
	1-subject		1/32
	1-object	2/4	1/32
	1-dative	1/4	2/32
	Other	1/4	3/32

of speech and language difficulties, we can decipher whether the profile of 22q11.2DS is distinctive to the syndrome or not.

With regard to our first aim, we will describe the findings based on the pertinent literature outlined in the Introduction. Overall, global language ability as probed by the DVIQ is impaired. This finding supports what is reported so far (Persson *et al.*, 2006), namely that language impairment is evident at the pre-school stage in 22q11.2DS. Similarly, the receptive and expressive language abilities of our participant with 22q11.2DS are differentiated based on the single-word tools used: expressive vocabulary (measured on the EVT) appeared intact for his chronological age, but *receptive vocabulary* (measured on the PPVT) lagged behind. This noticeable difference between receptive and expressive vocabulary abilities has not been described in the literature for the large cohorts of children with 22q11.2DS, neither in research from the US (Solot *et al.*, 2000) nor from Sweden (Persson *et al.*, 2006).

In relation to narrative retell production, P.I. neither showed difficulties retelling the information of the story nor using subordinate clauses or producing long sentences. This finding stands in stark contrast to what was reported for the Swedish cohort (Persson *et al.*, 2006), where the majority of children with 22q11.2DS showed a low information score, a lower number of subordinate clauses and shorter sentence length than expected, according to the Swedish BST norms. However, P.I. also produced a significantly smaller *number of sentences* on the BST retell task. In our search of the literature, we have not found reported deficits in sentence productivity for 22q11.2DS pre-schoolers, so we cannot classify P.I. with respect to a cross-linguistic profile for 22q11.2DS on this aspect of language abilities.

Taking into consideration our second aim, P.I. was significantly more impaired in comparison to his typically developing, chronological age-matched peers on global language performance (total DVIQ score), and specifically on the two subtests *comprehension of morphosyntax* and *sentence repetition*. He was also significantly different on *receptive vocabulary* abilities, scoring way below his TLD peers. On the other hand, no such difference was evident for expressive vocabulary. On the narrative retell task, only the *number of sentences produced* was significantly lower for P.I. as compared to his TLD peers. In addition, he performed significantly worse than his TLD peers on the *CIT*. In other words, P.I. showed similar performance to the TLD group for comprehension of metalinguistic concepts (DVIQ), production of morphosyntax (DVIQ), retell information (BST), MLU-word (BST), A5LS (BST), number of subordinate clauses produced (BST) and expressive vocabulary (DVIQ and EVT). Finally, P.I. showed a significantly worse performance on comprehension of subject and object *which*-questions compared to TLD peers but performed similarly on subject and object *who*-questions. With regards to comprehending exhaustivity, his only difficulty lay with *who all*-questions. However, he had significant difficulties with responding to paired and triple Wh-questions. Without achieving any correct target response in paired Wh-questions (Type 3), P.I. responded with 1-object responses for a total of six out of eight target questions. It is important to note that P.I. avoided exhaustive responses (the production of lists) in contrast to the TLD group who responded, erroneously, with subject lists on 19 occasions out of a total of 64 response items. The TLD children's responses made for a variety of errors: from the production of 1-triple-responses and the most common error type (the production of subject list) to the least common error types (1-subject, 1-object, 1-dative, and other response types). However, P.I. is in line with four-year-old Cypriot Greek-speaking children, who avoid the production of lists but mostly prefer 1-object responses (see Varnava & Grohmann, 2014).

Our third aim was to compare P.I. with a group of chronological age-matched children with SLI. Global language abilities (total DVIQ score) did not differentiate P.I. from the SLI group. In a similar vein, comprehension of metalinguistic concepts (DVIQ), production of morphosyntax (DVIQ), retell information (BST), MLU-word (BST), A5LS (BST), number of subordinate clauses produced (BST), expressive vocabulary (DVIQ and EVT) and receptive language abilities (PPVT) did not differentiate P.I. with 22q11.2DS from the SLI group. He was significantly worse compared to the children with SLI (i) on the subtest *comprehension of morphosyntax* (DVIQ), (ii) on the subtest *sentence repetition* (DVIQ), (iii) on the *Clitics-in-Islands Test* (CIT) and (iv) on the *total number of sentences produced* (BST). At age 6;5, P.I.'s responses show a delayed age of acquisition pattern for exhaustivity in paired and triple Wh-questions. His performance on paired and triple Wh-questions was similar to the pattern exhibited by German children with SLI, who also avoid the production of lists but mostly prefer to respond with 1-item answers, of the subject-type (Schulz, 2010; Schulz & Roeper, 2011). At this point, no (Cypriot) Greek-speaking children with SLI have yet been tested on these tools to compare P.I.'s performance with. This will be done in future research.

Putting both group results together, those of children with TLD and those of ones with SLI, P.I. was significantly worse on comprehension of subject and object *which*-questions, comprehension of *who all*-questions, the number of sentences produced on the BST retell task, on comprehension of morphosyntax, on sentence repetition, responding to paired and triple Wh-questions and on the clitic production task. The last three tasks probe structural language (morphosyntactic and language complexity). Unfortunately, we do not yet have a solid analytical knowledge base for the relevance of complex language stemming from the BST and the DVIQ as markers of language difficulties. This is to say that we can describe the performance by individuals and groups, but we cannot yet pinpoint the source of deviations from the norm.

The relevance of clitic productions and their placement in the context of first language acquisition of Cypriot Greek has been highlighted in work from our research group since Grohmann (2011); see, for example, recent summaries by Grohmann (2014) and Grohmann and Kambanaros (2016). P.I. clearly behaves differently from both children with TLD and children with SLI by producing significantly fewer clitics than both. However, his clitic placements resembled more those of his typically developing peers, while he showed more omissions than either group, a phenomenon which is rare even for children with SLI (Theodorou & Grohmann, 2015). Clitic production *vis-à-vis* omission has been taken as a clinical marker for SLI in other languages, although it is unlikely to be a clinical marker for SLI in Cypriot Greek (Theodorou & Grohmann, 2015; see also Theodorou, 2013, for further discussion and references).

Our final aim is to tentatively use our findings to shed light on the 22q11.2DS ± SLI debate as reported in the 22q11.2DS literature and outlined in the Introduction section (see Table 8.1). One informative approach for a more general notion of language impairment is to compare non-verbal intelligence and the linguistic performance outcomes of the children with SLI to P.I., our participant with 22Q11.2DS. Following Rice (2016), a first conceptualization can be summarized as a 2 × 2 design with four cells of interest identified as 'A', 'B', 'C' or 'D' (Table 8.7). If P.I. has concurrent SLI (Cell A)

Table 8.7 2 × 2 design comparison for 22q11.2DS and specific language impairment (22q11.2DS ± SLI)

		22Q11.2DS	
		+	–
SLI	+	A	B
	–	C	D

he could be compared with SLI children who do not have 22q11.2DS (Cell B), 22q11.2DS children who do not have SLI (Cell C), and typically developing children without either condition (Cell D). At this point in time, based on our assessment results and comparison groups, we are able to weigh P.I.'s linguistic performance against children with SLI but without 22q11.2DS (Cell B) and to children with TLD (Cell D). This allows us to speculate that if $A = C$ and $A \neq B$, it would suggest a distinctive linguistic profile contributing to 22q11.2DS but not SLI. In our view, P.I.'s language-specific symptoms suggest that the 22q11.2DS variant is the common element and this variant is not diagnostic of SLI (Cell C).

Conclusion

The purpose of the present study was to provide evidence for the language profile of 22q11.2DS. Based on our findings of a single case, we opt for a *distinctive language profile of 22q11.2DS* for our participant, as he appeared significantly impaired on receptive and expressive measures of complex language, not evidenced by the chronological age-matched group with SLI in our study. While similar in terms of below-TLD performance, his inferior abilities in complex language also do not match those of SLI qualitatively. However, future work will have to decide on the final outcome. In that respect, we do hope that our findings provide awareness of 22q11.2DS. They surely constitute a first contribution to the knowledge base of the behavioural language phenotype for (Cypriot) Greek, even if only based on a single case.

This study was a preliminary investigation of the language profile of 22q11.2DS compared to children with SLI (as well as a typically developing control group). While the study presents data that support further research using a comparison group of children with SLI, several limitations were apparent based on the small number of participants. This precludes big generalizations for the different populations as a whole. However, the results of this study indicate the potential benefits of research with larger numbers of children with 22q11.2DS and SLI in order to tease apart the linguistic profiles of each group.

Seen from the perspective of a larger research agenda, further exploring the exact deficits in language and cognition presented by pathologies like 22q11.2DS contributes to the growing research interest in *comparative biolinguistics* (Benítez-Burraco & Boeckx, 2014; Boeckx, 2013; Boeckx & Grohmann, 2013; Kambanaros & Grohmann, 2015). This research programme investigates similarities and, especially, differences in specific tasks and abilities across different pathologies, from developmental language impairment and acquired language disorders to apparently non-linguistic pathologies, that is, those that are not primarily connected to language. By so doing, we present language pathology from the perspective of the underlying system: what non-intact language can tell us about universal grammar (cf. also Tsimpli *et al.*, 2016), perhaps even 'uncover the locus of variation (and its constraints) across genotypes, pathologies, or across species' (Leivada, 2014: 54).

Finally, the clinical relevance of the present research is for speech and language therapists to recognize the communication symptoms of children with 22q11.2DS, and to be aware of differentiating characteristics between 22q11.2DS, SLI and TLD. This will facilitate improved clinical guidelines for the identification and treatment of children with 22q11.2DS. Given the limited research regarding language function in 22q11.2DS to date, this is not only a first case study for (Cypriot) Greek; it also addresses larger issues of language ability in 22q11.2DS with respect to adaptive functioning. Concerning our participant, P.I., the next step is to test his linguistic performance over time in order to determine the effects of speech-language therapy and special education services on continued language growth.

Note

(1) Greek here is transcribed into IPA, with added normal punctuation.

References

Benítez-Burraco, A. and Boeckx, C. (2014) Universal Grammar and biological variation: An EvoDevo agenda for comparative biolinguistics. *Biological Theory* 9, 122–134.

Bishop, D.V.M. (2014) Ten questions about terminology for children with unexplained language problems. *International Journal of Language & Communication Disorders* 49 (4), 381–415.

Bishop, D.V.M. and Leonard, L.B. (2000) *Speech and Language Impairments in Children: Causes, Characteristics, Intervention and Outcome*. Hove: Psychology Press.

Boeckx, C. (2013) Biolinguistics: Forays into human cognitive biology. *Journal of Anthropological Sciences* 91, 1–28.

Boeckx, C. and Grohmann, K.K. (2013) *The Cambridge Handbook of Biolinguistics*. Cambridge: Cambridge University Press.

Crawford, J.R. and Howell, D.C. (1998) Comparing an individual's test score against norms derived from small samples. *Clinical Neuropsychologist* 12, 482–486.

Dunn, L.M. and Dunn, L.M. (1981) *Peabody Picture Vocabulary Test*. Circle Pines, MN: American Guidance Service.

European Social Survey (2010) *Round 5 Source Showcards*. London: Centre for Comparative Social Surveys, City University London.

Goorhuis-Brouwer, S.M., Dikkers, F.G., Robinson, P.H. and Kerstjens-Frederikse, W.S. (2003) Specific language impairment in children with velocardiofacial syndrome: Four case studies. *Cleft Palate-Craniofacial Journal* 40 (2), 190–195.

Grohmann, K.K. (2011) Some directions for the systematic investigation of the acquisition of Cypriot Greek: A new perspective on production abilities from object clitic placement. In E. Rinke and T. Kupisch (eds) *The Development of Grammar: Language Acquisition and Diachronic Change* (pp. 179–203). Amsterdam: John Benjamins.

Grohmann, K.K. (2014) CAT research on object clitic placement: Where we are now. In K.K. Grohmann and T. Neokleous (eds) *Developments in the Acquisition of Clitics* (pp. 1–40). Newcastle-upon-Tyne: Cambridge Scholars.

Grohmann, K.K. and Kambanaros, M. (2016) The gradience of multilingualism in language development: Positioning bilectalism within comparative bilingualism. *Frontiers in Psychology: Language Sciences* 7 (37); doi:10.3389/fpsyg.2016.00037.

Kambanaros, M. and Grohmann, K.K. (2015) Grammatical class effects across impaired child and adult populations. *Frontiers in Psychology: Language Sciences* 6, 1670; doi: 10.3389/fpsyg.2015.01670.

Kambanaros, M., Grohmann, K.K., Michaelides, M. and Theodorou, E. (2013) Comparing multilingual children with SLI to their bilectal peers: Evidence from object and action picture naming. *International Journal of Multilingualism* 10, 60–81.

Kambanaros, M., Grohmann, K.K., Michaelides, M. and Theodorou, E. (2014) On the nature of verb–noun dissociations in bilectal SLI: A psycholinguistic perspective from Greek. *Bilingualism: Language and Cognition* 17 (1), 169–188.

Leivada, E. (2014) From comparative linguistics to comparative (bio)linguistics: Reflections on variation. *Biolinguistics* 8, 53–66.

Mastropavlou, M., Petinou, K. and Tsimpli, I.M. (2011) The role of morpho-phonological salience in tense marking: A comparison between Greek and Cypriot-Greek SLI children. In A. Tsangalides (ed.) *Selected Papers from the 19th International Symposium on Theoretical and Applied Linguistics, Thessaloniki, 3–5 April 2009* (pp. 313–328). Thessaloniki: Monochromia.

Niklasson, L., Rasmussen, P., Óskarsdóttir, S. and Gillberg, C. (2001) Neuropsychiatric disorders in the 22q11 deletion syndrome. *Genetics in Medicine* 3 (1), 79–84.

Persson, C., Niklasson, L., Óskarsdóttir, S., Johansson, S., Jönsson, R. and Söderpalm, E. (2006) Language skills in 5–8 year old children with 22q11 deletion syndrome. *International Journal of Language & Communication Disorders* 41 (3), 313–333.

Petinou, K. and Okalidou, A. (2006) Speech patterns in Cypriot-Greek late talkers. *Applied Psycholinguistics* 27, 335–353.

Raven, J., Raven, J.C. and Court, J.H. (2000) *Manual for Raven's Progressive Matrices and Vocabulary Scales*. San Antonio, TX: Harcourt Assessment.

Renfrew, C. (1997) *The Renfrew Language Scales* (4th edn). Milton Keynes: Speechmark.

Rice, M. (2016) Specific language impairment, nonverbal IQ, attention-deficit/hyperactivity disorder, autism spectrum disorder, cochlear implants, bilingualism, and dialectal variants: Defining the boundaries, clarifying clinical conditions, and sorting out causes. *Journal of Speech, Language, and Hearing Research* 59 (1), 122–132.

Rowe, C. and Grohmann, K.K. (2013) Discrete bilectalism: Towards co-overt prestige and diglossic shift in Cyprus. *International Journal of the Sociology of Language* 224, 119–142.

Scandurra, V., Scordo, M.R., Canitano, R. and de Bruin, E.I. (2013) 22q11 deletion syndrome and multiple complex developmental disorder: A case report. *Journal of Clinical Medical Research* 5 (2), 135–139.

Schulz, P. (2010) Some notes on semantics and SLI. In J. Costa, A. Castro, M. Lobo and F. Pratas (eds) *Language Acquisition and Development: Proceedings of GALA 2009* (pp. 391–406). Newcastle-upon-Tyne: Cambridge Scholars.

Schulz, P. and Roeper, T. (2011) Acquisition of exhaustivity in *wh*-questions: A semantic dimension of SLI? *Lingua* 121, 383–407.

Shprintzen, R.J. (2008) Velocardiofacial syndrome: 30 years of study. *Developmental Disability Research Reviews* 14 (1), 3–10.

Sideridis, G., Antoniou, F., Mouzaki, A. and Simos, P. (2015) *Raven's Coloured Progressive Matrices and Vocabulary* [in Greek]. Athina: Motivo.

Simos, P.G., Kasselimis, D. and Mouzaki, A. (2011) Age, gender, and education effects on vocabulary measures in Greek. *Aphasiology* 25, 475–491.

Solot, C.B., Handler, S.D., Gerdes, M., *et al.* (2000) Communication disorders in the 22q11.2 microdeletion syndrome. *Journal of Communication Disorders* 33, 187–204.

Solot, C.B., Gerdes, M., Kirschner, R.E., *et al.* (2001) Communication issues in 22q11.2 deletion syndrome: Children at risk. *Genetics in Medicine* 3 (1), 67–71.

Stavrakaki, S. and Tsimpli, I.M. (2000) Διαγνωστικό Τεστ Γλωσσικής Νοημοσύνης για παιδιά σχολικής και προσχολικής ηλικίας: στάθμιση, στατιστική ανάλυση, ψυχομετρικές ιδιότητες [Diagnostic Verbal IQ Test for Greek Preschool and School Age Children: Standardization, statistical analysis, psychometric properties]. In M. Glykas and G. Kalomiris (eds) *Proceedings of the 8th Symposium of the Panhellenic Association of Logopedists* [in Greek] (pp. 95–106). Athens: Ellinika Grammata.

Theodorou, E. (2013) Specific language impairment in Cypriot Greek: Diagnostic and experimental investigations. PhD dissertation, University of Cyprus.

Theodorou, E. and Grohmann, K.K. (2010) Narratives in Cypriot Greek mono- and bilingual children with SLI. In A. Botinis (ed.) *Proceedings of ISCA Tutorial and Research Workshop on Experimental Linguistics 2010 – 25–27 August 2010, Athens, Greece* (pp. 185–188). Athens: ISCA & University of Athens.

Theodorou, E. and Grohmann, K.K. (2015) Object clitics in Cypriot Greek children with SLI. *Lingua* 161, 144–158.

Theodorou, E., Kambanaros, M. and Grohmann, K.K. (2016) Diagnosing bilectal children with SLI: Determination of identification accuracy. *Clinical Linguistics & Phonetics* 30 (12), 925–943; doi:10.1080/02699206.2016.1182591.

Tsimpli, I.M., Kambanaros, M. and Grohmann, K.K. (2017) Language pathology. In I. Roberts (ed.) *The Oxford Handbook of Universal Grammar* (pp. 486–508). Oxford: Oxford University Press.

Varlokosta, S., Belletti, A., Costa, J., *et al.* (2015) A crosslinguistic study of the acquisition of pronoun and clitic production. *Language Acquisition* 23 (1), 1–26; doi:10.1080/10489223.2015.1028628.

Varnava, M. and Grohmann, K.K. (2014) The development of the comprehension of *wh*-questions and the notion of exhaustivity in Cypriot Greek. *Linguistic Variation* 14 (1), 69–108.

Vogindroukas, I., Protopapas, A. and Sideris, G. (2009) *Word-finding Test* [in Greek]. Chania: Glafki.

Woodin, M., Wang, P.P., Aleman, D., McDonald-McGinn, D., Zackai, E. and Moss, E. (2001). Neuropsychological profile of children and adolescents with the 22q11.2 microdeletion. *Genetics in Medicine* 3 (1), 34–39.

9 The Emergence and Development of Self-repair: A Longitudinal Case Study of Specific Language Impairment from 3;0 to 6;10 Years

Mª Isabel Navarro-Ruiz and Lucrecia Rallo Fabra

Introduction

In a broad sense, a child whose speech is coherent and complex can be considered a *fluent speaker*. When a child speaks fluently, the listener has the impression that the psycholinguistic processes of speech planning and speech production are functioning easily and efficiently (Lennon, 1990). Whereas fluent speech is an 'automatic procedural skill that does not require much attention or effort from the speaker' (Schmidt, 1992: 358), non-fluent speech requires substantial effort and attention. As a consequence, the speech of non-fluent speakers exhibits a considerable number of hesitations and other manifestations of groping for words as well as unsuccessful attempts to combine them into utterances.

Self-repairs: Self-monitoring versus metalinguistic competence

There is no agreement in the literature as how to label the set of pauses, repetitions, revisions and abandoned utterances that characterize a non-fluent speaker. This lack of consensus often responds to different interpretations of the functions, purposes and processes associated with disfluencies (see MacLurg, 2014, for a review). For instance, Postma *et al.* (1990) propose a classification of these processes on the basis of three criteria: (i) *speech errors* or deviations of speech planning (e.g. phoneme substitutions); (ii) *disfluencies* or disruptions of speech planning (e.g. pauses, repetitions, sound lengthening); and (iii) *self-repairs*, which represent the knowledge a speaker has of their linguistic system to fix errors (self-monitoring). Children's self-repairs are based in their capacity to monitor their role in the conversation, adjust their speech acts and remediate potential problems or mismatches between the child's and the adult's linguistic systems (Morgenstern *et al.*, 2013).

In the present study, we adopt the taxonomy proposed by Fletcher (1990), which in turn is based on Levelt's (1989) model of speech production. According to this taxonomy, self-repairs are a subclass of mazes and they are part of the monitoring mechanism which has three main functions: (i) controlling the productions of a speaker, which must match his/her communicative intentions; (ii) controlling the potential ambiguity of the context in a given message; and (iii) controlling the establishment of the phonological and syntactic patterns. The monitoring system functions as a 'watch-out' system that detects errors and gives the instructions to fix these errors.

Self-repairs affect all language levels. The speaker detects a speech error and substitutes a given word with a more appropriate one. As a rule, it is the speaker who self-repairs his/her productions (Schegloff, 1979; Schegloff *et al.*, 1977), but occasionally the interlocutor may also repair speech through verbal or non-verbal communication (Forrester, 2008), using gestures that can be interpreted as asking for clarification. Speakers with a higher linguistic competence are more bound to initiate repair (Norrick, 1991). Error correction is often preceded by fillers (meaningless words such as *uhm* or *eh*) and hesitations. Self-repair involves a sequence of three phases (Levelt, 1989; Levelt & Cutler, 1983). First, the error is detected, secondly a filler or a pause is introduced immediately afterwards, and thirdly the error is corrected. Self-repairs may occur either at the articulatory or at the pre-articulatory stage. In the second case, the addressee may not detect the error. The speaker then resorts to hesitations or pauses to indicate to the recipient that he/she (the speaker) has chosen a better fit for his/her communicative intentions or discourse characteristics. Laakso (2010) suggests that repair at the pre-articulatory level functions like a self-monitoring system, an alert mechanism.

The complexity of self-repairs cannot just be accounted for in terms of monitoring but also in terms of metalinguistic competence (Levy, 1999; Levy *et al.*, 2003). According to the authors, the ability to locate an error and to repair it once the source of the error has been identified are separate processes. This claim is supported by evidence found in studies of agrammatic aphasia in which patients were able to identify errors but could not correct them. Based on this evidence, the authors made a clear distinction between metalinguistic abilities and awareness. They argued that monitoring and repair do not rely on awareness and, as such, they may be performed unconsciously. To support this view, they reported the case of typically developing

(TD) children aged two who were able to monitor their productions, identify a series of linguistic errors and provide repair in 50% of the cases.

Following Levy and colleagues, we suggest that the relationship between self-repairs and metalinguistic competence must take into account three issues: (i) young children base their self-repairs on overall mental representations of linguistic knowledge; (ii) self-repairs are a consequence of the monitoring system (Levelt, 1983); and (iii) the monitor receives input from communicative intentions, not pure linguistic acts. Given these circumstances, we assume that children at an early age can perform these meta-operations because these levels are more accessible to young children whose communicative intentions surpass their linguistic structures. Self-repairs reflect their own system along with their age-related limitations.

The social role of self-repairs

Self-repairs thus allow the child to adapt and adjust socially to discourse (Laakso, 2010). Children aged 18–24 months have been found to monitor speech while they are delivering it (Clark, 1978). They may use repairs to interact with the interlocutor; that is, they do not just repair their own productions, but also the interlocutor's (Forrester & Cherington, 2009). Metalinguistic abilities allow the speaker to assess the accuracy of a given speech act, on the basis of various criteria such as the adequacy of their communicative intents, negotiation, self-analysis of the speech act, self-repair and additional information if needed.

Children and adults use similar self-repair strategies. However, some differences can be found depending on the child's stage of development. De Ruiter (2013) reports that children stall their productions if they detect an error but, unlike adults, they do not stop if the message they deliver is not appropriate in a given situation. Two different approaches may account for this behaviour. The first one claims that children distinguish both strategies as a function of context. The other approach associates this behaviour with different processing levels. Apparently, the child's ability to detect an inappropriate production requires a more complex level of processing than detecting an error.

Specific language impairment

Specific language impairment (SLI) is a developmental disorder characterized by an alteration of normal language development of receptive and productive skills at one or more linguistic levels. To date, the causes of this disorder have not been clearly established. Although in some cases the disorder has a genetic basis, it often involves an interaction of genetic and environmental factors (see Bishop, 2006, for a review). A child with SLI struggles to communicate and shows difficulties in understanding language if this requires complex vocabulary or syntax (Bishop, 2000). These difficulties affect various language levels, although individual variability in performance is often the rule. A child with SLI may also exhibit deficits in social interaction thus affecting relationships with peers. From the pragmatics perspective, Bishop and Adams (1989) reported difficulties in sentence formulation, semantic selection and use of stereotyped utterances with abnormal prosody.

Two types of hypothesis have attempted to account for SLI: the grammar-deficit hypothesis and the processing-deficit hypothesis (see Ullman & Pierpont, 2005, for a review). The first perspective posits that a substantial number of people with the disorder 'suffer from a deficit or delay that is specific to the domain of language, specifically to grammar – that is, to the capacity that underlies the rule-governed combination of words into complex structures' (Ullman & Pierpont, 2005: 400). The second theoretical perspective, claims that SLI is caused by a non-linguistic processing deficit. Children with SLI have been found to be slower at processing information relative to TD children. This delay could be attributed to deficits in verbal working memory, short-term memory and auditory attention (Duinmeijer *et al.*, 2012). More recently, Petersen and Gardner (2011) extended these difficulties to (i) speed processing impairment and (ii) poor phonological representations (Claessen & Leitão, 2012; Jackson *et al.*, 2016).

Empirical studies comparing the linguistic abilities of children with SLI to those of their TD peers have reported lexical processing deficits by the former. For instance, in a simple verbal repetition task, children with SLI were slower at repeating abstract verbs compared to concrete verbs (Hennessey *et al.*, 2010). This effect was not found in TD children. In more demanding cognitive tasks such as narratives and storytelling, school children with SLI (age range 7;6–9;0) have been reported to elicit stories of uneven strength, that is, stories with poor content but grammatically accurate or stories with complex content but grammatically inaccurate (Colozzo *et al.*, 2011). In the case of Spanish, Muñoz López and Carballo García (2005) reported that children with SLI experience difficulties in the development of verbal morphology and lexis. The authors attributed these difficulties to short-term memory deficits. These deficits are also responsible for poor phonological and lexical representations of new words and suggested that the linguistic and cognitive levels of processing of children with SLI are interrelated and, as such, they cannot be conceived as separate entities. It has also been shown that difficulties in information processing affect not only linguistic competence but also storage and lexical access (Gathercole & Baddeley, 1990), auditory perception (Bermeosolo, 2012) and executive dysfunction (Quintero *et al.*, 2013).

An alternative perspective to SLI, the procedural deficit hypothesis (PDH) proposed by Ullman and Pierpont (2005), posits that neither the grammar-deficit hypothesis nor the processing-deficit hypothesis can fully account for the wide range of variability of SLI profiles. The PDH is grounded on the evidence that a considerable number of children and adults with SLI suffer from 'abnormalities of brain structures that constitute a well-studied brain system known as the *procedural memory system*' (Ullman & Pierpont, 2005: 401). Through an extensive review of the grammatical profiles of SLI, the authors provided behavioural evidence that the PDH can fully explain the consistency and heterogeneity in the linguistic and non-linguistic deficits exhibited by different individuals. For instance, at the syntactic level, deficits include difficulties in following appropriate word order patterns, assigning reference to pronouns or reflexives and performing syntactic acceptability judgements. At the morphological level, children and adults with SLI show difficulties in producing complex words, specifically in verbal and nominal inflectional morphology (past tense formation, agreement, pluralization) and in generalizing grammatical rules. All these skills are hypothesized to depend on procedural memory.

At the pragmatics level, Navarro-Ruiz (1997) showed that the language processing and abstraction skills of a child with SLI are comparable to those of TD children at an earlier stage of development. They also exhibit differential metalinguistic abilities such as a general delay in the emergence of self-repairs, which at onset affect the more preserved language levels (Navarro-Ruiz & Rallo-Fabra, 2001). Children with SLI have shown a preference for adult–child interactions. In peer-to-peer interactions, they often miss their turn in discourse and hardly ever start conversational events. Further to this, the slower rate of delivery triggers frequent interruptions by their peers.

Empirical work examining speech disruptions in typically developing and specifically language-impaired children

Studies comparing disfluencies in TD and SLI populations are scarce and cover mostly English-speaking children. For instance, an early study by Nettelbladt and Hansson (1999) compared the distributional patterns of mazes in two clinical groups of Swedish schoolchildren, a group of children with SLI and another group of children with phonological impairment (PI) for control purposes. The children of both groups were matched in mean length of utterance (MLU). Maze rates were calculated per 100 fluent words, and they included four dependent variables, namely, filled and empty pauses, repetitions and revisions. Overall, children with SLI used significantly more mazes per 100 fluent words than the MLU-matched controls. Examination of the data revealed that children with SLI showed a trend of repeating initial phonemes and syllables, rather than whole words. In addition, the nature of these repetitions differed between the two groups: the PI group tended to repeat mainly function words, whereas the SLI group repeated function and lexical words equally. All in all, the SLI children showed a pattern of asynchronous development relative to their MLU-matched peers; in other words, the amount and distribution of mazes correspond to the syntactic development of younger TD children. These findings had relevant implications for Levelt's (1989) speech production model in that they suggested that speech planning by the SLI group did not run smoothly.

Thordardottir and Weismer (2002) investigated the use of mazes[1] by TD English children and children with SLI aged 5;5–9;8 years. Specifically, the authors compared the use of filled pauses and 'content mazes' operationalized as semantic and syntactic revisions in a narrative task. The comparison was performed at two levels. At the first level, the number of filled pauses and content mazes used by SLI children was compared with the number of mazes used by age-matched TD children. At the second level, the group comparison involved matching SLI and TD children on the basis of MLU. In the age-matched comparison, the results indicated that overall both groups of TD and SLI children used more content mazes than filled pauses; however, whereas this difference was small and non-significant for TD children, the difference was significantly larger for the SLI group. Interestingly, in the MLU-matched comparison, SLI children were found to use significantly more content mazes than their MLU-matched peers. These findings suggested that the use of content mazes reflected processing difficulties and their use increased as a function of utterance length.

Rispoli *et al.* (2008) examined the developmental trends in stall rate (pauses) and revision rate (repair) of a group of TD children aged 1;9 to 2;6 years. The category of 'stalls' included silent and filled pauses and repetitions and insertions; revisions included morphosyntactic corrections and message revisions. The children were tested at five three-month intervals. The language samples were obtained during adult–child interactions in a playroom. The disruption rates were calculated from the mono-clausal sentences produced by the children. The authors reported strong revision trends of stall rate at 27 months. The rate was 1%, that is, one revised sentence in every 100 active declarative sentences. Conversely, children did not exhibit a strong developmental trend for stall rate. Surprisingly, sentence length did not seem to affect revision rate. These results were interpreted in light of Levelt's model of speech production and reflected the children's ability to monitor language production at a very early age.

In sum, the studies just reviewed show that in TD children, mazes are related to language development, specifically to syntactic and lexical development. A high level of sentence complexity triggers a high rate of speech disruptions (Rispoli & Hadley, 2001). On these grounds, one would expect that, as the child's syntax and lexicon become enriched, children should have less difficulty in building complex sentences or retrieving lexical items and, consequently, the number of speech disruptions would decrease. In the case of atypical language development, we could predict that children with SLI will exhibit higher rates of speech disruptions than their age-matched peers. However, as Guo *et al.* (2008) argue, the relationship between speech disruptions and language impairment is not a simple one. The studies just reviewed show inconsistencies across results, probably due to the different approaches used for the taxonomy and calculation of the disruption rates (see MacLurg, 2014, for a comprehensive review). Nevertheless, in their concluding remarks, most authors make a plea for developmental data in sentence production to form a basis of comparison between impaired and typical language development.

Specific language impairment and bilingualism

The development of language abilities in bilingual children with language impairment is a challenging one. Some authors have argued that coping with two languages puts additional pressure onto SLI children who already struggle to communicate and to be understood. In an extensive review, Paradis (2010) argued that limited processing capacity (LPC) theories posit that children with SLI need a considerable amount of extra exposure to each of the two languages, and thus predict 'double delay' in the acquisition of morphology (Leonard *et al.*, 2007). Other authors (Orgassa & Weerman, 2008) refer to a 'cumulative effect' or combination of dual language exposure and processing deficits, which would hinder learning of gender inflection by Dutch bilinguals. However, other studies comparing monolingual and bilingual children provided conflicting evidence. For instance, a study comparing performance in verb morphology by Spanish-English bilinguals and monolinguals with SLI (Gutiérrez-Clellen *et al.*, 2008) yielded similar levels of morphological acquisition by the two groups.

Paradis (2010) argued that the discrepancies of these studies are probably caused by the sociolinguistic status of the second language (L2). When one of the languages spoken by the bilingual children with SLI is a minority language only spoken in the household, children do not receive enough exposure and therefore it will take them several years to reach the same levels of performance as their monolingual language-impaired peers who are exposed to only one language. Paradis also recommended that to test the 'cumulative effects' of SLI and bilingualism, adequate statistical methods, such as effect sizes, must be applied. Developmental data of TD and SLI monolingual and bilingual children performing a morphology task were compared. The developmental trends indicated that the magnitude of the difference between TD monolingual children and language-impaired bilingual children at eight years was the same as the magnitude of the difference between TD bilingual children and language-impaired bilingual children. These findings were interpreted as evidence against the LPC theories and in favour of the 'compensatory' benefits of bilingualism to overcome the processing deficits of children with SLI, namely, lower working memory and executive function.

Thus, the present study gives a descriptive approach to the emergence of self-repairs in a child with SLI and compares the results with his/her age-matched peers. Specifically, we provide quantitative data of self-repairs classified as a function of the language level affected at different stages of development in TD children. These data have been used as baseline to place the developmental age of the child with SLI. The self-repair patterns of this child are discussed in the light of findings of prior studies.

Method

Given the methodological limitations of testing a large group of TD children over a period of nine years, this study combined a cross-sectional design with a longitudinal design. The cross-sectional design allowed us to obtain data of typically-developing children's linguistic profiles at different stages of development, which served as baseline in order to compare the linguistic profile of the child with SLI with their age-matched peers.

Participants

A total number of 40 TD children (20 males, 20 females) aged 2 to 10 years and a child with SLI participated in the study. The choice of the age span was based on the findings of prior work (Navarro & San Martín, 2007, 2009), which documented that the early emergence of self-repairs occurs around two years. Since one of the purposes of the study was to create an instrument that would also serve as baseline to better diagnose cases of SLI, testing TD children from a wide age span was essential. All the children lived in Catalonia, a bilingual region in Northeastern Spain, and came from households of a mid socio-economic status (SES). Although all participants were sequential bilinguals exposed to both Spanish and Catalan at home, only participants who came from Spanish-dominant households were selected. Following Stark and Tallal (1981), the recruitment requirements were as follows:

- auditory threshold levels of 25 dB at conversational frequencies;
- non-verbal or performance IQ of 85 or higher;
- normal emotional and behavioural indicators;
- no signs of neurologic disorders;
- normal speech motor skills.

In order to participate in the study, the TD children could not exhibit a linguistic deficit, neither a psychopathologic, social, neurologic, sensitive or cognitive disorder. To be included in the TD group, the participants' family history should not have any cases of pathology. All the children in the TD group had a IQ of 90 or higher.

The SLI child also came from a Spanish-dominant household of a mid-SES. The family had a history of language delay and auditory impairment. The child's parents sought counselling because at the age of three he still did not talk. They reported a similar case of language delay in their eldest child, but this was solved when the child under study was born. The child started nursery school at two years. The school reports described him as a happy and affectionate child albeit active. The report also noted that the SLI child exhibited attention deficit and rejection of any tasks that did not arouse his interest. His play habits were monotonous and bound to few changes. He accepted the participation of the adult but play sessions were always silent. The adult often needed to change activities to keep his attention.

As for his communication strategies in child–adult interactions, the SLI child used gestures to express himself and was persistent in his attempts until he was sure that the adult had understood him. He showed difficulty in turn-taking when establishing communication. His receptive language was impaired; he could understand simple commands if these were related to the present situation. In addition, the child had trouble with understanding most of the words produced by the adult. More importantly, his active vocabulary was reduced to two-syllable words and he also showed difficulty in discriminating phonemes. His utterances had not more than two constituents but holophrases were the rule.

Procedure

The children interacted with the experimenter in a playroom inside the school premises, which contained a wide selection of toys and story-books. Children were not prompted to make use of their metalinguistic abilities through specific questions posed by the experimenter for two reasons: (i) to preserve the ecological validity of the study, and (ii) to control the frequency of use of these abilities in a child–adult interaction. It was also deemed appropriate to control the discursive style of the interviewer. Therefore, the experimenter's role was that of an external participant in a natural playing situation. This role was preserved throughout all the interviews conducted with the TD children and the child with SLI.

Each interview lasted about 45 minutes approximately. The child and the adult interacted playing and talking about topics of general interest to all the children. The language used in the play sessions was Spanish, since this was the language that all the children used in the playground with their peers. The experimenter had an informal meeting with the children prior to the audio-/video-recording sessions. A total of 20 developmental times were established, starting at 1;10 years. The time interval between each developmental time was four months for the 1;10–4;4-year-old children. Children up to four years are known to make significantly faster progress in terms of linguistic competence than older children. Older children (over 4;4 years) were recorded at six-month intervals. Since we used a cross-sectional design for the TD children, we recorded two different children (a boy and a girl) at each developmental time. The child with SLI was recorded at 12 developmental times: 3;0, 3;4, 3;7, 3;10, 4;2, 4;6, 4;10, 5;2, 5;6, 5;9, 6;2 and 6;10 years.

Transcription of language samples

The language elicitations were audio-/video-recorded and transcribed using the SALT system (Systematic Analysis of Language Transcript; Miller & Chapman, 1985). Utterances of two words or longer were taken as the unit of analysis. Following Crystal *et al.* (1983), falls in intonation were considered as utterance boundaries in case of ambiguity. The first five minutes of each sample were discarded. At the beginning of each recording session, children tend to be nervous and/or easily distracted. After the first five minutes had elapsed, the next 100 utterances were considered for the analysis. The corpus was coded by the first author plus two additional transcribers, who coded 10% of the language sample for reliability purposes. Cohen's kappa coefficient showed a high inter-rater agreement ($\kappa = 0.87$ and $\kappa = 0.90$) indicating that the coding of the language categories was reliable. The taxonomy of language categories used for the self-repairs was based on the five language levels: phonology, morphology, lexis, syntax and pragmatics.

Results

Typically developing children

The ages of emergence and frequencies of maximum use of self-repairs by TD children and the child with SLI are shown in Table 9.1 and Figure 9.1, respectively. Phonological self-repairs are the first to emerge as early as 1;10 and disappear around four years. The first language sample corresponds to a phonological self-repair by a TD child aged 1;10. The target Spanish word *pequeñas* /pe'keɲas/ is first replaced with [pe'tenas] showing a fronting of both the velar stop and the palatal nasal. Immediately afterwards, the child

Table 9.1 Age of emergence and frequency of maximum use of self-repairs in the normal-speaking children (TD) and the child with SLI as a function of the language level affected

Language level	*Emergence TD*	*Emergence SLI*	*Maximum use TD*	*Maximum use SLI*
Phonology	1;10	3;0	1;10	X
Morphology	2;2	4;2	3;4	4;6
Syntax	2;2	4;6	6;6	4;6
Lexis	2;2	5;2	7;6	5;2
Pragmatics	2;2	4;10	3	2;2

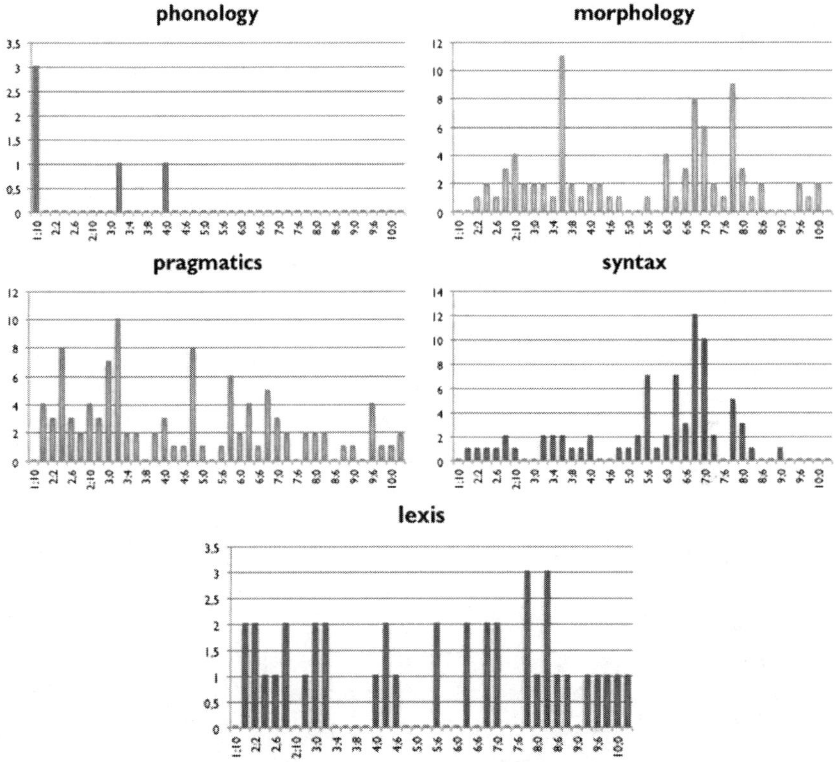

Figure 9.1 Frequency of maximum use of self-repairs by typically developing children as a function of language level

self-repairs her first attempt and elicits a second word much closer to the target [pe'kjeɲas]:

(1) {the child points to a pair of small trainers}
Niño: *son petenas pequieñas*
Child (1;10): *they are tiny, tiny*

Sample 2 shows an instance of pragmatic self-repair by another TD 22-month-old child. The child is describing a picture with various stars. She mentions the *star*, and later realizes she has not talked about the *star* yet. Therefore she substitutes the definite article for the undefinite article:

(2) {the 22-month-old child describes a picture with various stars}
Niña: *l'estel (:) una estel*
Child (1;10): *the star (:) one star*

Morphological self-repairs appear a bit later, around 2;2 years, and they reach the maximum frequency in the three to four years age span. Overall, morphological self-repairs are the most frequent followed by syntactic and lexical self-repairs. In the case of morphology, children often repair genre, tense marking and subject/verb agreement. Samples 3–9 show instances of morphological and lexical self-repairs:

(3) **Niña:** *si, pero yo tengo (un, un) una muñeca*
Child (2;10): *yes, but I have (a, a) a doll* (repairs morphology: genre)

(4) **Niño:** *(:2) (un) (:2) ¿oto cochesito?*
Child (2;6): *(:2) (a) (:2) another small car?* (repairs lexis)

(5) **Niño:** *aquest es el cochecito (:) era*
Child (3;4): *this is the small car (:) was* (repairs morphology: tense marking)

(6) **Niña:** *(un) una muñeca, ala mira!*
Child (2;10): *(a) a doll, look!* (repairs morphology: genre)

(7) **Adulto:** *¿y qué más juguetes tienes?*
Adult: *and which other toys have you got?*
Niño: *tengo (una) un helicóptero*
Child (3;10): *I have got (a) a helicopter* (repairs morphology: genre)

(8) **Niña:** *muchas cosas (vivía) ellas vivían en la tienda*
Child (6;0): *many things (she lived) they lived in the shop* (repairs morphology: subject/verb agreement)

(9) **Niña:** *una (bic* una a, a) una moto*
Child (4;6): *a (bik* one, a, a) a moto* (repairs lexis)

From four years onwards, there is an increase in syntactic and morphological self-repairs (see Samples 10–13). For instance, in Sample 13, the child produces some false starts and then he abandons the first utterance to produce a better fit to his communicative intentions. This is partially in line with an earlier study reporting self-repairs by Finnish-speaking children aged four (Salonen & Laakso, 2009), who found that syntactic and lexical self-repairs were the most frequent among four-year-olds. As shown in Sample 9, lexical repairs often involve semantically related primes.

(10) **Niño:** *si, ahora (van, va) siempre va empatando a cero*
Child (8;6): *yes, now (they are, he is) he is always tying on cero* (repairs morphology: subject/verb agreement).

(11) **Niña:** *y el tenia que pegar cuando, cuand* ven* cuando estaban parados*
Child (3;0): *and he had to hit when, whe* see* when they stopped*

(12) **Niño:** *(yo yo no tengo) yo tengo helicóptero*
Child (3;10): *(I I don't have) I have helicopter* (repairs syntax)

(13) **Niño:** *(y mi) mi tito, yo ya se me a a ir a a los > a casas de mi tito Manolo ya se ir solo.*

Child (4;8): *(and my) my uncle, I already know me to to go to to the > to houses of my uncle Manolo I already go on my own*

The graphs in Figure 9.1 show the frequency of maximum use of self-repairs produced by TD children. The bars represent the number of self-repairs produced by each child in a sample of 100 utterances. An inspection of the data in terms of the language level affected reveals that, in TD children, phonological self-repairs reach the maximum frequency at 1;10 years of age. Pragmatic self-repairs reach the highest frequency of use at three years, followed by morphological self-repairs at 3;4 years and lexical self-repairs at 7;6–8 years. Except for lexical self-repairs, all language levels exhibit a U-shape pattern of usage at different developmental stages. Bowerman (1982) suggested that this pattern responds to a 'developmental process from onset to expertise in an ability' and it involves successive reorganizations when a category has its maximum frequency at more than one age.

Child with specific language impairment

A summary of the self-repairs elicited by the child with SLI classified by language level is shown in Figure 9.2. The only phonological self-repair tracked in the child with SLI appeared at three years (see Sample 8). No further instances of phonological self-repairs are tracked at later stages of development. However, the child exhibits many instances of simplification such as **qui* instead of *aquí (here)*, **ta* instead of pelota and **ta* instead of *patata* 'potato', *papa* 'dad' or *tata* (informal for 'sister'). The absence of phonological self-repairs could be traced down to the fact that the child with SLI was first recorded at the age of three years. We speculate that the child might have repaired phonology prior to this age but, unfortunately, these data were not available.

(14) **Child with SLI aged 3:** *do ado* (he refers to his friend Fernando)

Self-repairs of morphology and syntax are the most common in the speech of the child with SLI. They emerge at 4;2 years and persist until age 10 (see Samples 15–16). As for the frequency of maximum use, morphological self-repairs increase around six years of age. The child starts to repair pragmatics at 4;6 and 4,10 years, respectively (see Sample 17). This is a considerable delay relative to TD children, who start repairing pragmatics very early at 1;10 years. At this age, pragmatics is paramount to develop the child's communicative and linguistic abilities. Lexical self-repairs are the last to emerge at 5;2 years and no other instances are found at later stages of development (see Sample 17).

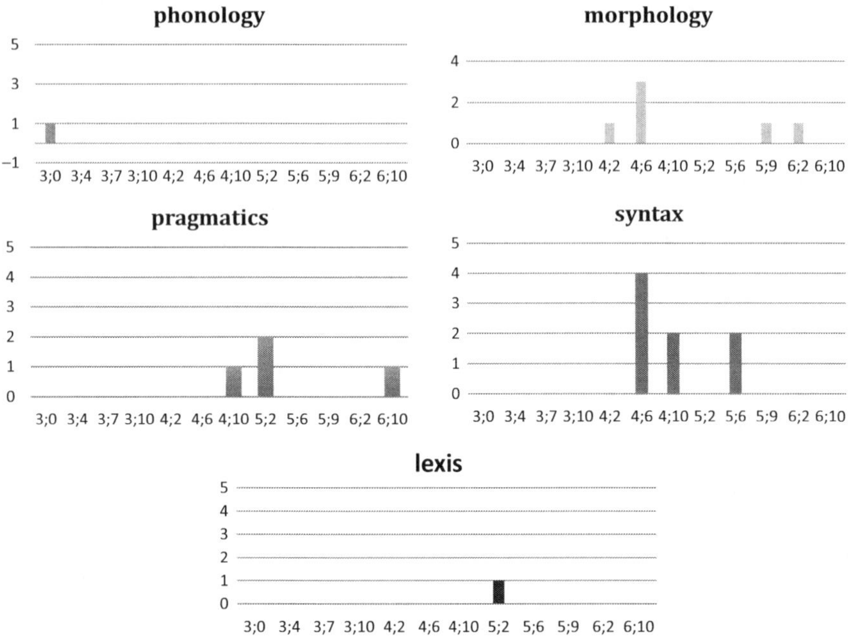

Figure 9.2 Frequency of maximum use of self-repairs by the child with specific language impairment

(15) **Niño:** *(el) los animales van aquí*
Child with SLI (5;9): *(the) animals go here* (repairs morphology: number)

(16) **Niño:** *igual es que >*
Child with SLI (5;6): *maybe it's that*
Niño: *igual >*
Child: *maybe >*
Niño: *igual el que viste.*
Child: *same you saw* (repairs syntax)

(17) Child with SLI aged 6;10 (the child attends a story-telling activity in the local library)
Niño (dirigiéndose a la bibliotecaria): *¿señora, cuando empieza el cuento?*
Child with SLI (6;10) (addressing the librarian): *Miss, when does the story start?*
Niño: *¿(me das) da uno?*

Child: *can you give me one?* (repairs pragmatics: the child self-corrects register and replaces the verb form *das* with the courtesy form *da*)

(18) **Niño:** *el caba* (caballo) no la cebra*
Child with SLI (5;2): *the hor* (horse) not the zebra* (repairs lexis)

A comparison of self-repairs by the TD children and the child with SLI reveals that the child with SLI's behaviour corresponds to a child at a lower stage of development. Morphological self-repairs emerge at 2;2 years in TD children, whereas in the child with SLI they do not emerge until 4;2 years. TD children start to repair syntax and lexis before they turn two years of age, specifically at 1;10 years. In contrast, the child with SLI does not start to repair syntax until two years later. Similarly, lexical and pragmatic self-repairs by the child with SLI are late in the stage of development. They do not emerge until past five years of age, a considerable delay in comparison to TD children, who use pragmatic repairs before age 2.

Frequencies of maximum use also exhibit a delay (see Figure 9.2). The child with SLI produces very few phonological self-repairs. Among TD children pragmatic self-repairs reach maximum frequency at three years, whereas the maximum frequencies for the child with SLI appear much later, at 5;2 years. The frequency of morphological self-repairs reaches the highest values at 3;4 years among TD children, but for the child with SLI a delay of more than one year is found (4;6 years). Surprisingly, the child with SLI elicits the most syntactic and lexical self-repairs earlier, at 4;6 and 5;2, respectively. In contrast, TD children self-repair syntax and lexis much later, between the ages of 6;00 and 8;00.

Discussion and Conclusions

The present study has provided cross-sectional data of self-repairs by 40 Spanish-Catalan TD children. These data have been used as a baseline for determining the developing age of a child with SLI. Overall, the frequency of self-repairs is considerably lower in the child with SLI's utterances relative to his TD peers. Unlike TD children, self-repairs are absent at some developmental stages of the child with SLI, specifically at ages 3;4, 3;7 and 3;10. Early emergence of self-repairs in the child with SLI involves the better preserved language levels. In line with prior work (Merrison, 2005), self-repairs involving the more affected language levels emerge later. We hypothesized that the child exhibited deficits in metalinguistic competence and was thus unable to detect his own errors.

As the child made progress in linguistic competence, the number of self-repairs increased, which is especially noticeable at 4;6 years. At this age, there was an abrupt peak in the use of morphological and syntactic repairs, showing that his metalinguistic abilities improved and the child had acquired new strategies. This interpretation of the results would be in line with Hirchman (2000), who suggested that the metalinguistic function helps the child to overcome a potential neurological deficit in that they become aware of the rules that govern language. She refers to a metalinguistic 'bridge effect' which facilitates the building of linguistic knowledge despite impaired functionality of the brain area involved.

The data of the TD children do not exhibit a linear model of development; that is, the number of self-repairs does not decrease as a function of age. Instead, they exhibit a U-shaped pattern of behaviour (Bowerman, 1982), which has different peaks and decreases that change across language levels. For instance, morphological repairs show a clear U-shaped pattern from ages 3;4 to 7;6. Pragmatic self-repairs show various U-shaped patterns at three age ranges: 2;2–3;0, 3;0–4;6 and 4;6–5;6. From age 5;6 onwards, TD children gradually decrease in repairing pragmatics. In the case of syntax, the U-shaped pattern is visible between ages 5;6 and 7;0 and then there is a gradual slope, suggesting that TD children rarely repair syntax from seven years onwards and are in line with prior work comparing speech disruptions in TD and SLI populations (Guo *et al.*, 2008) which relates a decrease in speech disruptions to syntactic development.

In addition, U-shaped patterns signal the child's mastering of the linguistic system and their metalinguistic abilities. This universal pattern follows three stages and responds to reorganization processes (Bowerman, 1982). At the first stage, the child produces a given linguistic form correctly, at a later stage of development they produce the same form incorrectly (or deviated from the norms of adult usage) and, at the final stage, they produce the correct form again. A typical example is the over-regularization of verbal inflectional morphology in Spanish. In this case, the child would produce a correct instance of the past tense of the verb *tener* ('to have got') such as *tenía*. At the next stage, they would elicit the incorrect form because it conforms to the general pattern **teniba (tenia)* ('he had'). In the end, the correct form will generalize. The interpretation of this sequence of events assumes that, at the first stage, the child learns the correct forms as individual cases. Later, when they have already acquired some instances that meet the general pattern, the child 'comes to recognize their systematicity and to abstract rules that allow her to create new exemplars at will' (Bowerman, 1982: 104). When the new rules come into play, the child applies them on a regular basis, ignoring exceptions. Eventually the irregular forms will be integrated into the child's linguistic system.

By contrast, reorganization processes are absent in the child with SLI, who uses a considerably lower number of repairs relative to their age-matched peers.

Like younger TD children, language-impaired children have general mental representations, more communicative intentions but fewer linguistic structures (see Levy, 1999; Levy *et al.*, 2003). In line with Kamhi and Koenig (1985), SLI children not only need more time to understand and produce certain linguistic structures, but they also need more time to access newly acquired linguistic knowledge. This explains why the child under study shows a slower access to the metalinguistic function than his age-matched peers.

The low frequency of phonological self-repairs in both the TD and SLI data might be a combination of two factors. On the one hand, phonology was not particularly impaired in this child; on the other hand, the possibility exists that the child had started to repair phonology prior to the data collection (3;0 years). The data from the TD children showed that phonological repairs emerged as early as 1;10 years. These outcomes replicate findings by previous studies (Clark, 2014; Laakso, 2010) which also reported early emergence of phonological repairs.

Social factors

In line with recent work which highlights the role of social factors in helping children adjust their discourse (Morgenstem *et al.*, 2013), we have found evidence that the child with SLI attempts to adjust to the system of his environment or social group. More importantly, the environment plays a crucial role in the development of the child with SLI as well as in his self-esteem. In our case study, the child's attitude changed when his peers at school accepted him as one of their members. At some point in the interview he reported that he now played with the other children. When asked whether he had not played with his peers before, the child responded by asking why he should bother playing with the other children if they could not understand each other.

The interaction of the child with his environment is also paramount to improving their knowledge of the language. A recent study by Barachetti and Lavelli (2014) investigated repair by mothers of children with SLI in mother–child interactions, in which both participants used story books with images and text. This format facilitates joint attention of mother and child towards one object. In these interactions, the participants have very clear roles and the language they use is repetitive, thus facilitating the active participation of the child. The results suggested that mothers of children with SLI adjust repairs to their children's linguistic limitations. This has a supportive effect on the SLI child's productions, in that they obtain the information they need to generate correct answers and, more importantly, the repair provided by adults is the first step in helping the child self-repair his own errors. These aspects should be considered in designing intervention programmes that highlight the relevance of the context as well as the interlocutor's implication. Eventually, the SLI child will acquire strategies to produce his own self-repairs and generate introspection about his own language.

Limitations and further research

The present study has explored the emergence and development of self-repairs in TD Spanish-Catalan bilingual children and a Spanish-Catalan bilingual child with SLI, a subgroup that has not received much attention in the literature (see Verhoeven *et al.*, 2012, for a review). The authors argued that this population suffers 'restricted language input'. At the first developmental stages they are mostly exposed to the L1 spoken in the household but once children start school a drastic change occurs. Most curricula in immersion programmes in bilingual communities involve massive exposure to the L2. It is hypothesized that the abrupt transition from L1 to L2 may slow down the linguistic development of bilingual children with SLI. Conversely, it has also been suggested that bilingualism could actually have a compensatory effect from the cognitive perspective, helping them to overcome their processing deficits, i.e. lower working memory or executive function. The case study of SLI reported here did not exhibit any instances of transfer from the L1 (Spanish) to the L2 (Catalan). We are unsure whether the fact that the interviewer addressed him in Spanish ruled out any chance that the SLI child used Catalan in the interaction. Further, the child with SLI was a sequential bilingual from a Spanish-dominant household, which poses limitations to any influence of the L1 onto the L2 or any shift of language dominance over time. Further research should consider the possibility of recording adult–child interactions in two different language conditions (Spanish and Catalan) to explore any possible differences in the use of self-repairs as a function of language.

We acknowledge that the developmental trends in the use of self-repairs exhibited by TD children do not allow for generalization because they are based on the speech samples of two TD children per age. However, these trends have diagnostic potential in that they provide valuable information to the speech practitioner to design a more customized intervention plan, focusing on the linguistic areas that are more impaired. In our case, using the ages of emergence of self-repairs by TD children, we could infer that the child with SLI exhibits a delay of four years in the onset of syntactic repair and a delay of three years in the onset of lexical repair. Based on this comparison, the intervention plan for this client should give priority to these two linguistic levels.

We can also speculate that, at the first stages of literacy development, the child's written language will probably be a reflection of his oral language. Soon, written language will surely guide the child's thoughts about oral language. At this stage, self-repairs will probably emerge in the written language. In cases of older children with SLI who are poor readers, Zwitserlood *et al.* (2015) recommend intervention approaches that are less dependent on literacy skills, combining metalinguistic and multimodal methods to treat morphology and syntax, which are the most impaired affected language levels of our case study examined here.

Acknowledgements

This research was partly funded by Research Grant FFI2013-48640-C2-2-P by the Spanish Ministry of Economy and Competitiveness to the second author. The authors would like to thank the editors and the two anonymous reviewers for their insightful comments on earlier versions of this chapter.

Note

(1) The reader must be reminded that the term 'maze' must be understood as a large class and it includes repetitions, pauses and repairs.

References

Barachetti, C. and Lavelli, M. (2014) Maternal input to children with specific language impairment during shared book reading: Is mothers' language in tune with their children's production? *International Journal of Language & Communication Disorders* 49 (2), 204–214.

Bermeosolo, J. (2012) Memoria de trabajo y memoria procedimental en las dificultades específicas del aprendizaje y del lenguaje: algunos hallazgos [Working memory and procedural memory in specific learning and language impairment: some findings]. *Revista Chilena de Fonoaudiología* 11, 57–75.

Bishop, D.V.M. (2000) Pragmatic language impairment: A correlate of SLI, a distinct group or part of the acoustic continuum? In D.V.M. Bishop and L.B. Leonard (eds) *Speech and Language Impairments in Children: Causes, Characteristics, Intervention and Outcome* (pp. 99–113). Hove: Psychology Press.

Bishop, D.V.M. (2006) What causes specific language impairment in children? *Current Directions in Psychological Science* 15 (5), 217–221.

Bishop, D.V.M. and Adams, C. (1989) Conversational characteristics of children with semantic-pragmatic disorder. II. What features lead to a judgement of inapropriacy? *British Journal of Disorders of Communication* 24, 241–263.

Bowerman, M. (1982) Starting to talk worse: Clues to language acquisition from children's late speech errors. In S. Strauss (ed.) *U-shaped Behavioral Growth* (pp. 101–145). New York: Academic Press.

Claessen, M.E. and Leitão, S. (2012) Phonological representations in children with SLI. *Child Language Teaching and Therapy* 28 (2), 211–223.

Clark, E.V. (1978) Awareness of language: Some evidence from what children say and do. In A. Sinclair, R.J. Jarvella and W.J.M. Levelt (eds) *The Child's Conception of Language* (pp. 17–44). Berlin: Springer Verlag.

Clark, E.V. (2014) Pragmatics in Acquisition. *Journal of Child Language* 41 (S1), 105–116.

Colozzo, P., Gillam, R.B., Wood, M., Schnell, R.D. and Johnston, J.R. (2011) Content and form in the narratives of children with specific language impairment. *Journal of Speech, Language, and Hearing Research* 54 (6), 1609–1627.

Crystal, D., Fletcher, P. and Garman, M. (1983) *Análisis Gramatical de los Trastornos del Lenguaje: un Procedimiento de Evaluación y Reeducación [The Grammatical Analysis of Language Disability: A Procedure for Assessment and Remediation]*. Barcelona: Editorial Médica y Técnica.

de Ruiter, L. (2013) Self-repairs in German children's peer interaction – initial explorations. In R. Eklund (ed.) *DiSS 2013: Proceedings of Disfluency in Spontaneous Speech, TMH-QPSR* 54 (1), 29–32.

Duinmeijer, I., de Jong, J. and Scheper, A. (2012) Narrative abilities, memory and attention in children with a specific language impairment. *International Journal of Language & Communication Disorders* 47 (5), 542–555.

Fletcher, P. (1990) Sub-groups of school-age language impaired children. *Child Language Teaching and Therapy* 6 (1), 47–58.

Forrester, M.A. (2008) The emergence of self-repair: A case study of one child during the early preschool years. *Research on Language and Social Interaction* 41 (1), 99–128.

Forrester, M.A. and Cherington, S.M. (2009) The development of other-related conversational skills: A case study of conversational repair during the early years. *First Language* 29, 166–191.

Gathercole, S.E. and Baddeley, A.D. (1990) Phonological memory deficits in language disordered children: Is there a causal connection? *Journal of Memory and Language* 29, 336–360.

Guo, L., Tomblin, J.B. and Samelson, V. (2008) Speech disruptions in the narratives of English-speaking children with specific language impairment. *Journal of Speech, Language, and Hearing Research* 51, 722–738.

Gutiérrez-Clellen, V., Simon-Cereijido, G. and Wagner, C. (2008) Bilingual children with language impairment: A comparison with monolinguals and second language learners. *Applied Psycholinguistics* 29, 3–20.

Hennessey, N.W., Leitão, S. and Mucciarone, K. (2010) Verbal repetition skill in language impaired children: Evidence of inefficient lexical processing? *International Journal of Speech-Language Pathology* 12 (1), 47–57.

Hirchman, M. (2000) Language repair via metalinguistic means. *Journal Language Communication Disorders* 35 (2), 251–268.

Jackson, E., Leitao, S. and Claessen, M. (2016) The relationship between phonological short-term memory, receptive vocabulary, and fast mapping in children with specific language impairment. *International Journal of Language Communication Disorders* 51, 61–73.

Kamhi, A. and Koenig, L. (1985) Metalinguistic awareness in normal and language disordered children. *Language, Speech, and Hearing Services in Schools* 16, 199–221.

Laakso, M. (2010) Children's emerging and developing self-repair practices. In H. Gardner and M. Forrester (eds) *Analysing Interactions in Childhood: Insights from Conversation Analysis* (pp. 74–99). Oxford: Wiley-Blackwell.

Lennon, P. (1990) Investigating fluency in EFL: A quantitative approach. *Language Learning* 40, 387–417.

Leonard, L., Ellis Weismer, S., Miller, C.A., Francis, D., Tomblin, B. and Kail, R. (2007) Speed of processing, working memory, and language impairment in children. *Journal of Speech, Language, and Hearing Research* 50, 408–428.

Levelt, W.J.M. (1983) Monitoring and self-repair in speech. *Cognition* 14, 41–104.

Levelt, W.J.M. (1989) *Speaking: From Intention to Articulation*. Cambridge, Mass: MIT Press.

Levelt, W.J.M. and Cutler, A. (1983) Prosodic marking in speech repair. *Journal of Semantics* 2, 205–217.

Levy, Y. (1999) Early metalinguistic competence: Speech monitoring and repair behavior. *Developmental Psychology* 35 (3), 822–834.

Levy, Y., Tennebaum, A. and Ornoy, A. (2003) Repair behavior in children with intellectual impairments: Evidence for metalinguistic competence. *Journal of Speech, Language, and Hearing Research* 46, 368–381.

MacLurg, A. (2014) Mapping mazes: Developing a taxonomy to investigate mazes in children's stories. MA thesis, University of Alberta.

Merrison, S. (2005) Repair in speech and language therapy interaction: Investigating pragmatic language impairment of children. *Child Language Teaching and Therapy* 21(2), 191–211.

Miller, G. and Chapman, J. (1985) *Systematic Analysis of Language Transcript (SALT)*. Madison, WI: University of Wisconsin.

Morgenstem, A., Leroy-Collombel, M.L. and Caët, S. (2013) Self- and other-repairs in child–adult interaction at the intersection of pragmatic abilities and language acquisition. *Journal of Pragmatics* 56, 151–167.

Muñoz López, J. and Carballo García, G. (2005) Alteraciones lingüísticas en el trastorno específico del lenguaje [Language deviations in specific language impairment]. *Revista de Neurología* 41 (1), 57–63.

Navarro-Ruiz, M.I. (1997) Estructuras lingüísticas y déficit de lenguaje [Language structures and language deficit]. Unpublished PhD dissertation, Universitat de Barcelona.

Navarro, M.I. and San Martín, C. (2007) Desarrollo de las habilidades metalingüísticas en la edad escolar [Development of metalinguistic abilities at school age]. In P. Pequito and A. Pinheiro (eds) *Quem aprende mais? Reflexoes sobre educaçao de infància* (pp. 326–344). Oporto: Ediçoes Gailivro.

Navarro, M.I. and San Martín, C. (2009) Emergencia y desarrollo de las habilidades metalingüísticas relacionadas con la regulación de la información: Un estudio transversal en niños de edades comprendidas entre los 22 meses y los diez años [Emergence and development of metalinguistic abilities related to information regulation. A cross-sectional study in children aged 22 months to 10 years. *RLA Revista de Lingüística Teórica y Aplicada* 47, 61–82.

Navarro-Ruiz, M.I. and Rallo-Fabra, L. (2001) Characteristics of mazes produced by SLI children. *Clinical Linguistics and Phonetics* 15 (1–2), 63–66.

Nettelbladt, U. and Hansson, K. (1999) Mazes in Swedish pre-school children with specific language impairment. *Clinical Linguistics and Phonetics* 13, 483–497.

Norrick, N.R. (1991) On the organization of corrective exchanges in conversation. *Journal of Pragmatics* 16 (1), 59–83.

Orgassa, A. and Weerman, F. (2008) Dutch gender in specific language impairment and second language acquisition. *Second Language Research* 24, 333–364.

Paradis, J. (2010) The interface between bilingual development and specific language impairment. *Applied Psycholinguistics* 31, 227–252.

Petersen, D.B. and Gardner, C.M. (2011) Trastorno específico del lenguaje: una revisión [Specific language impairment: A revision]. *Revista Chilena de Fonoaudiología* 10, 19–32.

Postma, A., Kolk, H. and Povel, D.J. (1990) On the relation among speech errors, disfluencies, and self-repairs. *Language and Speech* 33 (1), 19–29.

Quintero, I., Hernández, S., Verche, E., Acosta, V. and Hernández, A. (2013) Disfunción ejecutiva en el trastorno específico del lenguaje [Executive dysfunction in specific language impairment]. *Revista de Logopedia, Foniatría y Audiología* 33, 172–178.

Rispoli, M. and Hadley, P. (2001) The leading-edge: The significance of sentence disruptions in the development of grammar. *Journal of Speech Language, and Hearing Research* 44, 1131–1143.

Rispoli, M., Hadley, P. and Holt, J. (2008) Stalls and revisions: A developmental perspective on sentence production. *Journal of Speech, Language, and Hearing Research* 51, 953–966.

Salonen, T. and Laakso, M. (2009) Self-repair of speech by four-year-old Finnish children. *Journal of Child Language* 36 (4), 855–882.

Schegloff, E.A. (1979) The relevance of repair to syntax-for-conversation. In T. Givón (ed.) *Syntax and Semantics, Vol. 12* (pp. 261–286). New York: Academic Press.

Schegloff, E.A., Jefferson, G. and Sacks, H. (1977) The preference for self-correction in the organization of repair in conversation. *Language* 53 (2), 361–382.

Schmidt, R. (1992) Psychological mechanisms underlying second language fluency. *Studies in Second Language Acquisition* 14, 357–385.

Stark, R.E. and Tallal, P. (1981) Selection of children with specific language deficits. *Journal of Speech and Hearing Disorders* 46 (2), 114–122.

Thordardottir, E. and Weismer, S. (2002) Content mazes and filled pauses in narrative language samples of children with specific language impairment. *Brain and Cognition* 48, 587–592.

Ullman, M.T. and Pierpont, E.I. (2005) Specific language impairment is not specific to language: The procedural deficit hypothesis. *Cortex* 41, 399–433.

Verhoeven, L., Steenge, J. and van Balkom, H. (2012) Linguistic transfer in bilingual children with specific language impairment. *International Journal of Language & Communication Disorders* 2 (47), 176–183.

Zwitserlood, R., Wijnen, F., Weerdenburg, M. and Verhoeven, L. (2015) 'MetaTaal': Enhancing complex syntax in children with specific language impairment. A metalinguistic and multimodal approach. *International Journal of Language Communication Disorders* 50 (3), 273–297.

10 Local Assimilation in Children Acquiring Farsi: A Study of Typical versus Atypical Phonological Development

Froogh Shooshtaryzadeh

Introduction

There are two types of assimilation: *local assimilation*, which is the modification that makes a segment identical to or more similar to another segment in its neighbourhood, and *reciprocal assimilation*, which is the modification of two sounds that makes them more akin to each other (e.g. Katamba, 1991; Lass, 1984; Miccio & Scarpino, 2008). Assimilation can occur in two directions. If a segment turns out to be more like the segment that precedes it, the process is called *progressive* or *perseverative* assimilation. However, if assimilation causes a sound to become more like the sound that follows it, the process is called *regressive* or *anticipatory* assimilation (e.g. Katamba, 1991; Lass, 1984). Furthermore, assimilation can be total or partial. Total assimilation leads to identical adjacent segments, while partial assimilation can occur with respect to any one feature of the target segment, i.e. place, voice and manner.

There are some studies on local assimilation in adult language (e.g. Beckman, 2004; Boersma, 1998; Cho, 1990; Dvorak, 2010; Jun, 1995, 2002, 2004; Lombardi, 2004; Rose & Walker, 2004; Pater, 2002; Winters, 2002) and a few in child language (e.g. Akpan, 2006; Bernhardt & Stemberger, 1998; Cho & Lee, 2014; Martinez & Diez-Itza, 2012). Bernhardt and Stemberger (1998) studied assimilation in word-initial sonorant and /s/ clusters using the data from a child, named Charles. This study concluded that default features are often subject to assimilation; however, sometimes a particular feature can be the target of assimilation, regardless of its relative specification status.

Bernhardt and Stemberger (1998: 434) also investigated the development of medial and final clusters in several children. The data revealed both total as well as partial assimilation. Total assimilation in medial nasal clusters was argued to be a function of [voice]: /mb, nd, ng/ clusters were reduced to a long nasal (e.g. /nʌmbɹ/ → [nʌm:ɤ]), while /mp, nt, nk/ clusters were reduced to a long stop (e.g. /dɑŋki/ → [dɑk:i]). In other words, the direction of assimilation in these productions was determined by the voice feature of the following stops.

Akpan (2006) investigated the process of assimilation in 50 children (aged 2;6–4;6) learning Ibibio language. He investigated place and manner assimilation in nasal clusters. The study showed that nasals usually assimilate to the place of articulation of a following segment. Overall, the direction of assimilation can be both regressive and progressive, depending on the type of assimilation. Cho and Lee (2014) studied place assimilation in children acquiring Korean and concluded that consonants, irrespective of their place of articulation, can be both targets and triggers of local assimilation. Moreover, they maintained that the dominant direction observed in local assimilation is regressive. Kirk (2008) studied the errors occurring in consonant clusters in 11 English-speaking TD children (aged 1;5–2;7). She found that ease of articulation provides the most convincing explanation for within-cluster assimilation in these children. Martinez and Diez-Itza (2012) studied assimilation in 240 Spanish-speaking children with a focus on directionality, distance and the type of phoneme involved in the process. They concluded that progressive assimilation is much less frequent than regressive assimilation, and that it tends to disappear earlier. Szreder (2011) also studied the phonological processes which affected consonant clusters in the speech of a Polish child (aged 1;5–1;9). She concluded that the nature of the processes and the mode of their application reveal that articulatory and attentional factors are the major source of the child's errors.

Furthermore, several studies on adult languages (e.g. Jun, 1995, 2004; Kohler, 1990; Ohala, 1990; Steriade, 2000) investigated the assimilation of nasals to the place of articulation of plosives in nasal-plosive clusters. They claimed that perceptual factors provide a primary motivation for nasals to assimilate to the place of articulation of plosives. However, Winters (2000, 2001, 2002) and Hura *et al.* (1992), who also examined assimilation in nasal and plosive clusters in adult languages, have questioned this claim.

With these findings in mind, the present study aims to investigate the patterns of assimilation in typically developing (TD) children and children with phonological disorder (PD) acquiring Farsi as their first language. The goal is to discover the assimilation patterns that generally occur in their productions and to compare them with previous findings in the literature. In addition, this study discusses the similarities and/or differences found in the assimilation patterns during typical and atypical phonological development. In the remaining part of the chapter, the theoretical framework employed in this study, namely optimality theory (McCarthy & Prince, 1993a, 1993b; Prince & Smolensky, 1993), is briefly introduced, followed by some pertinent information on Farsi, which is the investigated language in this study. Subsequently, the chapter discusses the methodology used here, presents the data and discusses the results of this investigation.

Optimality Theory

Optimality theory (henceforth OT) was developed in the early 1990s (McCarthy & Prince, 1993a, 1993b; Prince & Smolensky, 1993). It is a theoretical approach in phonology which resorts to mental procedures to explain linguistic processes. Recent versions, however, have attempted to incorporate phonetic (articulatory) aspects within the phonological (abstract) framework (Boersma, 1998; Jun, 1995, 2004), as well. OT differs from earlier theoretical frameworks in that it dispenses with the notion of rules applied in the explanation of different linguistic patterns in the grammar. It is based instead on the notion of the presence of a constraint, i.e. 'a limit on what constitutes a possible pronunciation of a word' (Bernhardt & Stemberger, 1998: 211). The OT framework utilizes three basic mechanisms: the *generator* (GEN), *constraints* (CON) and *evaluator* (EVAL). GEN presents a ranking of the constraints in CON and EVAL evaluates the outputs of GEN taking into consideration universal constraints, and their ranking for a certain language. Based on this evaluation, EVAL chooses the *optimal output* that is the candidate which violates the smallest number of high-ranked constraints within the grammar and it emerges therefore as the winner among productions (Prince & Smolensky, 1993). There are two types of constraints in OT: *markedness constraints* and *faithfulness constraints*. Markedness constraints are formulated solely in terms of output properties and are against marked segment types, sequences and structures. Faithfulness constraints insist on the identity between corresponding constituents in input and output representations.

Constraints are assumed to be both universal and language specific (Barlow, 2001; Barlow & Gierut, 1999; Gierut & Morrisette, 2005; Kager, 1999). Except for those constraints that participate in a fixed universal ranking, all other constraints can rank in different ways across languages (Bernhardt & Stemberger, 1998; Dinnsen & O'Connor, 2001a, 2001b). OT maintains that diversities in different linguistic productions originate from differences in the relative ranking of markedness and faithfulness constraints in speakers' grammars. Moreover, according to OT, in the child's system, contrary to the adult's system, markedness constraints dominate faithfulness constraints. OT represents the input, output candidates, markedness and faithfulness constraints, their ranking, and violations in a *tableau*. OT has been widely used in investigations on phonology, and in typical and atypical phonological development (e.g. Barlow & Gierut, 1999; Bernhardt & Stemberger, 2000; Dinnsen & O'Connor, 2001a, 2001b; Gilbert, 2001; Jesney, 2007; Ueda & Davis, 2001). The present study also applies the OT framework to the similarities and/or differences observed in the assimilation patterns of typically versus atypically developing children participating in this study.

The Farsi Language

As argued above, the present study investigates assimilation in TD children and children with a PD learning Farsi as their first language. Farsi has six vowels, i.e. /e, æ, o, i, a, u/ and 23 consonants, i.e. /b p t d s z ʧ ʤ g k q ʔ r ʃ x ʒ v f h m n l j/. Three types of syllable structures are attested in adult Farsi: CV, CVC and CVCC, e.g. *ta* /ta/ 'up to', *bar* /bar/ 'load', *sang* /sæng/ 'stone'. There are no word-initial clusters in Farsi; therefore, local assimilation can only take place in word-medial and word-final clusters and at word boundaries. Samare (1999) explains collocation restrictions in final clusters; however, for the restrictions on medial clusters, which are the main focus of this study, no source has been found to compare with the results here. Some of the restrictions on final clusters are:

- the members of a cluster cannot be identical;
- the members of a cluster cannot have the same place of articulation;
- sibilants and spirants never appear in a cluster;
- /p/ never appears in C_1 position in final clusters or medial clusters).

Furthermore, there is no /ŋ/ sound in Farsi; therefore, the cluster /ng/ is not phonetically [ŋg], with an allophonic assimilation to the velar. It is phonetically an anterior coronal nasal.

Some common regressive assimilation patterns are observed in Standard Farsi, both in word-medial clusters and at word boundaries, such as the assimilation of coronal nasal /n/ to the place of articulation of labial plosive /b/ in /nb/ clusters (e.g. /pænbe/ is pronounced as [pæmbe] 'cotton') and the assimilation of /d/ to the voiceless phoneme /t/ in /dt/ (e.g. /sæd.ta/ is pronounced as [sæt.ta] 'hundred'). Stress normally falls on the last syllable of a noun and the first syllable of a verb. The majority of assimilation errors observed in the present study involve medial clusters, because final clusters mainly display deletion rather than assimilation. Therefore the discussion and results of this study are mainly related to assimilation in medial clusters. There are different types of medial clusters in Farsi such as plosive-liquid, nasal-plosive, fricative-plosive, etc., which will be examined in following sections.

Method

Participants

The participants in this qualitative cross-sectional study are five children (three girls and two boys) diagnosed with a functional PD, whose age ranges from 4;6 to 6;0, and 10 TD children (four girls and six boys), whose age ranges from 2;3 to 4;0. The reason for the age difference among the groups participating in this study is that the PD children were purposefully chosen to be older than four years, since a child is generally considered phonologically disordered if his/her speech remains unintelligible past the age of 4;0, which is when TD children are generally intelligible to strangers (Adams *et al.*, 1997). However, TD children aged 4;0 and above usually make few assimilation errors in clusters, so the speech of TD children younger than 4;0 were examined in this study to account for this.

To identify the PD children from the TD children, the candidates were assessed in terms of their speech, hearing and cognitive/mental abilities by a speech therapist, an audiometrist and a psychologist. Furthermore, the children's medical profiles were checked and their parents filled out related questionnaires. There were also interviews with parents and teachers. The results of these enquiries indicated that the PD children are physically and mentally healthy, and that their speech problem is due to *functional/nonorganic phonological disorder*. All children come from middle-class families. They are primarily monolingual and speak standard Farsi (the Tehrani accent) in most social settings, including at home and in school.

Speech assessment tools

The children participating in this study were tested using a picture-naming task, which was devised based on known standards in research methodology, and the features of the Farsi language. The task contained pictures of 132 familiar objects and served to elicit the spontaneous production of the corresponding 132 target words. The word types used in the task included a good number of all types of consonants, i.e. 167 plosives, 14 affricates, 108 fricatives, 75 nasals, 73 liquids, and 16 glides. Except for the phoneme /ʔ/ which is only pronounced in word-initial and medial positions in Farsi, all other consonants are present in initial, medial, and final word positions. There are different types of clusters in the test, as outlined next:

Liquid clusters: /2rb, 2br, rt, tr, 2rd, rk, rg, 3rq, rv, rf, 2rs, rʧ, rx, rj/; /lf, 2lv, fl, bl, tl, lk/
Nasal clusters: /nb, 6nd, 5ng , nk, zn, jn/; /2mp, sm, ʃm, xm, 3rm, 2jm/
Plosive, Fricative: /bz, sb, tf, st, 3ʃt , 2xt, dʃ, 2sk, ʃq/

Fricatives, Fricatives: /sv, sʃ, fʃ, sf/
Plosive, Plosive: /2dk, bt, kp/
Others: /jk, jʧ, xʧ/

The numbers preceding some of the clusters in the above list (e.g. 2 in 2rb) indicate the frequency of each cluster in the test. The word types targeted in the test were simple, complex or compound words, featuring all syllable types licensed in Farsi, i.e. CV, CVC and CVCC, and they were between one and six syllables long.

Data Elicitation

Each child was guided through the procedures of the test in plain language. Each picture was presented to the child separately, and he/she was asked to label the picture. On some occasions, the data were collected from a single child over two or three different sessions, depending on his/her age and the child's willingness to respond to questions. As well as recording each child's productions during picture elicitation, there were 15–30 minutes of free speech recording. Recordings took place in a quiet room using a Samsung 4 GB digital recorder (*YP-VP1*) with an external directional microphone that was at a consistent distance from the participant's mouth (about 20–25 cm). The format used for recording was MP3 with 44,100 Hz sampling rate and 192 kps resolution.

Data Processing

The recorded data were listened to carefully by three judges and were transcribed using the IPA. In the case of disagreements, the consensus method was used, taking the transcription agreed upon by two of the three judges. The errors in the children's productions were analyzed to determine the phonetic inventories of each child and to identify cases of assimilation. To separate context-free substitutions (quasi-assimilation errors) from real assimilation errors, all utterances produced as a result of the child's articulatory limitations were deleted from the list. Such cases are mainly observed in some PD children that have problems in the articulation of fricatives and/or back consonants. For example, one of the children, named Me, cannot produce /x/ and generally substituted the glottal fricative (in a single instance) and the glottal stop in word-initial position. Me uses plosives for /x/ in word-medial and word-final positions or deletes it (e.g. /nax/ → [tat] 'thread'; /xorus/ → /ʔojut/ 'rooster'; /xæmir/ → [hæmiz] 'paste'). Therefore, her production [dæddebal] for /tæxtexab/ is not considered to be assimilation.

Results

The data elicited from the picture naming task were analyzed and the phonetic inventories of the TD and PD children participating in this study were determined. Such inventories help determine if production errors are due to phonetic limitations or evidence of an abstract phonological process, like assimilation (Tables 10.1 and 10.2). In the acquisition literature, the conventional criterion for including a phone in the phonetic inventory of a child is a two-time occurrence of the phone independently of its target or context (e.g. Stoel-Gammon & Dunn, 1985). The same convention is followed in the present study.

The analyses, here, addressed the quantity and quality of the assimilation processes occurring in the TD and PD groups, as well as the differences between the assimilation processes occurring in these two groups and the assimilation processes occurring in adults and children acquiring other languages. As indicated in earlier studies, the main trend observed for local assimilation in adult and child language is towards regressive assimilation (e.g. Beckman, 1998; Cho & Lee, 2014; Dvorak, 2010; Jun, 2002, 2004; Lombardi, 2004; Martinez & Diez-Itza, 2012). However, the data from this study do not only include progressive assimilation (see Appendix), but also to what extent progressive assimilation in TD children is significantly higher

Table 10.1 The phonetic inventory of the TD group

Ay	/m n b p t d k g q ʔ f v s z ʃ x h j l r ʤ/	Sy	/m n b p t d k g q ʔ f v s z ʃ x h j l r ʧ ʤ ʒ/
Ms	/m n b p t d k g q ʔ f v s ʃ x h j l r ʤ ʧ ʒ/	Ma	/m n b p t d k g q ʔ f v s z ʃ x h j l r ʧ ʤ/
Ni	/m n b p t d k g q ʔ f v s z ʃ x h j l r ʤ ʒ/	Sh	/m n b p t d k g q ʔ f v s z ʃ x h j l r ʧ ʤ ʒ/
El	/m n b p t d k g q ʔ v f s z ʃ x h j l r ʧ ʤ/	Sm	/m n b p t d k g q ʔ f v s z ʃ x h j l r ʧ ʤ/
Al	/m n b p t d k g q ʔ f v s z ʃ x h j l r ʧ ʤ/	Ro	/m n b p t d k g q ʔ f v s z ʃ x h j l r ʧ ʤ ʒ/

Table 10.2 The phonetic inventory of the PD group

Se	/ m n b p t d g k q ʔ f v s z ʃ x h l r j /
Ti	/ m n b p t d g k q ʔ f v z x h l r j ʧ ʤ /
Ze	/ m n b p t d g ʔ f v s z h l r j ʧ ʤ /
Me	/ m n b p t d g k q ʔ f v s z h x l r j ʧ ʤ /
Hi	/ m n b p t d g k q ʔ f v s z ʃ x h l r j ʧ ʤ ʒ /

than regressive assimilation: 41 errors of progressive assimilation versus 21 errors of regressive assimilation. The following examples display regressive and progressive assimilation in TD children acquiring Farsi. Acronyms T.A. and P.A., used below, refer to total assimilation and partial assimilation, respectively.

Example 1

	Clusters	*Target word*	*Child pronunciation*	*Gloss*	*Direction*
T.A.	/mp/ → [pp]	/dæmpai/	[næppaji]	slipper	regressive
	/rq/ → [qq]	/ʤarubærqi/	[ʤarubæqqi]	vacuum cleaner	regressive
	/nd/ → [dd]	/hendune/	[heddune]	watermelon	regressive
	/rt/ → [tt]	/porteqal/	[potteqal]	orange	regressive
	/br/ → [bb]	/ʔæbru/	[næbbu]	eyebrow	progressive
	/st/ → [ss]	/bæstæni/	[bæssæni]	ice cream	progressive
P.A.	/kp/ → [bp]	/lakpoʃt/	[labpoʃ]	turtle	regressive
	/dk/ → [dt]	/badkonæk/	[badtonæk]	balloon	progressive
	/xʧ/ → [xʃ]	/jæxʧal/	[jæxʃal]	refrigerator	progressive
	/sk/ → [st]	/biskujit/	[bistujit]	biscuit	progressive
	/ng/ → [nd]	/?ængoʃt/	[?ændoʃ]	finger	progressive
	/ʃq/ → [dt]	/boʃqab/	[pudtap]	plate	progressive
	/sv/ → [dt]	/mesvak/	[pedtap]	toothbrush	progressive
	/fl/ → [fp]	/qofl/	[qufp]	lock	progressive

Both directions of assimilation are also observed in the PD group; however, the number of instances of regressive assimilation is considerably higher than that of progressive assimilation in this group: 41 regressive assimilation errors versus 17 progressive assimilation errors. Figure 10.1 shows the number of progressive and regressive assimilation errors in the PD and TD groups. The figure is read from left to right, starting with the results on the 10 TD children and continues with the results on the 5 PD children (from younger children to older ones). It is seen that while both progressive and regressive assimilation errors occur in the speech of TD children, in seven out of nine TD children the number of progressive assimilation errors is greater than that of regressive assimilation errors. Moreover, some of the older children in the study show evidence of only progressive assimilation (this is the case for children Sy, Ro and Hi), while one of them (Sh) only makes regressive assimilation errors. For the PD children, the balance between the regressive versus the progressive assimilation errors depends on the severity of the PD; i.e. the more severe the disorder, the more evidence there is of regressive assimilation and less evidence for progressive assimilation.

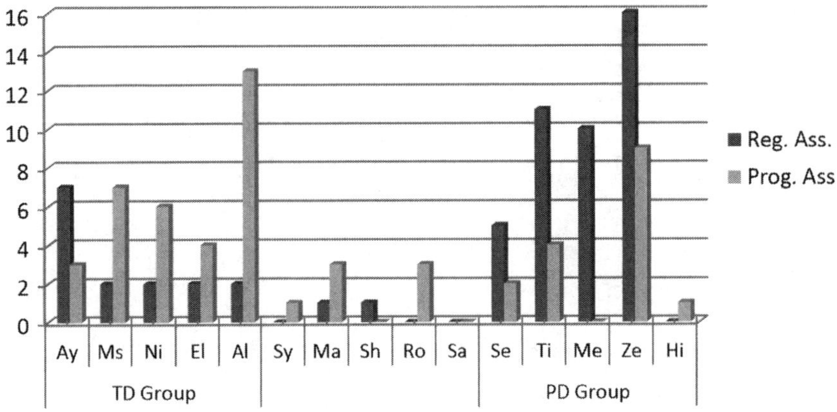

Figure 10.1 Progressive and regressive assimilation errors in the PD and TD groups

Overall, errors of progressive assimilation are more frequent than errors of regressive assimilation in the TD group, while errors of regressive assimilation are more frequent than errors of progressive assimilation in the PD group (Figure 10.2).

Place and manner assimilations are also observed in both the TD and PD groups, although there are both qualitative and quantitative differences between them (see Appendix). Tables 10.3 and 10.4 present the numerical information on the place and manner assimilatory errors found in the groups of the TD and PD children, respectively. Two types of manner assimilation account for most of the errors in the TD group: plosive assimilation and fricative assimilation. There are 12 cases of plosive assimilation (with 44 relevant target words produced by 10 children: 2.7% of tokens) and seven cases of

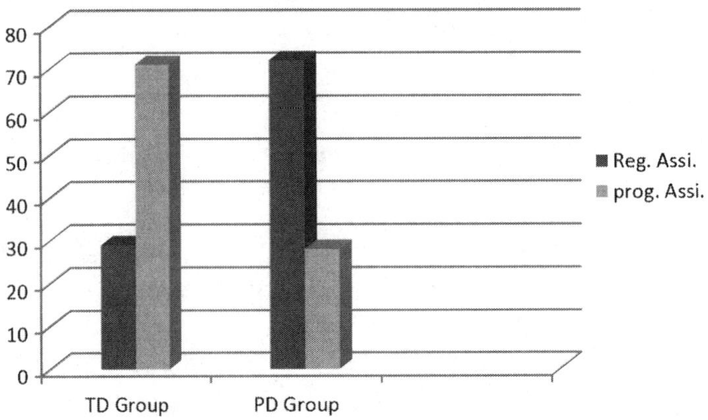

Figure 10.2 Comparing progressive and regressive assimilation in the TD and PD groups

Table 10.3 Numerical information on manner and place assimilation in the TD group

	Potential context	*Ay 2;3*	*Ms 2;4*	*Ni 2;7*	*El 2;11*	*Al 3;3*	*Sy 3;4*	*Ma 3;6*	*Sh 3;6*	*Ro 4*	*Sm 4*
Manner assimilation	59	5	1	4	2	3	–	3	1	1	–
Place assimilation	43	2	7	3	4	13	1	1	–	2	–

fricative assimilation (with 22 relevant words produced by 10 children: 3.2% of tokens). However, in spite of the 23 relevant target words for nasal assimilation, there are no instances of assimilation of nasality in the data. Examples are:

Example 2

(a) Plosive assimilation

	Clusters	*Target word*	*Child pronunciation*	*Gloss*
T.A.	/nd/ → [dd]	/hendune/	[heddune]	watermelon
	/nd/ → [dd]	/sændæli/	[sæddæli]	chair
	/mp/ → [pp]	/dæmpaji/	[næppaji]	slippery
	/nb/ → [bb]	/zænbur/	[sæbbur]	bee
	/br/ → [bb]	/ʔæbru/	[næbbu]	eyebrow
	/rt/ → [tt]	/porteqal/	[potteqal]	orange
	/rq/ → [qq]	/ʤarubærqi/	[ʤarubæqqi]	vacuum cleaner
P.A.	/sk/ → [tk]	/biskujit/	[mitkujid]	biscuit

(b) Fricative assimilation

	Clusters	*Target word*	*Child pronunciation*	*Gloss*
T.A.	/st/ → [ss]	/bæstæni/	[bæssæni]	ice cream
	/sk/ → [ss]	/biskujit/	[bessuji]	biscuit
	/tf/ → [ff]	/tutfærængi/	[tuffærængi]	strawberry
P.A.	/ʃq/ → [xʃ]	/boʃqab/	[boxʃap]	plate
	/xʧ/ → [xʃ]	/jæxʧal/	[jæxʃal]	freezer

Table 10.4 Numerical information on manner and place assimilation in the PD group

	Potential context	*Se 4;5*	*Me 4;8*	*Ze 4;10*	*Ti 4;10*	*Hi 5;6*
Manner assimilation	59	4	11	9	13	–
Place assimilation	43	3	4	1	13	1

It should be noted that all examples in (a) above, and /bæstæni/, /biskujit/, /tutfærængi/ and /boʃqab/ in (b) can also be considered as samples of total assimilation. In /zænbur/, /ʔæbru/, and /ʤarubærqi/ in (a) and /biskujit/ and /tutfærængi/ in (b), the total assimilation involves both manner and place assimilations; therefore, they are taken to be evidence of both types of assimilation.

Two types of place assimilation were observed in the TD children: labial assimilation and coronal assimilation. There are seven cases of labial assimilation (with 24 relevant words: 2.9% of tokens) and 26 cases of coronal assimilation (with 41 relevant words: 6.3% of tokens). However, there are only two cases of dorsal assimilation in the TD children despite the 23 relevant words where dorsal assimilation could occur (0.86% of tokens). The most frequent place assimilation type observed in the TD children in this study is coronal place assimilation; coronal assimilation is about twice as frequent as labial assimilation. Coronals and labials usually trigger assimilation, and dorsals are usually the target of assimilation in these children acquiring Farsi. Examples are:

Example 3

(a) Coronal place assimilation

	Clusters	*Target word*	*Child pronunciation*	*Gloss*
P.A.	/rg/ → [rd]	/xærguʃ/	[xærduʃ]	rabbit
	/ng/ → [nt]	/sæng/	[sænt]	stone
	/ng/ → [nd]	/naxongir/	[naxondir]	nail cut
	/ʃq/ → [sʃ]	/boʃqab/	[bosʃap]	plate
	/dk/ → [dt]	/badkonæk/	[badtonæk]	balloon
	/sk/ → [st]	/susk/	[sust]	cockroach
	/lf/ → [ls]	/telfon/	[telson]	telephone
	/sv/ → [st]	/mesvak/	[mestat]	toothbrush
	/sk/ → [st]	/biskujit/	[bistujit]	biscuit
	/lk/ → [lt]	/dæsmalkaqæsi/	[dæsmaltaqæsi]	tissue
	/dk/ → [dt]	/xodkar/	[xodtar]	pen
T.A.	/rv/ → [rr]	/pærvane/	[pærrame]	butterfly
	/sk/ → [ss]	/biskuit/	[bessuji]	biscuit

(b) Labial place assimilation

	Clusters	*Target word*	*Child pronunciation*	*Gloss*
P.A.	/kp/ → [bp]	/lakpoʃt/	[labpoʃ]	turtle
	/kp/ → [fp]	/lakpoʃt/	[dæfpos]	turtle
T.A.	/nb/ → [bb]	/zænbur/	[sæbbur]	bee
	/br/ → [bb]	/ʔabru/	[ʔabbu]	eyebrow
	/tf/ → [ff]	/tutfærængi/	[tuffærængi]	strawberry

What has been described as coronal place assimilation may arguably be instances of velar fronting (e.g. /badkonæk/ → [badtonæk]). However, it is worth noting that the children producing these assimilated sounds are also able to produce all phonemes that are targeted in the assimilation process in singleton contexts, including singleton /g/ and /k/ in a number of different words. However, in cluster contexts and depending on the adjacent phoneme, the sounds are changed. For example, as displayed in part (a), a child produces /k/ as [t] in /badkonæk/ [badtonæk], where /k/ is adjacent to /d/; however, the same child produces /k/ as [b] in /lakpoʃt/ [labpoʃ], where /k/ is adjacent to /p/. These examples and other similar ones confirm that the change of dorsals to coronals in the Persian children studied here is due to an assimilatory process. Similarly, the greatest amount of manner assimilation evidenced in the PD group involves plosive assimilation: out of 35 manner assimilation errors occurring in four out of five PD children, 32 errors involve plosive assimilation (14.5% of tokens) versus only two involving nasal assimilation (1.7% of tokens), and one involving fricative assimilation (0.9% of tokens). Examples are:

Example 4 Plosive assimilation

	Clusters	*Target word*	*Child pronunciation*	*Gloss*
P.A.	/nk/ → [dʔ]	/ʔænkæbut/	[ʔædʔæput]	spider
	/nd/ → [dt]	/hendune/	[ʔedtune]	watermelon
	/sk/ → [tk]	/biskujit/	[mitkujid]	biscuit
	/mp/ → [bp]	/dæmpaji/	[dæbpaji]	slipper
	/nb/ → [bp]	/zænbur/	[tæbpur]	bee
	/ng/ → [dt]	/ʔængur/	[ʔædtur]	grape
	/ng/ → [dt]	/ʔængoʃt/	[ʔædtot]	finger
	/ng/ → [qg]	/ʔængur/	[ʔæqgur]	grape
	/ng/ → [qg]	/ʔængoʃt/	[ʔæqgot]	finger
	/ng/ → [qk]	/sæng/	[tæqk]	stone
T.A.	/ng/ → [gg]	/tutfærængi/	[dudfæʔæggi]	strawberry
	/nd/ → [dd]	/sændæli/	[tæddæni]	chair
	/nd/ → [tt]	/dændun/	[dættun]	tooth
	/ng/ → [dd]	/naxongir/	[tatoddi]	nailclipper
	/ng/ → [dd]	/ʧængal/	[tæddal]	fork
	/ng/ → [dd]	/tutfærængi/	[dotfæʔæddi]	strawberry
	/nd/ → [dd]	/xæmirdændun/	[qæmidæddun]	toothpaste

The data of the PD group, similarly to those of the TD group, show evidence of both labial and coronal place assimilation. However, the data of the PD group show instances of dorsal assimilation as well. Examples are:

Example 5

(a) Coronal assimilation

	Clusters	*Target word*	*Child pronunciation*	*Gloss*
P.A.	/ng/ → [nd]	/ʔængoʃt/	[ʔændoʃ]	finger
	/sk/ → [zt]	/biskujit/	[biztuji]	biscuit
	/dk/ → [dt]	/badkonæk/	[badtonæk]	balloon
	/ʃq/ → [dt]	/boʃqab/	[pudtap]	plate
	/sv/ → [dt]	/mesvak/	[pedtap]	toothbrush

(b) Labial assimilation

	Clusters	*Target word*	*Child pronunciation*	*Gloss*
P.A.	/kp/ → [bp]	/lakpoʃt/	[dabpot]	turtle
	/nb/ → [bp]	/zænbur/	[tæbpur]	bee
	/fl/ → [fp]	/qofl/	[qufp]	lock
T.A.	/sf/ → [bb]	/gusfænd/	[gubbæt]	sheep
	/sm/ → [bb]	/dæsmalkaqæzi/	[dæbbalkaqædi]	tissue
	/sm/ → [mm]	/dæsmalkaqæzi/	[dæmmaʔaʔædi]	tissue

(c) Dorsal assimilation

	Clusters	*Target word*	*Child pronunciation*	*Gloss*
P.A.	/ng/ → [qg]	/ʔængoʃt/	[ʔæqgot]	finger
	/ng/ → [qg]	/ʔængur/	[ʔæqgur]	grape
	/dk/ → [qk]	/xodkar/	[qoqkal]	pen
	/ng/ → [qk]	/sæng/	[tæqk]	stone
T.A.	/ng/ → [gg]	/tutfærængi/	[dudfæʔæggi]	strawberry

There are eight cases of coronal assimilation (3.9% of tokens) and eight cases of labial assimilation (6.7% of tokens) in the PD children, plus six cases of dorsal assimilation (5.2% of tokens). Notably, while out of 23 relevant words for dorsal assimilation only seven of them include nasal-dorsal plosive clusters, five out of six dorsal assimilation errors occur in nasal-plosive clusters (assimilation in 14.3% of tokens). These results indicate the strong tendency for dorsal assimilation in nasal-plosive clusters in the PD children. In this group, considering the potential contexts for each type of assimilation, labial and dorsal assimilation is more frequent than coronal assimilation.

Discussion

In the following discussion, first the results on the direction of assimilation in the data of the TD and PD groups are considered, and then manner and place assimilations are discussed. Since the two groups indicate differences in place and manner assimilations between the clusters with or without nasal segments, the assimilation data from this study are discussed first in non-nasal segments and then in nasal segments.

Direction of assimilation

As argued in the results section, both directions of assimilation, i.e. progressive and regressive, are observed in the typical and atypical developing children in the study. Nevertheless, with the exception of the youngest child in the group of the TD children, progressive assimilation is much more frequent than regressive assimilation. The opposite holds for the group of PD children. Notably, partial assimilations are mostly progressive whereas total assimilations are mostly regressive in both groups (see Appendix). These findings contradict the results in previous studies (e.g. Ito, 1986, 1989; Jun, 2004; Ohala, 1990; Padgett, 1995; Selkirk, 1994), where it is predicted that the direction of place assimilation in adjacent clusters is typically regressive. Theoretical explanations view the phenomenon in terms of positional faithfulness (Beckman, 1998; Lombardi, 1999; Padgett, 1995; Selkirk, 1994), coda condition (Beckman, 2004; Ito, 1986, 1989), or perceptual cues (Jun, 1995, 2004; Kohler, 1990; Ohala, 1990). In addition, the findings of this study are different from the findings of some other studies on child language which maintain that the dominant direction observed in local assimilation is regressive (e.g. Cho & Lee, 2014; Martinez & Diez-Itza, 2012).

The results of this study indicate that regressive assimilation is not necessarily the dominant direction of the assimilatory process. It is argued that assimilation depends on a number of factors, such as the language targeted, the stage at which the children are in their phonological development, and whether the children are typically or atypically developing. The difference in the direction of assimilation observed between the TD group and the PD group (i.e. more instances of regressive assimilation in the PD children and the reverse for the TD children) may imply that there is a specific relationship between the direction of assimilation and the acquisition level in these children acquiring Farsi, i.e. the earlier they are in their phonological development, the more regressive assimilation there is, and vice versa. It seems that the direction of assimilation is also affected by the phonological context of the trigger segment within a cluster. For instance, labials can trigger both progressive and regressive assimilation depending on the phonological context in clusters (see Appendix). This recalls the feature-based directionality mentioned by Bernhardt and Stemberger

(1998). The majority of instances of regressive assimilation in the TD and PD children studied here involve nasal-plosive clusters, to be discussed in a later section.

Assimilation in the clusters without nasals in the TD and PD groups

In clusters without nasals, assimilation was detected in both place and manner features in the TD and PD groups.

Place assimilation

As the results of this study have indicated (Example 3), the most frequent place assimilation type observed in the TD children is the dorsal to coronal or labial assimilation, i.e. dorsals are likely to be the target of place assimilation rather than its trigger. This pattern also holds for the PD children targeting clusters without nasals, i.e. dorsals generally assimilate to coronals or labials in the assimilation process. However, these findings are different from the findings of Cho and Lee (2014) who studied Korean-speaking children. They maintained that consonants, irrespective of their place of articulation, can be both targets and triggers of local assimilation.

Assimilation of dorsal place to coronal place in developing phonologies in Farsi cannot be explained based on Jun's (1995, 2004) hypothesis that coronals are vulnerable to assimilate to non-coronals because of place cues being better perceived in dorsals and labials rather than in coronals. Also, the place of dorsal segments in abutting clusters cannot account for the assimilation patterns; dorsals, either in onset or coda position, assimilate to their labial or coronal neighbour. Similarly, word stress seems to be irrelevant in these assimilation patterns. In Farsi, word stress is a predictable feature; stress usually falls in the last syllable in nouns. Again, the assimilation pattern does not show any difference in stressed syllables versus non-stressed syllables. The only criterion that may be able to explain the assimilation errors in Persian children is markedness criteria. In the majority of place assimilation errors occurring in this study, a marked place of articulation (dorsal) is assimilated to an unmarked place of articulation (coronal or labial). This result matches the OT's prediction that in child language the constraints which need outputs to be unmarked in structure dominate the constraints that need output to be marked. The OT constraints inferred from the input and output forms in these assimilation errors are AGREE(place), FAITH[COR], FAITH[LAB] and FAITH[DOR] which are defined below:

FAITH[X]: An Input segments specifications of feature X must be preserved in its Output correspondent
Where X ϵ {CORONAL, DORSAL, LABIAL) (Pater & Werle, 2003)
AGREE(place): Obstruent clusters should agree in place (Kager, 1999)

The assimilation outputs propose the following ranking in these constraints:

FAITH[COR], FAITH[LAB] >> FAITH[DOR]

This analysis is illustrated in Tableau 10.1, which ranks AGREE(place) and FAITH[COR] and FAITH[LAB] higher than FAITH[DOR].

As Tableau 10.1 illustrates, candidates a. and d. fatally violate the highest ranked constraint AGREE(place), and candidates b. and e. violate the higher ranked constraints FAITH[LAB] and FAITH[COR], respectively. However, candidates c. and f., in which dorsals are assimilated to the less marked labial and coronal place of articulation, violate the lowest ranked constraint FAITH[DOR]. Therefore, they are the optimal output in the production of the children acquiring Farsi in this study.

Manner assimilation

Another type of assimilation observed in clusters without nasals is manner assimilation to plosives and fricatives (see Examples 2 and 4). As results show for the PD group (see Example 4), liquids and fricatives (the more marked segments) assimilate to plosives (the less marked segments). In the TD group, liquids (the more marked segments) assimilate to plosives (the less marked segments) (see Example 2(a)); however, plosives (the less marked segments) generally assimilate to fricatives (the more marked segments) (see Example 2(b)). The difference in the assimilation patterns between the PD and TD children can be explained considering the articulatory and perceptual features of fricatives. On the one hand, fricatives are more difficult to articulate than plosives; the production of fricatives needs finer grained coordination of articulators compared to that for plosives which are produced by

Tableau 10.1 Place assimilation in consonant clusters without nasals in the TD and PD groups

Input: /lakpoʃt/	AGREE(place)	FAITH[LAB]	FAITH[DOR]
a. [lakpoʃt]	*!		
b. [lakgoʃt]		*!	
c. ☞ [labpoʃ]			*
Input: /badkonæk/	AGREE(place)	FAITH[COR]	FAITH[DOR]
d. [badkonæk]	*!		
e. [bagkonæk]		*!	
f. ☞ [badtonæk]			*

complete closure and open cycles. On the other hand, the perceptual cues of fricatives are more prominent than those of plosives (Jun, 2004; Wright, 2004). Therefore, PD children, who usually have articulation problems, have a tendency to produce the articulatorily easier segments in a cluster. This finding is similar to the finding of Kirk (2008), who investigated assimilation in TD young children. Nevertheless, the TD children, with few or no articulatory problems, tend towards the production of more perceptually prominent segments. As explained before within the OT perspective, children's errors involve a mismatch between output and input which is the result of the violation of some faithfulness constraint. The constraint violated by assimilation is FAITH[X] which requires a full realization of all input features in the output. The formal statement of this constraint is given below:

FAITH[X]: An Input segments specifications of feature X must be preserved in its Output correspondent
Where X ϵ {PLOSIVE, FRICATIVE, NASAL) (Pater & Werle, 2003)

The violation of FAITH[X] is forced by its being ranked beneath AGREE(manner) which requires clusters to agree in manner.

AGREE(manner): Obstruent clusters should agree in manner (Kager, 1999)

Moreover, the different outputs observed between the PD and TD children (plosive assimilation versus fricative assimilation) assumes the presence of two different FAITH[X] constraints in the assimilation patterns, i.e. FAITH[PLO] which requires plosives in clusters to be maintained, and FAITH[FRI] which requires fricatives to be preserved. The featural differences between plosives and fricatives, and the different tendencies observed in PD and TD children lead to difference in the ranking of FAITH[PLO] and FAITH[FRI] between PD and TD children and, accordingly, lead to different outputs. Tableaux 10.2 and 10.3 illustrate how the different rankings of the constraints lead to different assimilation patterns.

As illustrated in Tableaux 10.2 and 10.3, the high ranking of AGREE(manner) leads to assimilation in the clusters. Moreover, though the same constraints

Tableau 10.2 Assimilation of fricatives to plosives in the PD and TD groups

Input: /biskujit/	AGREE(manner)	FAITH[PLO]	FAITH[FRI]
a. [biskujit]	*!		
b. ☞ [mitkujid]			*
c. [besxuji]		*!	

Tableau 10.3 Assimilation of plosives to fricatives in the TD children

Input: /boʃqab/	AGREE(manner)	FAITH[FRI]	FAITH[PLO]
a. [boʃqab]	*!		
b. [botqab]		*!	
c. ☞ [boxʃap]			*

are applied in the PD and TD children's grammar, the difference in their ranking results in different assimilation patterns (e.g. /sk/ → [st] versus /ʃq/ → [xʃ]).

Assimilation in the clusters with a nasal segment in the TD and PD groups

When nasals are involved in clusters with the adjacent segment differing in terms of manner or place of articulation, they show different assimilation patterns. In such environments, nasals may trigger assimilation (Examples 3(a), 5(a) and 5(b)). In these assimilation errors, the place or manner features in the nasal consonants are generally less marked than those of the adjacent consonant in the cluster; consequently, the nasal triggers assimilation in the adjacent consonant. OT analyzes these assimilation patterns through the related AGREE and FAITH constraints. For example, regarding place assimilation, it is maintained that in such cases markedness constraints, AGREE(place) and FAITH[COR], outrank the faithfulness constraint FAITH[DOR], which is what typically happens to the children participating in this study (as illustrated in Tableau 10.4).

While there are a few examples in which nasals trigger assimilation in this study, there are many cases in which nasals are the target of place and/or manner assimilation. This type of assimilation is observed mostly in the

Tableau 10.4 Place assimilation in coronal nasal-dorsal plosive in the TD and PD groups

Input: /ʔængoʃt/	AGREE(place)	FAITH[COR]	FAITH[DOR]
a. [ʔængoʃt]	*!		
b. ☞ [ʔændoʃ]			*
c. [ʔæggoʃ]		*!	

PD children (Examples 4 and 5(c)). The assimilation of the nasal to the manner of articulation of the plosive, observed in the present study, can be explained taking into consideration articulatory properties specific to nasals. As earlier work has shown (Ladefoged, 2001; Samare, 1999; Winters, 2002), the articulatory mechanics involved in the production of nasals are more complex than those needed for the articulation of plosives. As a result, nasals are usually acquired after the corresponding plosives and they are assumed to be more marked than plosives. The relative markedness of nasals when compared to plosives is also observed in the data of the PD children in this study; /m/ is absent from the phonetic inventories of three out of five PD children, and /n/ is absent from the phonetic inventories of two out of five PD children. The corresponding plosives, on the other hand, are present in all these children's phonetic inventories. Therefore, what motivates plosive assimilation in nasal-plosive clusters seems to be ease of articulation (e.g. Locke, 1983; MacNeilage & Davis, 1990; Smit, 1993). That is, the articulatory markedness of nasals relative to plosives results in the assimilation of nasals to plosives in the PD and younger TD children. Tableau 10.5 illustrates the constraint ranking inferred from the assimilation data in this study.

As illustrated by Tableau 10.5, Candidate a. fatally violates the higher ranked constraint AGREE (manner) and Candidate c. fatally violates FAITH[PLO]. Candidate b., however, only shows the violation of the lower ranked constraint, FAITH[NAS]. Consequently, Candidate b. is optimal output.

Another case of assimilation is evidenced in the data whereby the coronal nasal in a nasal-plosive cluster assimilates to the place and manner of articulation of the dorsal plosive, resulting in a total assimilation error (e.g. /-ng/ → [gg] in /tutfærængi/ → [dudfæʔæggi]). The assimilation of coronal place to dorsal place is uncommon in TD children, though it is evidenced in the PD children (see Examples 4 and 5(c)). Total assimilation is well known in the literature on phonological acquisition (e.g. Bernhardt & Stemberger, 1998; Vihman & Majorano, 2016) and is explained by the enactment of two processes: deletion and gemination or elongation. The nasal segment in a nasal-plosive cluster is deleted because it is more difficult to produce than the plosive, and the following plosive segment undergoes compensatory lengthening. Although the articulatory markedness of

Tableau 10.5 Manner assimilation in nasal-plosive clusters in the PD and younger TD children

Input: /ʔængur/	AGREE(manner)	FAITH[PLO]	FAITH[NAS]
a. [ʔængul]	*!		
b. ☞ [ʔædkul]			*
c. [ʔænnul]		*!	

nasals, when compared to plosives, is able to explain the tendency of nasals to assimilate to the manner of articulation of plosives in nasal-plosive clusters, it cannot explain the assimilation of the coronal place in nasal to the dorsal place of plosive in these clusters. If, on an articulatory basis, it is plausible that nasals assimilate to plosives in a nasal-plosive cluster, on the same articulatory basis it is not plausible that coronals assimilate to dorsals. It is noted that coronal place of articulation is the unmarked default, thus easier to produce. Lastly, another question that remains is why coronal nasals assimilate to the marked dorsal place in coronal nasal-dorsal plosive clusters in the PD children acquiring Farsi, when it could be produced as the geminated form [dd], which would be less marked, and is found in TD phonologies.

Some scholars have explained this assimilation process with reference to the perceptual cues of the segments in clusters (e.g. Jun, 1995, 2004; Kohler, 1990; Ohala, 1990; Padgett, 1995; Steriade, 2000). Jun (1995, 2004) argued that the place cues for nasals, especially in the first member position in clusters, is weaker than those of plosives, because nasals lack a burst. Jun's assumption implies that it is difficult to perceive the place cues of coronal nasal in nasal-plosive clusters, especially by children in atypical phonological development who generally face more difficulty than TD ones, in terms of both the perception and production of speech. This difference in the perception of coronal place of nasals versus the dorsal place of plosives can lead to the assimilation of coronal place of the nasal to dorsal place of the plosive resulting in the geminated form [gg], rather than [dd].

An OT analysis of this assimilation pattern further explains the preference for [gg] over [dd] in the PD children's productions. Tableau 10.6 displays the constraints participating in this process and their hierarchy. The constraints involved are given below:

*Cnasal: no nasal/nasalized consonants (Campos-Astorkiza, 2003)
MAX-IO Every segment of the input has a correspondent in the output (Kager, 1999)
*LONG-C: no long consonants (Holt, 1997)
IDENT-IO: Correspondents in input and output have identical values for feature (McCarthy & Prince, 1995)

Candidates a. and c. fatally violate *Cnasal constraint, while candidate d. exhibits two violations of IDENT-IO as well as a violation of *LONG-C. Therefore, Candidate b., which only violates the lowest constraint IDENT-IO, is the optimal output. According to Prince and Smolensky (1993), faithfulness constraints aim to preserve distinctions among different lexical items, while markedness constraints are designed to confine structural complexity and decrease the probable contrasts between words. Accordingly, Boersma (1998) stated that faithfulness constraints assess the similarity between

Tableau 10.6 Place assimilation in coronal nasal-dorsal plosive in the PD children

Input: /tutfæræ ngi/	*Cnasal	MAX-IO	*LONG-C	IDENT-IO
a. [dudfæʔængi]	*!			
b. ☞ [dudfæʔæggi]			*	*
c. [dudfæʔnni]	**!		*	*
d. [dudfæʔæddi]			*	**

perceptual input specification and perceptual output representation. Therefore, the lesser violation of the faithfulness constraint IDENT-IO in b. means more similarity between the perceptual output representation and perceptual input specifications. Thus, the assimilation of nasals to both the manner and place of articulation of dorsal plosives (as evidenced in many nasal clusters in the PD group) minimizes the articulatory effort and maximizes the perceptual adequacy, which is the ideal condition for the less phonologically developed children. From this analysis, it is concluded that both articulatory and perceptual adequacy are the motives of the assimilation patterns observed in the PD children. However, the TD children's productions (i.e. [dd] versus [gg] for coronal nasal-dorsal plosive clusters) are motivated mainly by articulatory adequacy.

Conclusion

The present study examined local assimilation in children with typical and atypical phonological development, acquiring Farsi and found differences in the data of the children studied here and the results of studies available in some other languages. The findings suggest that, in the TD children acquiring Farsi, coronals and labials (less marked segments) are usually the trigger of place assimilation, while dorsals (more marked segments) are the target of place assimilation. These findings match the results of Kirk (2008). Nevertheless, the results are different from the findings of Cho and Lee (2014), who argued that consonants can be both targets and triggers of local assimilation, irrespective of their place of articulation. In addition, the data of the TD children in this study, unlike children speaking languages like Korean and Spanish, show evidence of more progressive assimilation rather than regressive assimilation. Based on this, it is suggested that the direction of assimilation and its triggers and targets can vary from language to language in TD phonologies.

The assimilation patterns in the PD group exhibit some differences from the assimilation patterns in the TD group, i.e. the PD children have demonstrated instances of dorsal assimilation, which is not common, by and large, in TD children. Also, the PD children in the study, contrary to the TD children, show evidence of more regressive assimilation than progressive assimilation. Interestingly, the direction of assimilation in the PD group notably shows similarities with the assimilation patterns observed in TD children acquiring Korean and Spanish. Accordingly, these findings lead to the assumption that different assimilation patterns are available to child speakers of different languages. A decision on which particular pattern is selected may rely on which specific language is targeted and whether typical or atypical development is involved.

Moreover, the differences observed in the assimilation patterns of fricative-plosive and nasal-plosive clusters in the two groups can imply that the assimilatory productions in the TD children are motivated by both perceptual and articulatory factors while, in children with PD, these productions are mainly stimulated by articulatory factors. Furthermore, this study illustrates that differences in the assimilation patterns between the PD and TD children can sometimes originate from differences in constraint hierarchies in children's internal grammar. Such a conclusion is supported by the assertion in OT that diversities in different linguistic productions originate from differences in the relative ranking of markedness and faithfulness constraints in the developing grammars of children.

It is emphasized that this study aims to primarily contribute to the collection of phonological developmental data across languages in typically and atypically developing populations. The analysis of the data at hand does not seek to oppose the standing of findings in earlier studies. The extent to which conclusions here hold to be universally true with regard to the acquisition of Farsi as a first language needs to be corroborated by future studies on many more children, also taking into consideration differences in typical and atypical acquisition.

References

Adams, C., Byers Brown, B. and Edwards, M. (1997) Developmental disorders of language. London: Whurr.

Akpan, E.E. (2006) Assimilatory processes in Ibibio child phonology. In O.F. Arasanyin and M.A. Pemberton (eds) *Selected Proceedings of the 36th Annual Conference on African Linguistics* (pp. 27–36). Somerville, MA: Cascadilla Proceedings Project.

Barlow, J.A. (2001) Optimality theory and the assessment and treatment of phonological disorders. *Speech, Language, and Hearing Services in Schools* 32, 242–256.

Barlow, J.A. and Gierut, J. (1999) Optimality theory in phonological acquisition. *Journal of Speech, Language, and Hearing Research* 42, 1482–1498.

Beckman, J.N. (1998) Positional faithfulness: An optimality theoretic treatment of phonological asymmetries. PhD dissertation, University of Massachusetts-Amherst.

Beckman, J.N. (2004) Positional faithfulness. In J.J. McCarthy (ed.) *Optimality Theory in Phonology* (pp. 310–343). Malden, MA: Blackwell.

Bernhardt, B. and Stemberger, J. (1998) *Handbook of Phonological Development from the Perspective of Constraint-based Nonlinear Phonology*. San Diego, CA: Academic Press.

Bernhardt, B. and Stemberger, J. (2000) *Workbook in Nonlinear Phonology for Clinical Application*. Austin, TX: PRO-ED.

Boersma, P. (1998) Functional phonology: Formalizing the interaction between articulatory and perceptual drives. PhD dissertation, University of Amsterdam.

Campos-Astorkiza, R. (2003) Compensatory lengthening as root number preservation: Codas in Eastern Andalusian Spanish. In E. Hajicova, A. Kotesovcova and J. Miorvosky (eds) *Proceedings of the Seventeenth International Congress of Linguistics, Prague, 24–29 July* (pp. 1–11). CD-ROM. Prague: Matfyzpress & MFF UK.

Cho, M.-H. and Lee, S. (2014) Targets, triggers, and directionality in non-local and local place assimilation in child and adult language. *Poznan Studies in Contemporary Linguistics* 50 (3), 273–307.

Cho, Y.-M.Y. (1990) Parameters of consonantal assimilation. PhD dissertation, Stanford University.

Dinnsen, D.A. and O'Connor, K.M. (2001a) Implicationally related error patterns and the selection of treatment targets. *Language, Speech, and Hearing Services in Schools* 32, 257–270.

Dinnsen, D.A. and O'Connor, K.M. (2001b) Typological predictions in developmental phonology. *Journal of Child Language* 28, 597–628.

Dvorak, V. (2010) Voicing assimilation in Czech. In P.D. Staroverov, A. Altshuler, C. Braver, A. Fasola and S. Murray (eds) *Rutgers Working Papers in Linguistics, Vol. 3* (pp. 115–144). New Brunswick, NJ: LGSA, Rutgers University.

Gierut, J.A. and Morrisette, M.L. (2005) The clinical significance of optimality theory for phonological disorders. *Topics in Language Disorders* 25 (3), 266–280.

Gilbert, D. (2001) Conflicting phonologically based and phonetically based constraints in the analysis of liquid-nasal substitutions. *Clinical Linguistics & Phonetics* 15 (1/2), 23–28.

Holt, E.D. (1997) The role of the listener in the historical phonology of Spanish and Portuguese: An optimality theoretic account. PhD dissertation, Georgetown University.

Hura, S., Lindblom, B. and Diehl, R. (1992) On the role of perception in shaping phonological assimilation rules. *Language and Speech* 35, 59–72.

Ito, J. (1986) Syllable theory in prosodic phonology. PhD dissertation, University of Massachusetts-Amherst.

Ito, J. (1989) A prosodic theory of epenthesis. *Natural Language and Linguistic Theory* 7, 217–259.

Jesney, K. (2007) Child chain shifts as faithfulness to input prominence. In B. Alyona, M. Luisa and U. Mari (eds) *Proceedings of the 2nd Conference on Generative Approaches to Language Acquisition North America (GALANA)* (pp. 188–199). Somerville, MA: Cascadilla Proceedings Project.

Jun, J. (1995) Perceptual and articulatory factors in place assimilation: An optimality theoretic approach. PhD thesis, University of California, Los Angeles.

Jun, J. (2002) Positional faithfulness, sympathy, and inferred input. Unpublished manuscript, Yeungnam University. See http://ling.snu. ac. kr/jun/ work/inferred. pdf.

Jun, J. (2004) Place assimilation. In B. Hayes, R. Kirchner and D. Steriade (eds) *Phonetically Based Phonology*. Cambridge: Cambridge University Press.

Kager, R. (1999) *Optimality Theory*. Cambridge: Cambridge University Press.

Katamba, F. (1991) *An Introduction to Phonology*. Harlow: Longman.

Kirk, C. (2008) Substitution errors in the production of word-initial and word-final consonant clusters. *Journal of Speech, Language, and Hearing Research* 51, 35–48.

Kohler, K. (1990) Segmental reduction in connected speech in German: Phonological facts and phonetic explanations. In W.J. Hardcastle and A. Marchal (eds) *Speech Production and Speech Modelling* (pp. 69–92). Dordrecht: Kluwer.

Ladefoged, P. (2001) *Vowels and Consonants: An Introduction to the Sounds of Languages*. Malden, MA: Blackwell.

Lass, R. (1984) *Phonology: An Introduction to Basic Concepts*. Cambridge: Cambridge University Press.

Locke, J.L. (1983) *Phonological Acquisition and Change*. New York: Academic Press.

Lombardi, L. (1999) Positional faithfulness and voicing assimilation in optimality theory. *Natural Language and Linguistic Theory* 17 (2), 267–320.

Lombardi, L. (2004) Positional faithfulness and voicing assimilation in optimality theory. In J.J. McCarthy (ed.) *Optimality Theory in Phonology* (pp. 343–365). Malden, MA: Blackwell.

MacNeilage, P.F. and Davis B.L. (1990) Acquisition of speech production: Achievement of segmental independence. In W.I. Hardcastle and A. Marchal (eds) *Speech Production and Speech Modeling* (pp. 55–68). Dordrecht: Kluwer.

Martínez, V. and Diez-Itza, E. (2012) Assimilation processes in the late stages of phonological development. *Psicothema* 24 (2), 193–198.

McCarthy, J.J. and Prince, A.S. (1993a) Generalized alignment. In G.E. Booij and J. van Marle (eds) *Yearbook of Morphology 1993* (pp. 79–153). Dordrecht: Kluwer.

McCarthy, J.J. and Prince, A.S. (1993b) Prosodic morphology I: Constraint interaction and satisfaction. Linguistics Department Faculty Publication Series 14. University of Massachusetts-Amherst.

McCarthy, J.J. and Prince, A.S. (1995) Faithfulness and reduplicative identity. In J. Beckman, L. Walsh Dickey & S. Urbanczyk (eds) *Papers in Optimality Theory. University of Massachusetts Occasional Papers* 18. Amherst, MA.: Graduate Linguistic Student Association. pp. 249–384. [Rutgers Optimality Archive 60, http://roa.rutgers.edu]

Miccio, A.W. and Scarpino, S.E. (2008) Phonological analysis, phonological processes. In M.J. Ball, M.R. Perkins, N. Muller and S. Howard (eds) *The Handbook of Clinical Linguistics* (pp. 412–422). Oxford: Wiley-Blackwell.

Ohala, J.J. (1990) The phonetics and phonology of aspects of assimilation [And: A response to Pierrehumbert's commentary]. In J. Kingston and M. Beckman (eds) *Papers in Laboratory Phonology I: Between the Grammar and the Physics of Speech*. Cambridge: Cambridge University Press.

Padgett, J. (1995) Partial class behaviour and nasal place assimilation. In K. Suzuki and D. Elzinga (eds) *Proceedings of the South Western Optimality Theory Workshop 1995* (pp. 145–183). Tuscon, AZ: University of Arizona Coyote Papers.

Pater, J. (2002) Form and substance in phonological development. In L. Mikkelsen and C. Potts (eds) *WCCFL 21 Proceedings* (pp. 348–372). Somerville, MA: Cascadilla Press.

Pater, J. and Werle, A. (2003) Direction of assimilation in child consonant harmony. *Canadian Journal of Linguistics* 48 (3), 385–408.

Prince, A. and Smolensky, P. (1993) *Optimality Theory: Constraint Interaction in Generative Grammar*. Oxford: Blackwell.

Rose, S. and Walker, R. (2004) A typology of consonant agreement as correspondence. *Language* 80, 475–531.

Samare, Y. (1999) *The Phonetics of the Farsi Language*. Tehran: Markaze Nashre Daneshgahi.

Selkirk, E.O. (1994) Optimality theory and featural phenomena. Lecture notes, *Linguistics 730*, University of Massachusetts-Amherst.

Smit, A. (1993) Phonologic error distributions in the Iowa–Nebraska Articulation Norms Project: Word-initial consonant clusters. *Journal of Speech and Hearing Research* 36, 931–947.

Steriade, D. (2000) The phonology of perceptibility effects: The P-map and its consequences for constraint organization. Unpublished manuscript, University of California, Los Angeles.

Stoel-Gammon, C. and Dunn, C. (1985) *Normal and Disordered Phonology in Children*. Baltimore, MD: University Park Press.

Szreder, M. (2011) The acquisition of consonant clusters in Polish: A case study. *York Papers in Linguistics Series* 2, 88–102.

Ueda, I. and Davis, S. (2001) The acquisition of Japanese 'r'. *Gengo Kenkyu* 119, 111–138.

Vihman, M. and Majorano, M. (2016) The role of geminates in infants' early word production and word form recognition. *Journal of Child Language* 15, 1–27; doi:10.1017/S0305000915000793.

Winters, S. (2000) Turning phonology inside out, or testing the relative salience of audio and visual cues for place of articulation. In A. Miller-Ockhuizen, R. Levine and A.J. Gonsalves (eds) *Ohio State University Working Papers in Linguistics* 53, 168–199.

Winters, S. (2001) VCCV perception: Putting place in its place. *Ohio State Working Papers in Linguistics* 55, 70–87.

Winters, S. (2002) Perceptual influences on place assimilation: A case study. Unpublished manuscript, Ohio State University.

Wright, R.A. (2004) A review of perceptual cues and cue robustness. In D. Steriade, R. Kirchner and B. Hayes (eds) *Phonetically Based Phonology* (pp. 34–57). Cambridge: Cambridge University Press.

Appendix: List of Place and Manner Assimilation Errors for the TD and PD Groups

TD	*Assimilation*	*Gloss*	*Target word*	*Child pronunciation*	*Direction*
Ay	Place	telephone	/telfon/	[telson]	progressive
		turtle	/lakpoʃt/	[labpos]	regressive
		fork	/ʧængal/	[ʧæggal]	regressive
		bee	/zænbur/	[sæbbur]	regressive
		eyebrow	/ʔabru/	[ʔabbu]	progressive
	Manner	watermelon	/hendune/	[heddune]	regressive
		fork	/ʧængal/	[ʧæggal]	regressive
		chair	/sændæli/	[sæddæli]	regressive
		bee	/sænbur/	[sæbbur]	regressive
		eyebrow	/ʔabru/	[ʔabbu]	progressive
Ms	Place	balloon	/badkonæk/	[badtonæt]	progressive
		biscuit	/biskujit/	[bistujit]	progressive
		beetle	/susk/	[sust]	progressive
		tissue	/dæsmalkaqæzi/	[dæsmaltaqæsi]	progressive
		rabbit	/xærguʃ/	[xærdus]	progressive
		pen	/xodkar/	[xodtar]	progressive
		park	/park/	[part]	progressive
		vacuum cleaner	/ʤarubærqi/	[ʤarubæqqi]	regressive
	Manner	vacuum cleaner	/ʤarubærqi/	[ʤarubæqqi]	regressive
Ni		Place	/boʃqab/	[bosʃap]	progressive
		plate	/xodkar/	[xodtar]	progressive
		pen	/biskujit/	[bessuji]	progressive
		biscuit	/ʤarubærqi/	[ʤarubæqqi]	regressive
		vacuum cleaner			
	Manner	plate	/boʃqab/	[boxʃap]	progressive
		ice	/bæstæni/	[bæssæni]	progressive
		cream	/biskujit/	[bessuji]	progressive
		biscuit	/ʤarubærqi/	[ʤarubæqqi]	regressive
		vacuum cleaner			
El	Place	balloon	/bædkonæk/	[nædtonæk]	progressive
		turtle	/lækpoʃt/	[dæbpos]	regressive
		eyebrow	/ʔæbru/	[næbbu]	progressive
		finger	/ʔængoʃt/	[dæstos]	progressive
	Manner	eyebrow	/ʔæbru/	[næbbu]	progressive
		slipper	/dæmpaji/	[dæppaji]	regressive

(*Continued*)

TD	*Assimilation*	*Gloss*	*Target word*	*Child pronunciation*	*Direction*
Al	Place	biscuit	/biskujit/	[bistujit]	progressive
		balloon	/badkonæk/	[badtonæk]	progressive
		pen	/xodkar/	[xodtar]	progressive
		rabbit	/xærguʃ/	[xærduʃ]	progressive
		nailclipper	/naxongir/	[naxondir]	progressive
		stone	/sæng/	[ʃænt]	progressive
		beetle	/susk/	[ʃuʃt]	progressive
		turtle	/lakpoʃt/	[labpoʃ]	regressive
		washing	/maʃinlebasʃuji/	[maʃinleʔassuji]	progressive
		machine	/susk/	[sust]	progressive
		beetle	/ʔæbru/	[ʔæbbu]	progressive
		eyebrow	/mesvak/	[mestat]	progressive
		toothbrush			
	Manner	refrigerator	/jæxtʃal/	[jæxʃal]	progressive
		watermelon	/hendune/	[heddune]	regressive
		eyebrow	/ʔæbru/	[ʔæbbu]	progressive
Sy	Place	stone	/sæng/	[sænt]	progressive
	Manner		–	–	
Ma	Place	stone	/sæng/	[sæntʃ]	progressive
	Manner	ice	/bæstæni/	[bæssæni]	progressive
		cream	/boʃqab/	[boxʃap]	progressive
		plate	/porteqal/	[potteqal]	regressive
		orange			
Sh	Place		–	–	
	Manner	strawberry	/tutfærængi/	[tuffærængi]	regressive
Ro	Place	beetle	/susk/	[ʃuʃʃt]	progressive
		butterfly	/pærvane/	[pærrame]	progressive
	Manner	butterfly	/pærvane/	[pærrame]	progressive

PD	*Assimilation*	*Gloss*	*Target word*	*Child pronunciation*	*Direction*
Se	Place	finger	/ʔængoʃt/	[ʔændoʃ]	progressive
		tissue	/dæsmalkaqæzi/	[dæmmaʔaʔædi]	regressive
		strawberry	/tutfærængi/	[dudfæʔæggi]	regressive
	Manner	plate	/boʃqab/	[ʔoʃxar]	progressive
		biscuit	/biskujit/	[mitkujid]	regressive
		tissue	/dæsmalkaqæzi/	[dæmmaʔaʔædi]	regressive
		strawberry	/tutfærængi/	[dudfæʔæggi]	regressive
Me	Place	turtle	/lakpoʃt/	[dabpot]	regressive
		bee	/zænbur/	[tæbpur]	regressive
		finger	/ʔængoʃt/	[ʔænnot]	progressive

(*Continued*)

PD	*Assimilation*	*Gloss*	*Target word*	*Child pronunciation*	*Direction*
	Manner	slipper	/dæmpaji/	[dæbpaji]	regressive
		strawberry	/tutfærængi/	[dotfæʔæddi]	regressive
		finger	/ʔængoʃt/	[ʔænnot]	progressive
		bee	/zænbur/	[tæbpur]	regressive
		watermelon	/hendune/	[ʔeddune]	regressive
		tooth	/dændun/	[dættun]	regressive
		nailclipper	/naxongir/	[tatoddi]	regressive
		fork	/ʧængal/	[tæddal]	regressive
		grape	/ʔængur/	[ʔædtur]	progressive
Ze	Place	turtle	/lakpuʃt/	[gabpuʃt]	regressive
	Manner	spider	/ʔænkæbut/	[ʔædʔæput]	regressive
		toothpaste	/xæmirdændun/	[hæmitædtun]	regressive
		finger	/ʔængoʃt/	[ʔædtot]	regressive
		bee	/zænbur/	[dæbpoj]	regressive
		fork	/ʧængal/	[dædtan]	regressive
		chair	/sændæli/	[tæddæni]	regressive
		tooth	/dændun/	[dædtu]	regressive
		grape	/ʔængur/	[ʔædtor]	regressive
		slipper	/dæmpaji/	[dæbbaji]	regressive
Ti	Place	turtle	/lakpoʃt/	[dabpot]	regressive
		fork	/ʧængal/	[dæqqal]	regressive
		lock	/qofl/	[qufp]	progressive
		biscuit	/biskujit/	[biztuji]	progressive
		finger	/ʔængoʃt/	[ʔæqgot]	regressive
		grape	/ʔængur/	[ʔæqgur]	regressive
		pen	/xodkar/	[qoqkal]	regressive
		balloon	/badkonæk/	[badtonæk]	progressive
		plate	/boʃqab/	[pudtap]	progressive
		stone	/sæng/	[tæqk]	regressive
		sheep	/gusfænd/	[gubbæt]	progressive
		tissue	/dæsmalkaqæzi/	[dæbbalkaqædi]	progressive
	Manner	toothpaste	/xæmirdændun/	[qæmidæddun]	regressive
		bee	/zænbur/	[dæbbur]	regressive
		watermelon	/hendune/	[ʔedtune]	regressive
		fork	/ʧængal/	[dæqqal]	regressive
		chair	/sændæli/	[dæddæli]	regressive
		grape	/ʔængur/	[ʔæqgur]/	regressive
		tooth	/dændun/	[ʔædkul]	regressive
		finger	/ʔængoʃt/	[dædtur]	regressive
		stone	/sæng/	[ʔæqgot]	regressive
		toothbrush	/mesvak/	[tæqk]	progressive
		slipper	/dæmpaji/	[pedtap]	regressive
				[dæbbaji]	
Hi	Place	biscuit	/biskujit/	[biztuji]	progressive
	Manner		–	–	

Afterword

Elena Babatsouli, David Ingram and Nicole Müller

Admittedly, this edited volume, *Crosslinguistic Encounters in Language Acquisition: Typical and Atypical Development*, has undertaken a difficult task by attempting to merge together different themes of language acquisition into a single volume. As outlined in the Introduction, there is a focus on typical and atypical development; on crosslinguistic, bilingual and bidialectal research; on language assessment and research methodology; on phonology, the lexicon, morphology and syntax. By turning this very diversity into a core theme, the primary goal of the book has been a uniting one, nevertheless. The book seeks for threads in language acquisition research that better serve academic knowledge of what is typical and atypical in the linguistic development of children crosslinguistically. It intends to view the enormous diversity underlying language acquisition research (e.g. in terms of disparate languages, acquisition types, disorders, individual differences, ages and methodologies) as a motivation to continue searching for those links that unite these and permit comparisons across the board. Ensuing goals and actual steps were the following:

(a) to document some recent research developments by attempting to override differentiation between typical (Chapters 1, 2, 3, 4, 5) and atypical (Chapters 3, 4, 5, 6, 7, 8, 9, 10) language development in children, and how they compare (Chapters 6, 7, 8, 9, 10);
(b) to include language investigations that are less commonly represented in the literature, like Farsi (Chapter 10), Greek (Chapters 7, 8, 6), Icelandic (Chapter 4), isiXhosa (Chapter 1), Maltese (Chapter 5), Mandarin and Slovene (Chapter 5) without, however, excluding representative work in major languages like English (Chapters 1, 2, 3, 5) and Spanish (Chapters 4, 9);
(c) to permit accounts of different bilingual combinations (Chapters 1, 3, 5), bilectal combinations (Chapters 6, 7) and different single-language varieties, like those of English (Chapters 1, 3, 5), Greek (Chapters 6, 7, 8) and Spanish (Chapters 4, 9), which are under-represented in the literature;

(d) to incorporate studies which show that the language faculty is an integral part of human biology and, as such, that it is linked to human pathology (Chapters 6, 7, 8);
(e) to advance approaches in assessment and methodology that cut across the limitations imposed by the given diversity in language acquisition, so there can be more valid comparisons between them (Chapters 2, 3, 4, 5 and 6).

Each chapter in the volume has contributed towards at least one of these goals, complementing the existing language acquisition literature. Specifically: Chapter 1 filled a gap in knowledge on the acquisition of isiXhosa in South Africa by describing the phonetic inventory and phonological processes in three-year-old children acquiring English and isiXhosa. Chapter 2 provided an overview of the relationship between babbling and later language development, as well as on how parental behaviour impacts on pre-linguistic development. Chapter 3 took a closer look at the whole word measure (PWP, Ingram & Ingram, 2001), showing that detailed mathematical analyses of phonological measures can make a substantial contribution to our understanding of phonological development in typical and atypical language contexts. Chapter 4 provided significant information on methodological challenges in developing a large crosslinguistic project on typical and disordered phonological development, outlining problems related to transcription conventions and achieving consensus. Chapter 5 described the development of a bilingual English/Maltese speech assessment to test the additive bilingualism of children in Malta from the innovative methodological perspective of allowing children to respond in the language of their preference; results are compared to monolingual Maltese-speaking children and bilingual Maltese/English-speaking children, as well as a clinical sample, showing that bilinguals have superior phonological abilities compared to monolinguals in this particular setting.

Further, Chapter 6 presented findings on the norming procedure of the Cypriot adaptation of the MCDI with bilectal Cypriot Greek/Greek-speaking children, aged 18–36 months, examining the effects of age and gender and the relationship between vocabulary and morphological scores. Chapter 7 compared children suffering from Obstructive Sleep Apnoea Syndrome (OSAS) with a group of controls on a battery of language tests, with results alarmingly showing that these children receive significantly lower scores in all areas of language (semantics, phonology, morphosyntax). Chapter 8 compared the language profiles of three groups of children (one group with SLI and two control groups) with that of a child with 22q11.2 Deletion Syndrome on a comprehensive language assessment, revealing that the child with 22q11.2 DS has a distinctive language profile; the chapter also makes a final reference to the field of 'comparative biolinguistics' which is new and interesting. Chapter 9 examined the use of different types of self-repairs in a

Spanish-speaking child with SLI aged 3;0–6;10, also comparing with a group of 40 typically developing (TD) children aged two to 10 years; results showed that the frequency of self-repairs is lower in the child with SLI compared to the TD children. Chapter 10 focused on local assimilation in TD and phonologically disordered (PD) children acquiring Farsi – an innovative aspect since most studies in phonological acquisition have addressed long-distance assimilation; results showed differences between Farsi and other languages, as well as differences between the TD and PD children, which are accounted for within Optimality Theory (OT).

The ultimate goal of the volume has been to serve as a reminder that theoretical developments have significant practical relevance for guiding assessment and the ensuing early intervention in cases of language disorder. The studies in this volume have contributed towards charting norms and individual differences in both typical and atypical child language development. Such charting is expected to drive evaluation and intervention for children exhibiting a specific communication difficulty or combinations of them, also facilitating customized approaches where necessary. Ethical considerations with regard to typical and atypical language research suggest that theoretical postulations would better serve any ultimate humanitarian goals if the gap between linguists, language pathologists, therapists and children were better bridged. Assessment tools and batteries, like the ones presented in this volume and others elsewhere, are a constructive move in this direction, but future theoretical work may also assist this purpose by incorporating inferences and suggestions that are more directly applicable in assessment and intervention.

An all-encompassing comprehensive collection would include work covering all living languages and their multilingual/multidialectal combinations in typical and disordered contexts of language acquisition, but this is unrealistic at the moment and beyond the means of this volume. We feel that the present edited book has been effective in bringing the diverse themes of the contributed chapters together. It is our hope that there will be several readers who take an interest in various aspects of the contributed works, even though there may also be individual readers not concerned with certain aspects dealt with in the book.

Reference

Ingram, D. and Ingram, K. (2001) A whole-word approach to phonological analysis and intervention. *Language, Speech, and Hearing Services in Schools* 32, 271–283.

Index